Pancreatic Imaging

Guest Editors

DESIREE E. MORGAN, MD
KOENRAAD J. MORTELE, MD

RADIOLOGIC CLINICS OF NORTH AMERICA

www.radiologic.theclinics.com

Consulting Editor
FRANK H. MILLER, MD

May 2012 • Volume 50 • Number 3

SAUNDERS an imprint of ELSEVIER, Inc.

W.B. SAUNDERS COMPANY
A Division of Elsevier Inc.

1600 John F. Kennedy Boulevard • Suite 1800 • Philadelphia, Pennsylvania 19103-2899

http://www.theclinics.com

RADIOLOGIC CLINICS OF NORTH AMERICA Volume 50, Number 3
May 2012 ISSN 0033-8389, ISBN 13: 978-1-4557-3929-5

Editor: Sarah Barth
Developmental Editor: Donald Mumford

Radiologic Clinics of North America (ISSN 0033-8389) is published bimonthly by Elsevier Inc., 360 Park Avenue South, New York, NY 10010-1710. Months of issue are January, March, May, July, September, and November. Periodicals postage paid at New York, NY and additional mailing offices. Subscription prices are USD 421 per year for US individuals, USD 659 per year for US institutions, USD 202 per year for US students and residents, USD 491 per year for Canadian individuals, USD 827 per year for Canadian institutions, USD 606 per year for international individuals, USD 827 per year for international institutions, and USD 290 per year for Canadian and foreign students/residents. To receive student and resident rate, orders must be accompanied by name of affiliated institution, date of term and the signature of program/residency coordinatior on institution letterhead. Orders will be billed at individual rate until proof of status is received. Foreign air speed delivery is included in all *Clinics* subscription prices. All prices are subject to change without notice. **POSTMASTER:** Send address changes to *Radiologic Clinics of North America*, Elsevier Health Sciences Division, Subscription Customer Service, 3251 Riverport Lane, Maryland Heights, MO63043. **Customer Service: Telephone: 1-800-654-2452** (U.S. and Canada); **1-314-447-8871** (outside U.S. and Canada). **Fax: 1-314-447-8029. E-mail: journalscustomerservice-usa@ elsevier.com** (for print support); **journalsonlinesupport-usa@elsevier.com** (for online support).

Reprints. For copies of 100 or more of articles in this publication, please contact the Commercial Reprints Department, Elsevier Inc., 360 Park Avenue South, New York, New York 10010-1710. Tel.: (+1) 212-633-3812; Fax: (+1) 212-462-1935; E-mail: reprints@elsevier.com.

Radiologic Clinics of North America also published in Greek Paschalidis Medical Publications, Athens, Greece.

Radiologic Clinics of North America is covered in *MEDLINE/PubMed (Index Medicus), EMBASE/Excerpta Medica, Current Contents/Life Sciences, Current Contents/Clinical Medicine, RSNA Index to Imaging Literature, BIOSIS, Science Citation Index,* and *ISI/BIOMED.*

Printed and bound by CPI Group (UK) Ltd, Croydon, CR0 4YY

Transferred to Digital Print 2012

Contributors

CONSULTING EDITOR

FRANK H. MILLER, MD
Professor of Radiology; Chief, Body Imaging
Section and Fellowship Program and GI
Radiology, Medical Director MRI,
Department of Radiology, Northwestern
University Feinberg School of Medicine,
Chicago, Illinois

GUEST EDITORS

DESIREE E. MORGAN, MD
Professor and Vice Chair of Clinical Research,
Abdominal Imaging Section; Director Human
Imaging Shared Facility, Director, MRI; Chief,
GI Radiology, Department of Radiology,
University of Alabama at Birmingham,
Birmingham, Alabama

KOENRAAD J. MORTELE, MD
Director, Division of Clinical MRI; Staff
Radiologist, Abdominal Imaging and MRI;
Associate Professor of Radiology, Harvard
Medical School, Beth Israel Deaconess
Medical Center, Boston, Massachusetts

AUTHORS

LAUREN F. ALEXANDER, MD
Assistant Professor, Department of Radiology,
University of Alabama - Birmingham,
Birmingham, Alabama

MARIA CHIARA AMBROSETTI, MD
Istituto di Radiologia, Policlinico GB Rossi,
Azienda Ospedaliera Universitaria Integrata
Verona, Verona, Italy

APARNA BALACHANDRAN, MD
Associate Professor, Department of Diagnostic
Radiology, The University of Texas MD
Anderson Cancer Center, Houston, Texas

MUSTAFA R. BASHIR, MD
Department of Radiology, Duke University
Medical Center, Durham, North Carolina

PRIYA R. BHOSALE, MD
Associate Professor, Department of Diagnostic
Radiology, The University of Texas MD
Anderson Cancer Center, Houston, Texas

THOMAS L. BOLLEN, MD
Department of Radiology, St Antonius
Hospital, Nieuwegein, The Netherlands

DARWIN L. CONWELL, MD
Director for The Center for Pancreatic Disease,
Division of Gastroenterology, Hepatology,
and Endoscopy, Brigham and Women's
Hospital; Associate Professor of Medicine,
Harvard Medical School, Boston,
Massachusetts

**CATHERINE E. DEWHURST, MB BCh,
BAO, BMedSc**
Division of Abdominal Imaging and MRI,
Department of Radiology, Beth Israel
Deaconess Medical Center, Boston,
Massachusetts

MIRKO D'ONOFRIO, MD
Assistant Professor, Istituto di Radiologia,
Policlinico GB Rossi, Azienda Ospedaliera
Universitaria Integrata Verona, Verona, Italy

JASON B. FLEMING, MD
Associate Professor, Department of Surgical Oncology, The University of Texas MD Anderson Cancer Center, Houston, Texas

RAJAN T. GUPTA, MD
Department of Radiology, Duke University Medical Center, Durham, North Carolina

NAGARAJ-SETTY HOLALKERE, MD, DNB
Assistant Professor, Department of Radiology, Boston Medical Center, Boston, Massachusetts

MATTHEW H. KATZ, MD
Assistant Professor, Department of Surgical Oncology, The University of Texas MD Anderson Cancer Center, Houston, Texas

JEFFREY H. LEE, MD
Professor, Department of Gastroenterology, Hepatology & Nutrition, The University of Texas MD Anderson Cancer Center, Houston, Texas

LINDA S. LEE, MD
Director, Women's Health in GI and Endoscopic Education, Division of Gastroenterology, Hepatology, and Endoscopy, Brigham and Women's Hospital; Assistant Professor of Medicine, Harvard Medical School, Boston, Massachusetts

ALEC J. MEGIBOW, MD, MPH, FACR
Professor of Radiology, Department of Radiology, New York University Langone Medical Center, New York, New York

CHRISTINE O. MENIAS, MD
Associate Professor of Radiology, Washington University, St Louis, Missouri

DESIREE E. MORGAN, MD
Professor and Vice Chair of Clinical Research, Abdominal Imaging Section; Director Human Imaging Shared Facility, Director, MRI; Chief, GI Radiology, Department of Radiology, University of Alabama at Birmingham Birmingham, Alabama

KOENRAAD J. MORTELE, MD
Director, Division of Clinical MRI; Staff Radiologist, Abdominal Imaging and MRI; Associate Professor of Radiology, Harvard Medical School, Beth Israel Deaconess Medical Center, Boston, Massachusetts

ROCIO PEREZ-JOHNSTON, MD
Division of Abdominal Imaging and Intervention, Harvard Medical School, Massachusetts General Hospital, Boston, Massachusetts

ROBERTO POZZI MUCELLI, MD
Professor, Istituto di Radiologia, Policlinico GB Rossi, Azienda Ospedaliera Universitaria Integrata Verona, Verona, Italy

DUSHYANT V. SAHANI, MD
Director of CT, Massachusetts General Hospital; Associate Professor of Radiology, Division of Abdominal Imaging and Intervention, Harvard Medical School, Boston, Massachusetts

NISHA I. SAINANI, MD
Division of Abdominal Imaging and Intervention, Harvard Medical School, Brigham and Women's Hospital, Boston, Massachusetts

KUMARESAN SANDRASEGARAN, MD
Associate Professor of Radiology, Department of Radiology and Imaging Sciences, Indiana University School of Medicine, Indianapolis, Indiana

JORGE SOTO, MD
Professor, Department of Radiology, Boston Medical Center, Boston, Massachusetts

ERIC P. TAMM, MD
Professor, Department of Diagnostic Radiology, The University of Texas MD Anderson Cancer Center, Houston, Texas

TEMEL TIRKES, MD
Assistant Professor of Radiology, Department of Radiology and Imaging Sciences, Indiana University School of Medicine, Indianapolis, Indiana

GAURI R. VARADHACHARY, MD
Associate Professor, Department of GI Medical Oncology, The University of Texas MD Anderson Cancer Center, Houston, Texas

GIULIA A. ZAMBONI, MD
Istituto di Radiologia, Policlinico GB Rossi, Azienda Ospedaliera Universitaria Integrata Verona, Verona, Italy

Contents

MDCT Evaluation of the Pancreas: Nuts and Bolts   365

Mustafa R. Bashir and Rajan T. Gupta

> Multidetector-row CT (MDCT) imaging of the pancreas has important roles in diagnosis, staging, and treatment monitoring of a vast array of pancreatic diseases. Optimizing MDCT protocols not only requires an understanding of expected pathologies but also must take into account cumulative radiation dose considerations.

MR Imaging Techniques for Pancreas   379

Temel Tirkes, Christine O. Menias, and Kumaresan Sandrasegaran

> Pancreatic magnetic resonance (MR) imaging has become a useful tool in evaluating pancreatic disorders. Technical innovations in MR imaging have evolved over the last decade, with most sequences being performed in one or a few breath-holds. Three-dimensional sequences with thin, contiguous slices allow for improved spatial resolution on the postgadolinium images and MR cholangiopancreatography (MRCP). The diagnostic potential of MRCP is equivalent to endoscopic retrograde pancreatography, particularly when intravenous secretin is used to enhance the pancreatic duct assessment. This article highlights the advantages and disadvantages of state-of-the-art and emerging pulse sequences and their application to imaging pancreatic diseases.

Ultrasonography of the Pancreas   395

Giulia A. Zamboni, Maria Chiara Ambrosetti, Mirko D'Onofrio, and Roberto Pozzi Mucelli

> Although the pancreas is often thought of as an organ that is difficult to explore using ultrasound (US), because of its deep retroperitoneal location, with the appropriate technique it can be studied successfully in most patients. In this article, the authors discuss the use of available US techniques in the diagnosis of the most common pancreatic diseases, the use of US intraoperatively, and the use of sonographic guidance for diagnostic and therapeutic procedures. The authors also briefly discuss the potential use of elastosonography techniques in the evaluation of pancreatic disease.

Imaging of Pancreatic Adenocarcinoma: Update on Staging/Resectability   407

Eric P. Tamm, Aparna Balachandran, Priya R. Bhosale, Matthew H. Katz, Jason B. Fleming, Jeffrey H. Lee, and Gauri R. Varadhachary

> Because of the evolution of treatment strategies staging criteria for pancreatic cancer now emphasize arterial involvement for determining unresectable disease. Preoperative therapy may improve the likelihood of margin negative resections of borderline resectable tumors. Cross-sectional imaging is crucial for correctly staging patients. Magnetic resonance (MR) imaging and computed tomography (CT) are probably comparable, with MR imaging probably offering an advantage for

identifying liver metastases. Positron emission tomography/CT and endoscopic ultrasound may be helpful for problem solving. Clear and concise reporting of imaging
findings is important. Several national organizations are developing templates to
standardize the reporting of imaging findings.

Acute pancreatitis is an acute inflammatory process of the pancreatic gland with increasing incidence worldwide. Usually the clinical presentation and course are mild,
with an uneventful recovery. In 10% to 20% of patients, however, local and systemic
complications develop, resulting in significant morbidity and mortality. In 1992, the
Atlanta symposium provided definitions for acute pancreatitis and its severity. Insights into the pathophysiology of the disease, improved diagnostic imaging, and
implementation of minimally invasive techniques have led to classification updates.
This article reviews the cross-sectional imaging features of acute pancreatitis and
presents proposed definitions of the revised Atlanta classification.

Multiple disorders may cause chronic pancreatitis (CP) through recurrent inflammation
of the pancreatic parenchyma. Chronic calcifying pancreatitis caused by excessive
alcohol intake accounts for most cases of CP. However, there are multiple other causes
of CP, including obstructive chronic pancreatitis, autoimmune pancreatitis, groove
pancreatitis, tropical, and hereditary pancreatitis. This article reviews the multiple imaging techniques, some of which are accepted as first-line modalities in patients with
suspected CP, and the imaging features associated with the different causes of CP.

Cystic tumors of the pancreas are a subset of rare pancreatic tumors that vary from benign to malignant. Many have specific imaging findings that allow them to be differentiated from each other. This article (1) reviews the imaging features of the common
cystic pancreatic lesions, including serous microcystic adenoma, mucinous cystic tumor, intraductal papillary mucinous tumor, and solid pseudopapillary tumor, and including the less common lesions such as cystic endocrine tumors, cystic metastases, cystic
teratomas, and lymphangiomas; and (2) provides comprehensive algorithms on how to
manage the individual lesions, with recommendations on when to reimage patients.

Understanding pancreatic development and the congenital anomalies and variants
that result from alterations in normal development allows for better recognition of
these anomalies at diagnostic imaging. This article reviews normal pancreatic embryology and anatomy, and the appearance of the more common developmental
anomalies and ductal variants, with emphasis on computed tomography and magnetic resonance imaging. Common mimics of masses are also covered.

The vast array of possible histologies for a given pancreatic mass makes the specific
diagnosis of a solid pancreatic mass in an individual patient challenging. This article

discusses and reviews the imaging findings of those entities that are likely to be encountered in clinical practice, specifically pancreatic endocrine tumors, solid pseudopapillary tumor, secondary pancreatic masses, and heterotopic spleen.

GOAL STATEMENT

The goal of the *Radiologic Clinics of North America* is to keep practicing radiologists and radiology residents up to date with current clinical practice in radiology by providing timely articles reviewing the state of the art in patient care.

ACCREDITATION

The *Radiologic Clinics of North America* is planned and implemented in accordance with the Essential Areas and Policies of the Accreditation Council for Continuing Medical Education (ACCME) through the joint sponsorship of the University of Virginia School of Medicine and Elsevier. The University of Virginia School of Medicine is accredited by the ACCME to provide continuing medical education for physicians.

The University of Virginia School of Medicine designates this enduring material activity for a maximum of 15 *AMA PRA Category 1 Credit*(s)™ for each issue, 90 credits per year. Physicians should only claim credit commensurate with the extent of their participation in the activity.

The American Medical Association has determined that physicians not licensed in the US who participate in this CME enduring material activity are eligible for a maximum of 15 *AMA PRA Category 1 Credit*(s)™ for each issue, 90 credits per year.

Credit can be earned by reading the text material, taking the CME examination online at http://www.theclinics.com/home/cme, and completing the evaluation. After taking the test, you will be required to review any and all incorrect answers. Following completion of the test and evaluation, your credit will be awarded and you may print your certificate.

FACULTY DISCLOSURE/CONFLICT OF INTEREST

The University of Virginia School of Medicine, as an ACCME accredited provider, endorses and strives to comply with the Accreditation Council for Continuing Medical Education (ACCME) Standards of Commercial Support, Commonwealth of Virginia statutes, University of Virginia policies and procedures, and associated federal and private regulations and guidelines on the need for disclosure and monitoring of proprietary and financial interests that may affect the scientific integrity and balance of content delivered in continuing medical education activities under our auspices.

The University of Virginia School of Medicine requires that all CME activities accredited through this institution be developed independently and be scientifically rigorous, balanced and objective in the presentation/discussion of its content, theories and practices.

All authors/editors participating in an accredited CME activity are expected to disclose to the readers relevant financial relationships with commercial entities occurring within the past 12 months (such as grants or research support, employee, consultant, stock holder, member of speakers bureau, etc.). The University of Virginia School of Medicine will employ appropriate mechanisms to resolve potential conflicts of interest to maintain the standards of fair and balanced education to the reader. Questions about specific strategies can be directed to the Office of Continuing Medical Education, University of Virginia School of Medicine, Charlottesville, Virginia.

The faculty and staff of the University of Virginia Office of Continuing Medical Education have no financial affiliations to disclose.

The authors/editors listed below have identified no financial or professional relationships for themselves or their spouse/partner:

Lauren F. Alexander, MD; Maria Chiara Ambrosetti, MD; Aparna Balachandran, MD; Sarah Barth, (Acquisitions Editor); Mustafa R. Bashir, MD; Priya R. Bhosale, MD; Thomas L. Bollen, MD; Darwin L. Conwell, MD; Mirko D'Onofrio, MD; Catherine E. Dewhurst, MB BCh, BAO, BMedSc; Jason B. Fleming, MD; Rajan T. Gupta, MD; Nagaraj-Setty Holalkere, MD, DNB; Matthew H. Katz, MD; Jeffery H. Lee, MD; Linda S. Lee, MD; Christine O. Menias, MD; Frank H. Miller, MD (Consulting Editor); Desiree E. Morgan, MD (Guest Editor); Koenraad J. Mortele, MD (Guest Editor); Rocio Perez-Johnston, MD; Roberto Pozzi Mucelli, MD; Dushyant V. Sahani, MD; Nisha I. Sainani, MD; Jorge Soto, MD; Temel Tirkes, MD; Gauri R. Varadhachary, MD; and Gulia A. Zamboni, MD.

The authors/editors listed below have identified the following financial or professional relationships for themselves or their spouse/partner:

Klaus D. Hagspiel, MD (Test Author) is an industry funded research/investigator for Siemens Medical Solutions.
Alec J. Megibow, MD, MPH is a consultant for Bracco Diagnostics Inc.
Kumaresan Sandrasegaran, MD receives research grant support from Siemens Medical and Repligen Medical.
Eric P. Tamm, MD is a consultant for General Electric.

Disclosure of Discussion of Non-FDA Approved Uses for Pharmaceutical Products and/or Medical Devices

The University of Virginia School of Medicine, as an ACCME provider, requires that all faculty presenters identify and disclose any off-label uses for pharmaceutical and medical device products. The University of Virginia School of Medicine recommends that each physician fully review all the available data on new products or procedures prior to clinical use.

TO ENROLL

To enroll in the Radiologic Clinics of North America Continuing Medical Education program, call customer service at 1-800-654-2452 or sign up online at http://www.theclinics.com/home/cme. The CME program is available to subscribers for an additional annual fee USD 245.

RADIOLOGIC CLINICS OF NORTH AMERICA

DOWNLOAD Free App!

Review Articles
THE CLINICS

NOW AVAILABLE FOR YOUR iPhone and iPad

Preface

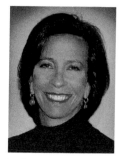
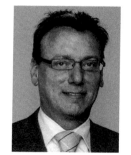

Desiree E. Morgan, MD   Koenraad J. Mortele, MD
Guest Editors

Imaging of the pancreas continues to evolve with both advances in diagnostic capabilities as well as improvement in image-guided therapeutic techniques for a variety of pancreatic diseases. Progressive understanding of the pathogenesis of common pancreatic diseases, such as acute pancreatitis, and discovery or enhanced recognition of pancreatic pathologies due to both broader applications of imaging strategies as well as improvements in imaging techniques requires a practicing radiologist to keep abreast of the latest information from the literature. This issue of *Radiologic Clinics North America* is devoted to the practice of Pancreatic Imaging. A fantastic group of internationally recognized pancreas imaging experts has been tapped to succinctly convey state-of-the-art imaging approaches for a vast array of pancreatic diseases. These categories of pancreatic disorders will be presented to the readers in familiar divisions, with some overlap of technical issues pertinent to the disease process being discussed. Articles on imaging as it relates to pancreatic surgery and endoscopic interventions are also included to enhance understanding of the complex interdisciplinary issues often required in caring for patients with pancreatic disorders. In addition to articles devoted specifically to the "nuts and bolts" of state-of-the-art pancreas diagnostic techniques, an emphasis on more advanced imaging applications, such as microbubble contrast-enhanced sonography, diffusion and perfusion magnetic resonance imaging, and low kVp and dual energy MDCT, are introduced. The latter allow practicing radiologists to familiarize themselves with these further advances in pancreatic imaging that will become mainstream and widely available to clinicians in the not too distant future.

The 1989 *Radiologic Clinics of North America* issue on Radiology the Pancreas sits on the shelf in my office, a nostalgic keepsake from the first year of my residency. It inspired me. Pat Freeny, MD, the guest editor of that volume, together with many other excellent abdominal imagers, surgeons, endoscopists, and oncologists, taught me a great deal about diseases of the pancreas. I would like to thank my co-editor, Koenraad Mortele, MD, for being on that list of enlightening colleagues. And to all of our contributing authors, I offer my sincere gratitude for your contributions to this issue on Pancreatic Imaging.—DM

The intent of this issue is to update practicing radiologists in efforts to enhance the care delivered to their patients suffering from pancreatic disorders. We also hope to excite aspiring pancreatologists to pursue and achieve further advances in diagnostic imaging of this fascinating organ.

Desiree E. Morgan, MD
Department of Radiology
University of Alabama at Birmingham
619 19th Street South, JT N452
Birmingham, AL 35249-6830, USA

Koenraad J. Mortele, MD
Abdominal Imaging and MRI
Division of Clinical MRI
Harvard Medical School
Beth Israel Deaconess Medical Center
330 Brookline Avenue, Ansin 224
Boston, MA 02115, USA

E-mail addresses:
dmorgan@uabmc.edu (D.E. Morgan)
kmortele@gmail.com (K.J. Mortele)

doi:10.1016/j.rcl.2012.03.013

MDCT Evaluation of the Pancreas: Nuts and Bolts

Mustafa R. Bashir, MD*, Rajan T. Gupta, MD

KEYWORDS

• Pancreas • Multidetector CT • Imaging protocols

Imaging with CT has become a frontline technique for initial diagnosis, evaluation of complications, and long-term follow-up of a variety of diseases of the pancreas. In the modern era of multidetector-row CT (MDCT) systems, CT offers high spatial resolution imaging with the ability to accurately detect pancreatic lesions as small as 2 to 3 mm. Detailed evaluation of the pancreatic duct, once the domain of endoscopic retrograde cholangiopancreatography (ECRP) and magnetic resonance cholangiopancreatography (MRCP), can now be performed using CT, with excellent depiction of the pancreatic ductal anatomy. Safe, high-quality imaging requires modern multiphasic protocols and an understanding of the strengths of each component of a CT examination, to maximize the yield of those examinations while delivering as low a radiation dose as possible.

CLINICALLY RELEVANT ANATOMY

The pancreas is a predominantly extraperitoneal organ with exocrine and endocrine functions. Most of the pancreas is located in the anterior pararenal space of the retroperitoneum; the pancreatic tail is located in the splenorenal ligament. The gland is nonencapsulated and normally has a lobulated feathery appearance because of the interdigitation of fat between its lobules.

The pancreatic parenchyma is divided anatomically into five parts: head, neck, body, tail, and uncinate process. The superior mesenteric vein (SMV) is considered the dividing point (neck) between the head and body of the pancreas, with the portion of the pancreas to the right of the SMV considered the head, and the portion to the left considered the body and tail. The uncinate process is located posterior to the superior mesenteric vessels and, along with the posterior portion of the pancreatic head, originates embryologically from the ventral pancreatic anlage. The neck, body, and tail of the pancreas lie ventral to the splenic vein, with the neck directly ventral to the SMV. No clear anatomic landmark is visible at imaging to separate the body of the pancreas from the tail.[1]

The main functional elements of the pancreas are divided into exocrine and endocrine components. The exocrine functions of the pancreas include production of digestive enzymes that travel from the pancreas to the duodenum through the pancreatic duct via the ampulla of Vater. The exocrine cells are arranged into acinar clusters. On the other hand, islet cells are responsible for the endocrine function of the pancreas, and produce hormones such as insulin, glucagon, and gastrin.

The major pancreatic duct, called the duct of Wirsung, extends from the pancreatic tail to the head and is supplied by numerous small side branches along its course. In general, the diameter of the main pancreatic duct can normally range from 1 mm in the tail to 3 mm in the head.[2] Detailed delineation of the pancreatic duct through imaging is important for a variety of reasons. First, the association of cystic pancreatic masses with the duct suggests the diagnosis of intraductal papillary mucinous tumor, and the prognosis of these lesions is partly related to their origin from the main duct or its side branches. Second, irregularity

Department of Radiology, Duke University Medical Center, DUMC 3808, Durham, NC 27710, USA
* Corresponding author.
E-mail address: mustafa.bashir@duke.edu

Radiol Clin N Am 50 (2012) 365–377
doi:10.1016/j.rcl.2012.03.012

and beading of the duct are important diagnostic features of chronic pancreatitis. Finally, anatomic variants of the pancreatic duct are common (occurring in up to 10% of individuals) and can be associated with pancreatitis.[3]

In addition to the more common congenital variants of the pancreatic duct, such as pancreas divisum, annular pancreas is important and occurs when a portion of descending duodenum is completely encircled by pancreatic parenchyma. This unusual variant can lead to symptomatic duodenal obstruction in children, but in adults is typically an incidental diagnosis. Although CT protocols designed to evaluate the pancreas do not typically include the administration of oral contrast material, an annular pancreas can mimic a pancreatic mass when the descending portion of the duodenum is collapsed. In these cases, oral contrast material administration can help in determining the diagnosis (Fig. 1).

Imaging Strategy

A variety of neoplastic and nonneoplastic conditions of the pancreas can be encountered, and the clinical potential for these entities to be present in an individual patient dictates the specific imaging techniques used. In CT, the benefit of acquiring multiple phases before and after the infusion of intravenous contrast material must be balanced against radiation dose considerations.

Unenhanced phase

Imaging before intravenous contrast material administration highlights pancreatic parenchymal and ductal calcifications, which are important features of chronic calcific pancreatitis.[4] Unenhanced imaging also provides baseline attenuation measurements for focal lesions, allowing comparison with contrast-enhanced imaging to determine lesion enhancement. In particular, lesions that are intermediate in attenuation (30–60 HU) after contrast administration can be more accurately characterized when an unenhanced image data set is acquired. Lesions with attenuation that does not change are likely proteinaceous or hemorrhagic cystic lesions, whereas those with attenuation that increases after contrast administration are solid masses. Finally, on the unenhanced phase, hemorrhage in patients with acute pancreatitis can be discerned as high attenuation material against a background of edema or inflammatory stranding; attenuation differences between hemorrhage and surrounding fluid may be less apparent on contrast-enhanced phases when images are windowed to optimize visualization of enhancing structures.[5]

Pancreatic parenchymal phase

This data set is obtained slightly later than the traditional hepatic arterial phase, at approximately 40 s after the initiation of intravenous contrast media infused at a rate of 3 mL/s.[6] This phase has been shown to improve visual contrast between hypoenhancing pancreatic adenocarcinomas and the surrounding pancreas, when compared with either the hepatic arterial or portal venous phases.[7] Visualization of the relationship between pancreatic masses and surrounding arterial structures is also optimized in this phase, which is critical when resection is contemplated.[7,8]

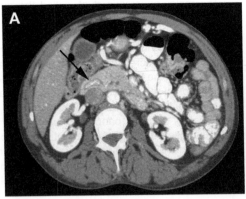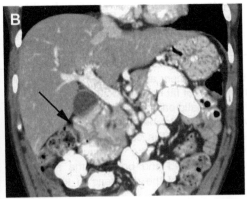

Fig. 1. Annular pancreas in a 45-year-old woman with abdominal pain. (A) Axial image in the pancreatic parenchymal phase and after oral ingestion of positive contrast material shows pancreatic parenchyma entirely surrounding the descending duodenum (arrow), compatible with a diagnosis of annular pancreas. This diagnosis is most often incidental in asymptomatic adult patients. Note the presence of enteric contrast material within the duodenum, which can be helpful in establishing this diagnosis. (B) Coronal reformatted image shows pancreatic parenchyma wrapping around both sides of the descending duodenum (arrow), compatible with diagnosis of annular pancreas.

Hypoenhancing adenocarcinomas can be subtle even under optimal imaging circumstances, and precise contrast bolus timing is important to maximize the likelihood of differentiating these masses from the surrounding parenchyma; even under ideal conditions, these tumor may be isoattenuating to the surrounding pancreatic parenchyma in all phases.[9] Mild acute pancreatitis, which presents with relative hypoenhancement of a portion of the gland without surrounding edema or fat stranding, may also be best seen in this phase.

Additionally, the inclusion of the pancreatic parenchymal phase is critical for identifying masses, which are hyperenhancing relative to the pancreatic parenchyma, because this finding confers a very different differential diagnosis than a hypoenhancing lesion (Fig. 2). Finally, this phase can be helpful to show early arterial enhancement in a pseudoaneurysm, a known complication of pancreatitis; this type of lesion may equilibrate and become less apparent in the portal venous phase.[10]

Some centers have advocated that image reconstruction of this phase should use a small field-of-view to improve in-plane spatial resolution and aid detection of small masses.[11] This strategy has two important drawbacks: (1) exclusion of portions of the liver, which must be evaluated for early-enhancing metastases when a pancreatic endocrine tumor (Fig. 3) is suspected, and (2) increased image noise as a result of small voxel size, which may hinder detection of subtle lesions.

The choice of small versus large field-of-view depends on the needs of the particular case and on reader preference.

Portal venous phase

Imaging in the portal venous phase (70–90 s after initiation of intravenous contrast infusion) provides optimal delineation of the portal, splenic, and superior mesenteric veins. Portal vein thrombosis is a common and important complication of pancreatitis and pancreatic adenocarcinoma, and patency versus invasion of the portal venous system has important implications for the resectability of pancreatic masses.[12] The portal venous phase also maximizes visual contrast between hypoenhancing hepatic metastases from pancreatic adenocarcinoma and the surrounding liver parenchyma (Fig. 4).[13] This phase provides a second opportunity to visualize low-attenuation masses in the pancreatic parenchyma, and may be complementary to the pancreatic parenchymal phase (Figs. 5–7). Finally, the portal venous phase is important for detecting pancreatic necrosis in cases of pancreatitis (Fig. 8); inflamed, hypoenhancing, but nonnecrotic pancreatic tissue may not have adequate time to enhance in the pancreatic parenchymal phase, whereas pancreatic tissue that has not enhanced by the time of the portal venous phase is most likely necrotic (Fig. 9).

The approximate timing and particular advantages of each contrast phase are summarized in Table 1.

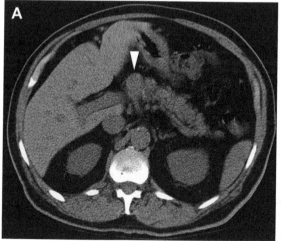 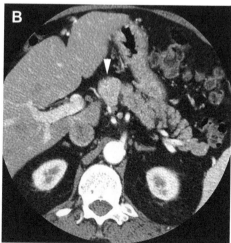

Fig. 2. Pancreatic endocrine tumor in a 40-year-old woman who presented for evaluation of a suspected pancreatic mass. (*A*) Unenhanced image through the upper abdomen shows the normal lobulated contour of the pancreas, with a focal contour abnormality suggesting a lesion in the pancreatic neck (*white arrowhead*). (*B*) Pancreatic parenchymal phase image obtained with a small field of view and 2.5-mm slice thickness shows a hyperenhancing mass in the pancreatic neck (*white arrowhead*), suggesting a pancreatic endocrine tumor. The smaller field of view and thinner sections used in this case (compared with standard 3- to 5-mm reconstructions) provide superior spatial resolution, which can aid in assessing vascular involvement.

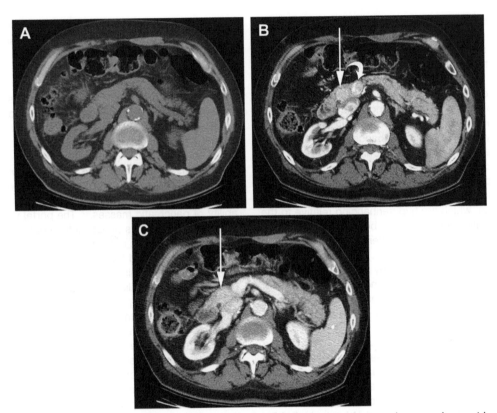

Fig. 3. Pancreatic endocrine tumor in a 74-year-old man. (*A*) Unenhanced CT image does not show evidence of a pancreatic mass. (*B*) Pancreatic parenchymal phase image at the same level shows a hypervascular mass in the head of the pancreas (*white arrow*), just to the right of the superior mesenteric vein (*curved white arrow*). (*C*) Portal venous phase image shows that the mass is much less conspicuous than on the pancreatic parenchymal phase (*white arrow*), illustrating the value of the pancreatic parenchymal phase in detecting hypervascular pancreatic lesions.

CONTRAST MEDIA INJECTION PROTOCOLS

The goal of administering iodinated contrast media intravenously in any CT examination is to provide optimal visual contrast between the anatomic structure of interest and pathologies it may harbor. While proper timing of enhancement is critical, the degree of enhancement of the organ in question is directly proportional to the amount of iodine present within the parenchyma and its associated microvasculature at any given time point. The amount of iodine delivered to the organ is, in turn, related to a number of patient factors (cardiac output, organ vascularity), as well as the injection protocol (contrast media iodine concentration, injection rate).[14] The use of a "saline chaser" has been shown to improve aortic enhancement in CT angiography, although the benefits are less pronounced in solid organ imaging (**Box 1**).[15]

Although the main controllable factor affecting pancreatic enhancement is iodine delivery to the organ, several other uncontrollable factors may influence the amount of visual organ enhancement

observed at CT, most commonly patient habitus. Large body habitus causes greater degrees of x-ray beam attenuation and may result in noisier CT images; increased image noise, in turn, may reduce the radiologist's ability to discern subtle differences in image contrast. Although the effects of body habitus can be mitigated at least partially through adjusting the imaging parameters of the CT system, weight-based contrast media bolus strategies have been described as alternative approaches to optimizing CT enhancement.[14] Although exact contrast media dosing can vary, a dose of 2.0 mL/kg of iohexol 300 (600 mg of iodine per kilogram body weight) has been shown to provide more consistent enhancement of the pancreas and liver across a range of patient body weights when compared with a fixed dose of 120 mL.

Finally, the use of oral contrast media in routine MDCT of the pancreas deserves careful consideration. In most cases, opacification of the gastrointestinal tract does not contribute to the evaluation

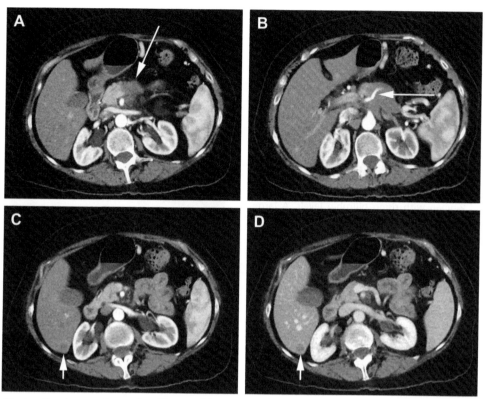

Fig. 4. Pancreatic adenocarcinoma in a 70-year-old woman with left upper quadrant pain lasting approximately 6 to 8 months. (A) Contrast-enhanced CT image in the pancreatic parenchymal phase shows a large low attenuation mass in the pancreatic body (white arrow), with normal enhancement of the parenchyma of the head and neck. This mass was proven at biopsy to be pancreatic adenocarcinoma. (B) The splenic artery (white arrow) is completely encased by the mass. (C) Pancreatic parenchymal phase images from the same patient shows a subtle hypoenhancing lesion in the posterior segment of the right hepatic lobe (white arrow). (D) Portal venous phase image shows improved conspicuity of the liver lesion (white arrow), indicating the importance of portal venous phase imaging in the detection of pancreatic adenocarcinoma metastatic to the liver.

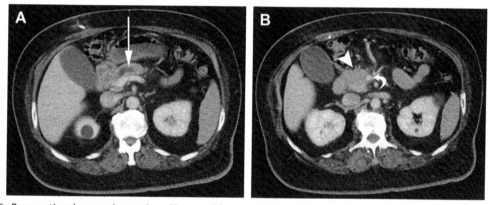

Fig. 5. Pancreatic adenocarcinoma in a 63-year-old man with jaundice and abnormally elevated serum bilirubin level. (A) Contrast-enhanced CT image in the portal venous phase of the upper abdomen shows dilation of the pancreatic duct in the body and tail (white arrow). (B) Axial CT image also in the portal venous phase shows a subtle low attenuation lesion in the pancreas (white arrowhead), pathologically proven to be pancreatic adeno-carcinoma. Note the 180° involvement of the superior mesenteric vein (white curved arrow) by the mass, and abutment without clear invasion of the extrahepatic main portal vein.

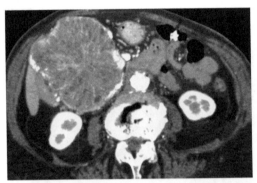

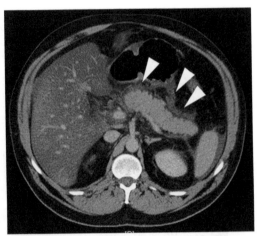

Fig. 6. Serous microcystic pancreatic adenoma in a 78-year-old woman with rising bilirubin levels. A large mass with small cystic components, peripheral calcifications, and a "spoke-wheel" pattern of enhancement is seen arising from the pancreatic head in the right upper quadrant in the pancreatic parenchymal phase of imaging. Serous microcystic pancreatic adenomas are characterized by the presence of small cysts and do not have malignant potential, unlike their mucinous counterparts. These tumors typically occur in older women and are generally asymptomatic; however, in this patient, mass effect from the lesion caused upstream biliary ductal dilation, and the lesion was ultimately resected.

of pancreatic disease. However, two important exceptions to this guideline should be noted. First, when annular pancreas is suspected, opacification of the duodenal lumen may improve delineation of the abnormal ring of pancreatic tissue encircling the descending portion of the duodenum. Second, when invasive pancreatic tumors extend anteriorly to the stomach, distension of the gastric lumen may

Fig. 8. Interstitial edematous acute pancreatitis in a 40-year-old man with acute onset of abdominal pain. Contrast-enhanced CT image of the upper abdomen in the portal venous phase shows peripancreatic fluid and inflammatory changes (white arrowheads). The pancreas appears enlarged and edematous, with some loss of the normal expected lobulated pattern, but the parenchyma enhances throughout. Fluid is seen extending into the perisplenic space. Diffuse hepatic steatosis is also present. Neither a formed retroperitoneal collection nor splenic vein thrombosis, two possible complications of this condition, were present in this case.

improve reader confidence in identifying invasion of the gastric wall. In these cases, a negative oral contrast agent such as water is preferable to a positive contrast agent for providing image optimal contrast between the gastric lumen and the enhancing gastric wall, and to avoid beam-hardening artifacts from pooled contrast material in the stomach.

SUGGESTED CT PROTOCOLS

The construction of practical imaging protocols from the available components requires anticipation of the pathologies that are likely to be encountered. A maximal amount of information could be obtained by performing a three-phase study on every patient. However, concerns regarding radiation dose, prior allergic reactions to iodinated contrast material, and renal impairment require the judicious use of both contrast media and multiphasic imaging. Several suggested imaging protocols are summarized in Table 2 and reviewed in the following sections.

Three-Phase Protocol

The three-phase imaging protocol includes unenhanced, pancreatic parenchymal, and portal venous phase acquisitions of the abdomen. It is

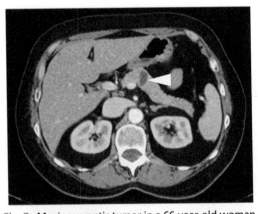

Fig. 7. Mucinous cystic tumor in a 66-year-old woman. Contrast-enhanced CT image obtained in the pancreatic parenchymal phase shows a unilocular cystic lesion in the pancreatic body (white arrowhead). Differential considerations included mucinous cystic tumor of the pancreas, pseudocyst, and intraductal papillary mucinous tumor. At resection, this lesion was found to be a mucinous cystic tumor with areas of high-grade dysplasia.

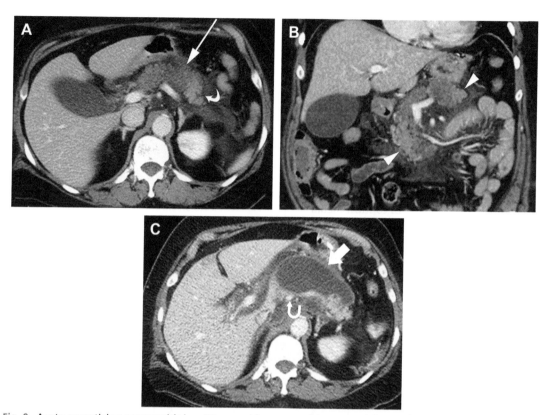

Fig. 9. Acute necrotizing pancreatitis in a 71-year-old woman with severe abdominal pain and a history of prior episodes of acute pancreatitis. (*A*) Contrast-enhanced CT image obtained in the pancreatic parenchymal phase shows large areas of nonenhancing pancreatic parenchyma (*straight white arrow*) and peripancreatic inflammatory changes, consistent with necrotizing pancreatitis. Note the area of preserved, normally enhancing parenchyma in the distal pancreatic body (*curved white arrow*). (*B*) Coronal reformatted image shows the extent of pancreatic necrosis, which extends from the head to the body. Some areas of preserved glandular enhancement are present in the uncinate process and distal pancreatic body (*white arrowheads*). (*C*) Follow-up contrast-enhanced CT in the portal venous phase obtained approximately 3 weeks later showed interval development of a large acute necrotizing collection (*white block arrow*) with minimal residual pancreatic parenchymal enhancement in the distal body/tail. The splenic artery courses directly adjacent to the large collection (*curved white arrow*); in these cases, close attention must be paid to the splenic artery to assess for pseudoaneurysm formation, and to the vein for thrombosis or occlusion.

Table 1
Timing and advantages of the contrast enhancement phases typically used in CT evaluation of the pancreas

Phase	Timing	Advantages
Unenhanced phase	Precontrast	Calcifications Baseline attenuation of cystic lesions Hemorrhagic pancreatitis
Pancreatic parenchymal phase	40 s postinfusion initiation	Hyperenhancing lesions Hypoenhancing lesions Hyperenhancing hepatic metastases Arterial patency and relationship to masses Pseudoaneurysms
Portal venous phase	70–90 s postinfusion initiation	Venous patency Pancreatic necrosis Hypoenhancing hepatic metastases

Box 1
Suggested characteristics of contrast media injection protocols optimized for imaging the pancreas

Contrast media iodine concentration	300–370 mg/mL
Injection rate	3 mL/s
Contrast media bolus volume	150–175 mL or weight-based volume (2 mL/kg)
Saline flush/chaser (optional)	20 mL total volume at same injection rate as contrast media bolus

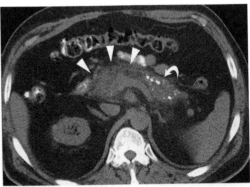

Fig. 10. Acute on chronic pancreatitis in a 69-year-old man with a history of multiple prior episodes of pancreatitis. (*A*, *B*) Unenhanced CT images show multiple calcifications in the body and tail of the pancreas (*curved white arrow*), consistent with chronic calcific pancreatitis. Peripancreatic inflammatory changes and fluid (*white arrowheads*) were new compared with a recent prior examination, and suggest acute on chronic pancreatitis.

an ideal initial evaluation of known or suspected pancreatic masses, and of chronic/recurrent pancreatitis (Fig. 10) when either an underlying mass or a complication (eg, venous thrombosis, pseudoaneurysm, hemorrhage) is suspected.

Two-Phase Protocol

A biphasic CT protocol consisting of pancreatic parenchymal and portal venous phases is ideally used when unenhanced imaging is not needed. This protocol is well suited for evaluating known solid pancreatic masses (for hyper/hypoenhancement and resectability). Known adenocarcinomas represent a special case in which evaluation of prior imaging is helpful; tumors that were well visualized in the portal venous phase can be assessed through follow-up portal venous phase imaging

only, whereas those that were best seen in the pancreatic parenchymal phase should be followed up with a biphasic examination in the pancreatic parenchymal phase (for the primary tumor) followed by the portal venous phase (for liver metastases).

Single-Phase Protocol

The single-phase protocol involves portal venous phase imaging only and is useful for evaluating

Table 2
Suggested indications for use of individual pancreatic imaging protocols

Imaging Protocol	Phases Included	Uses
Three-phase	UE, PP, PV	Evaluation of pancreatic and/or biliary ductal dilation New cystic pancreatic mass Chronic pancreatitis Recurrent pancreatitis (suspect complications)
Two-phase	PP, PV	New solid pancreatic mass Follow-up pancreatic endocrine tumor (resected or unresected)
Single-phase	PV	Follow-up known or resected adenocarcinoma Acute pancreatitis Recurrent pancreatitis (follow-up without complications suspected)
Unenhanced	UE	Chronic renal insufficiency Prior anaphylactic reaction to iodinated contrast material Prior breakthrough reaction to iodinated contrast material (despite premedication) Consider MRI with/without contrast or without contrast if possible

Abbreviations: PP, pancreatic parenchymal; PV, portal venous; UE, unenhanced.

acute pancreatitis. It also allows for evaluation of many of the complications of acute pancreatitis, including venous thrombosis and retroperitoneal collections. Although many pseudoaneurysms are visible in the portal venous phase, small pseudoaneurysms and lesions that enhance similarly to the hepatic parenchyma in this phase may be more easily discerned in the pancreatic parenchymal phase (Figs. 11 and 12).

Resected adenocarcinomas can also be followed up using portal venous phase imaging only, because in addition to liver metastases being optimally detected in this phase, local recurrence tends to present as a mass in the retroperitoneal fat or along the celiac or superior mesenteric arteries. These masses are typically equally conspicuous in the pancreatic parenchymal and portal venous phases, and a single phase is usually an adequate assessment for local recurrence. Follow-up of acute pancreatitis can also be performed with portal venous single-phase imaging.[16]

Unenhanced Protocol

For pancreatic indications, CT imaging should only be performed without intravenous contrast material when a specific contraindication to contrast material administration exists (eg, prior anaphylactic reaction to iodinated contrast material, acute renal failure, chronic renal insufficiency, lack of intravenous access). In these cases, MRI with contrast material, or even MRI without contrast, should be considered when feasible; unenhanced

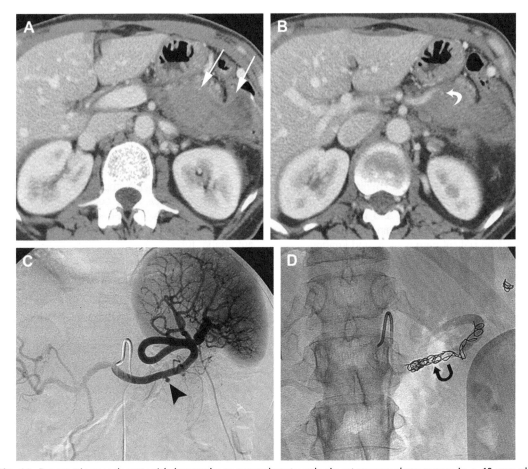

Fig. 11. Pancreatic pseudocyst with hemorrhage secondary to splenic artery pseudoaneurysm in a 40-year-old man with a history of pancreatitis and multiple pseudocysts presented with an acute decrease in hematocrit. (A, B) Images from a contrast-enhanced CT in the portal venous phase show a large collection (*white arrows*) with mixed attenuation contents compatible with hemorrhage. A possible pseudoaneurysm arising from the splenic artery was noted (*curved white arrow*). (C) Digital subtraction angiographic (DSA) image from a celiac axis injection shows a small pseudoaneurysm arising from the splenic artery (*black arrowhead*), corresponding to the CT findings. (D) Subsequent DSA image obtained after coiling of the splenic artery (*curved black arrow*). (*Courtesy of* Erik K. Paulson, MD, Durham, NC.)

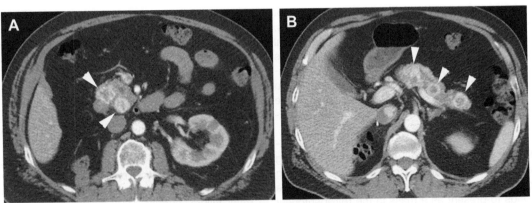

Fig. 12. Renal cell carcinoma with pancreatic metastases in a 63-year-old man with a history of right nephrectomy for renal cell carcinoma. (*A, B*) Pancreatic parenchymal phase CT images show multiple hyperenhancing lesions throughout the pancreas (*white arrowheads*). Differential considerations could include multiple pancreatic endocrine tumors; however, in a patient with a history of renal cell carcinoma, the most likely diagnosis is metastatic disease, especially in light of the multiplicity of lesions.

MRI offers superior tissue contrast compared with unenhanced CT, and is more sensitive for detecting findings of acute pancreatitis, complications of pancreatitis, and focal pancreatic lesions.

RADIATION DOSE CONSIDERATIONS

Public awareness of the potentially harmful effects of medical ionizing radiation has increased dramatically. The responsibility for minimizing radiation dose from imaging must be shared by the community of referring providers and medical imagers; referrers should order imaging tests when their impact on patient care is high, and imagers must carefully weigh dose concerns against issues of image quality.

The primary opportunity for imagers to minimize dose to individual patients is through limiting the number of imaging phases to only those that are necessary. In addition, several technologies are available on commercial CT systems that provide dose reduction. Automatic tube current modulation, which adjusts CT tube current according to preset measures of desired image quality, is available on all modern CT systems. In addition, first- and second-generation iterative reconstruction techniques can provide improved image quality from noisier source data sets, allowing further reductions in dose.[17–19] Spectral CT techniques may provide dose savings when combined with automatic tube current modulation and image postprocessing techniques that take advantage of redundancies in the data acquired at each tube

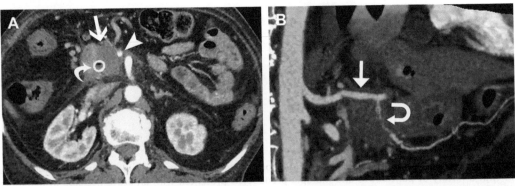

Fig. 13. Pancreatic adenocarcinoma in a 70-year-old woman with unresectable pancreatic ductal adenocarcinoma. (*A*) Axial contrast-enhanced CT image obtained during the pancreatic parenchymal phase shows a poorly defined low attenuation mass (*white arrow*) at the level of the pancreatic head. A metallic biliary stent is identified (*curved white arrow*) and the mass is noted to encase the superior mesenteric vein (*white arrowhead*). (*B*) Curved multiplanar reformatted images show tumor encasing portions of the celiac axis (*white arrow*) and complete encasement and diffuse irregular narrowing of the gastroduodenal artery (*curved white arrow*).

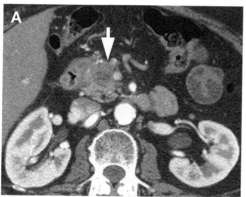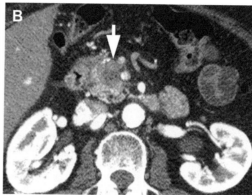

Fig. 14. Pancreatic adenocarcinoma in a 53-year-old man with history of abdominal pain. (*A*) Axial contrast-enhanced CT image obtained during the pancreatic parenchymal phase at 140 kVp and 385 mA shows a 1.5-cm hypoattenuating lesion (*arrow*) at the level of the uncinate process of the pancreas. (*B*) Axial contrast-enhanced CT image obtained during the pancreatic parenchymal phase at 80 kVp and 675 mA shows increased lesion conspicuity relative to the background pancreatic parenchyma (*white arrow*). Images are displayed with a preset soft-tissue window (window width, 350 HU; window level, 40 HU). (*Courtesy of* Daniele Marin, MD, Durham, NC.)

energy.[20,21] Additionally, the calculation of virtual unenhanced images from contrast-enhanced dual-energy CT data sets may allow elimination of the noncontrast phase from three-phase protocols, providing large dose savings.[6]

ADVANCED IMAGING TECHNIQUES

With the widespread availability of higher-order MDCT systems, multiplanar reformatted images (MPR) and three-dimensional renderings can be incorporated into routine pancreatic imaging protocols. MPR images can improve delineation of the association between focal lesions and the pancreatic duct, aid in staging pancreatic masses, and provide excellent visualization of anatomic variants and strictures of the pancreatic duct.[22–25] Moreover, MPR images can better show the relationship between pancreatic masses and the adjacent vasculature, and are vital for surgical planning (Fig. 13).

Even more recently, dual-energy CT systems have become commercially available and show great promise in pancreatic imaging. Low-tube-voltage technique (80 kVp) has been shown in small studies to improve apparent pancreatic enhancement and conspicuity of primary adenocarcinoma compared with higher tube voltage settings (Fig. 14).[26,27] Along with these gains in image quality, effective radiation dose can be reduced through using low-tube-voltage settings.[26] Total radiation dose may be further reduced through eliminating precontrast image acquisitions, and instead reconstructing virtual unenhanced image sets from dual-energy data.[6,27] In the near future, more-complex spectral analysis

techniques may become available for detecting subtle enhancement in both solid and cystic lesions, improving the sensitivity of CT for detecting malignant features of these lesions.

Finally, quantitative CT-based perfusion biomarkers have proven useful in differentiating adenocarcinoma from mass-forming pancreatitis, and in predicting tumor response to neoadjuvant therapy.[28,29] The combination of these dynamic data acquisition techniques with dual-energy technology may prove to be a powerful predictor of the biologic behavior of tumors, and is a promising new branch of oncologic imaging.

SUMMARY

A variety of techniques are available for MDCT imaging of the pancreas. Although specific protocol design and indications may be institution-dependent, multiphasic imaging has been well studied and shown to provide significant diagnostic advantages over single-phase protocols, particularly in evaluating pancreatic adenocarcinoma. As scanner acquisition and image processing techniques continue to evolve and the radiation dose required for these examinations decreases, CT remains an excellent tool for diagnosing pancreatic pathologies.

REFERENCES

1. Brant WE, Helms CA. Fundamentals of diagnostic radiology. 3rd edition. Philadelphia: Lippincott, Williams & Wilkins; 2007.

2. Chaya CT, Bhutani MS. Ultrasonography of the pancreas. 6. Endoscopic imaging. Abdom Imaging 2007;32(2):191–9.

3. Yu J, Turner MA, Fulcher AS, et al. Congenital anomalies and normal variants of the pancreaticobiliary tract and the pancreas in adults: part 2, Pancreatic duct and pancreas. AJR Am J Roentgenol 2006; 187(6):1544–53.

4. Campisi A, Brancatelli G, Vullierme MP, et al. Are pancreatic calcifications specific for the diagnosis of chronic pancreatitis? A multidetector-row CT analysis. Clin Radiol 2009;64(9):903–11.

5. Sahni VA, Mortele KJ. The bloody pancreas: MDCT and MRI features of hypervascular and hemorrhagic pancreatic conditions. AJR Am J Roentgenol 2009; 192(4):923–35.

6. Coursey CA, Nelson RC, Boll DT, et al. Dual-energy multidetector CT: how does it work, what can it tell us, and when can we use it in abdominopelvic imaging? Radiographics 2010;30(4): 1037–55.

7. Fletcher JG, Wiersema MJ, Farrell MA, et al. Pancreatic malignancy: value of arterial, pancreatic, and hepatic phase imaging with multi-detector row CT. Radiology 2003;229(1):81–90.

8. Lu DS, Vedantham S, Krasny RM, et al. Two-phase helical CT for pancreatic tumors: pancreatic versus hepatic phase enhancement of tumor, pancreas, and vascular structures. Radiology 1996;199(3): 697–701.

9. Prokesch RW, Chow LC, Beaulieu CF, et al. Isoattenuating pancreatic adenocarcinoma at multidetector row CT: secondary signs. Radiology 2002; 224(3):764–8.

10. Kim HC, Yang DM, Kim HJ, et al. Computed tomography appearances of various complications associated with pancreatic pseudocysts. Acta Radiol 2008;49(7):727–34.

11. Nishiharu T, Yamashita Y, Ogata I, et al. Spiral CT of the pancreas. The value of small field-of-view targeted reconstruction. Acta Radiol 1998;39(1): 60–3.

12. Jain P, Nijhawan S. Portal vein thrombosis: etiology and clinical outcome of cirrhosis and malignancy-related non-cirrhotic, non-tumoral extrahepatic portal venous obstruction. World J Gastroenterol 2007; 13(39):5288–9.

13. Valls C, Andia E, Sanchez A, et al. Dual-phase helical CT of pancreatic adenocarcinoma: assessment of resectability before surgery. AJR Am J Roentgenol 2002;178(4):821–6.

14. Yanaga Y, Awai K, Nakayama Y, et al. Pancreas: patient body weight tailored contrast material injection protocol versus fixed dose protocol at dynamic CT. Radiology 2007;245(2):475–82.

15. Marin D, Nelson RC, Guerrisi A, et al. 64-section multidetector CT of the upper abdomen: optimization of a saline chaser injection protocol for improved vascular and parenchymal contrast enhancement. Eur Radiol 2011;21(9):1938–47.

16. Kwon Y, Park HS, Kim YJ, et al. Multidetector row computed tomography of acute pancreatitis: utility of single portal phase CT scan in short-term follow up. Eur J Radiol 2011. [Epub ahead of print].

17. Schindera ST, Diedrichsen L, Muller HC, et al. Iterative reconstruction algorithm for abdominal multidetector CT at different tube voltages: assessment of diagnostic accuracy, image quality, and radiation dose in a phantom study. Radiology 2011;260(2): 454–62.

18. May MS, Wust W, Brand M, et al. Dose reduction in abdominal computed tomography: intraindividual comparison of image quality of full-dose standard and half-dose iterative reconstructions with dual-source computed tomography. Invest Radiol 2011; 46(7):465–70.

19. Singh S, Kalra MK, Hsieh J, et al. Abdominal CT: comparison of adaptive statistical iterative and filtered back projection reconstruction techniques. Radiology 2010;257(2):373–83.

20. Silva AC, Morse BG, Hara AK, et al. Dual-energy (spectral) CT: applications in abdominal imaging. Radiographics 2011;31(4):1031–46 [discussion: 47–50].

21. Leng S, Yu L, Wang J, et al. Noise reduction in spectral CT: reducing dose and breaking the trade-off between image noise and energy bin selection. Med Phys 2011;38(9):4946–57.

22. Fukushima H, Itoh S, Takada A, et al. Diagnostic value of curved multiplanar reformatted images in multislice CT for the detection of resectable pancreatic ductal adenocarcinoma. Eur Radiol 2006;16(8): 1709–18.

23. Gong JS, Xu JM. Role of curved planar reformations using multidetector spiral CT in diagnosis of pancreatic and peripancreatic diseases. World J Gastroenterol 2004;10(13):1943–7.

24. Kim HC, Yang DM, Jin W, et al. Multiplanar reformations and minimum intensity projections using multidetector row CT for assessing anomalies and disorders of the pancreaticobiliary tree. World J Gastroenterol 2007;13(31):4177–84.

25. Yun BL, Kim SH, Kim SJ, et al. Added value of multiplanar reformations to axial multi-detector row computed tomographic images for the differentiation of macrocystic pancreas neoplasms: receiver operating characteristic analysis. J Comput Assist Tomogr 2010;34(6):899–906.

26. Marin D, Nelson RC, Barnhart H, et al. Detection of pancreatic tumors, image quality, and radiation dose during the pancreatic parenchymal phase: effect of a low-tube-voltage, high-tube-current CT technique–preliminary results. Radiology 2010; 256(2):450–9.

27. Macari M, Spieler B, Kim D, et al. Dual-source dual-energy MDCT of pancreatic adenocarcinoma: initial observations with data generated at 80 kVp and at simulated weighted-average 120 kVp. AJR Am J Roentgenol 2010;194(1):W27–32.

28. Lu N, Feng XY, Hao SJ, et al. 64-slice CT perfusion imaging of pancreatic adenocarcinoma and mass-forming chronic pancreatitis. Acad Radiol 2011;18(1):81–8.

29. Park MS, Klotz E, Kim MJ, et al. Perfusion CT: noninvasive surrogate marker for stratification of pancreatic cancer response to concurrent chemo- and radiation therapy. Radiology 2009;250(1): 110–7.

MR Imaging Techniques for Pancreas

Temel Tirkes, MD[a],*, Christine O. Menias, MD[b],
Kumaresan Sandrasegaran, MD[a]

KEYWORDS

- Pancreas • Magnetic resonance imaging
- Magnetic resonance cholangiopancreatography (MRCP)
- New MRI techniques • Image optimization • Artifacts
- Secretin

The pancreas is one of the most challenging organs to image in the abdomen. The small size of the organ and its deep location require high-resolution imaging. Comprehensive magnetic resonance (MR) imaging of the pancreas should ideally show pancreatic and biliary ductal anatomy, help detect and characterize parenchymal disease, delineate extra pancreatic extension of a mass or inflammatory process, and evaluate the vascular anatomy. In the last few years, MR imaging scanners have become more sophisticated. Current MR imaging scanners have more than 100 integrated coil elements and more than 30 independent radiofrequency channels. Obese and claustrophobic patients can now be scanned easily in shorter scanners with wider bores. Higher field strength (3.0 T) scanners are increasingly used. New sequences have been introduced for performing pancreatic MR imaging, including 3-dimensional T1-weighted and MR cholangiopancreatography (MRCP) sequences. Secretin-enhanced MRCP (S-MRCP) protocols have been developed for a more complete assessment of pancreatic ducts and glandular function. MR imaging is used routinely in many centers as a problem-solving tool in patients with elevated liver function tests, acute pancreatitis, and pancreatic cancer. It is used as the primary imaging modality for suspected biliopancreatic pain,

staging of chronic pancreatitis, and diagnosis and follow-up of cystic pancreatic tumors. In this article, the authors discuss the techniques that contribute to a state-of-the-art MR imaging examination of the pancreas.

MR IMAGING SEQUENCES

To fully evaluate the pancreatic parenchyma and the pancreaticobiliary ductal system, it is useful to obtain the following sequences: dual-echo T1-weighted gradient-echo; T2-weighted axial and coronal sequences, turbo spin echo (TSE) or a variant of TSE; 2-dimensional and 3-dimensional MRCP; and fat-suppressed T1-weighted, 3-dimensional gradient-echo before and after gadolinium. S-MRCP is a useful, optional sequence. Tables 1 and 2 give the MR imaging parameters for these sequences on 1.5 T and 3.0 T scanners respectively. For most patients, it is possible to complete the core sequences and S-MRCP within 30 minutes. Different methods of performing these sequences are discussed in the following sections.

Patient Preparation

To ensure distension of the gallbladder and adequately assess the potential exocrine response to secretin, patients should fast for at least 4 hours before the MR imaging examination. Negative oral

[a] Department of Radiology and Imaging Sciences, Indiana University School of Medicine, 550 North University Boulevard, UH 0663, Indianapolis, IN 46202, USA; [b] Washington University, 510 South Kingshighway, St Louis, MO 63110, USA
* Corresponding author.
E-mail address: atirkes@iupui.edu

Radiol Clin N Am 50 (2012) 379–393
doi:10.1016/j.rcl.2012.03.003

Table 1
Parameters for pancreatic imaging on 1.5 T MR imaging scanners

	3D SPGR DIXON	T2 2D SSFSE	T2 2D STIR	T2 2D SSFSE	MRCP 2D Slab	MRCP 3D	MRCP Secretin[a]	3D SPGR FS
Plane of acquisition	Axial	Axial	Axial	Coronal	Coronal	Coronal	Coronal	Axial
TR/TE (msec)	7.47/4.76 (in), 2.38 (out)	1100/90	2900/132 (TI 150)	1100/90	2000/755	2500/691	2000/756	5.17/2.52
Flip angle (°)	10	130–50	180	130	180	Variable	1	12
ST/SG	3.4/-	4.0/4.0	7	4.0/4.0	40	1/-	40	3.0/-
NEX	1	1	1	1	1	2	1	1
RBW	290	475	250	476	300	372	300	300
Phase direction	A to P	A to P	A to P	R to L	R to L	R to L	R to L	A to P
Echo train length	1	160	33	192	320	189	256	1
Matrix	256 × 120	256 × 192	256 × 180	256 × 192	256 × 256	384 × 346	256 × 256	256 × 144
FOV	400	360	360	360	290	350	290	360
Respiration	BH	BH	BH	BH	BH	Navigator[b]	BH	BH
Fat saturation	No	No	IR	No	Fat sat	Fat sat	Fat sat	Fat Sat
Concatenation[c]	1	3	4	3	8	1	1	1
Parallel imaging[d]	2	No	No	No	No	3	No	2
Scan time[e] (min:sec)	0:12	0:44	0:58	0:31	0:18	3:55	0.03 (9:58)	0:18 (3:28)

Abbreviations: A to P, anterior-to-posterior; BH, breath-hold; Fat sat, spectral selective fat saturation; FOV, field of view in millimeters; IR, inversion recovery; NEX, number of excitations; RBW, receiver bandwidth in Hertz/pixel; R to L, right to left; SPAIR (see Table 2), spectral adiabatic inversion recovery (see text); SSFSE, half single-shot fast spin echo sequence; STIR, short tau inversion recovery; ST/SG, slice thickness and slice gap in millimeters; TE, echo time; 3D, 3-dimensional; 3D SPGR DIXON, 3-dimensional, nonfat-saturated, spoiled gradient-echo sequence for chemical shift imaging; 3D SPGR FS, fat-saturated, 3-dimensional, spoiled gradient-echo T1-weighted sequence for postcontrast; 2D, 2-dimensional.

a Secretin: presecretion and postsecretion MRCP as described in the text; 2D MRCP and secretin MRCP slabs are single slabs of 40-mm thickness. The 3D sequences do not have slice gap.
b Navigator refers to navigator-monitored respiratory triggering (see text).
c Concatenation is the number of interleaved acquisitions or number of breath-holds.
d Where parallel imaging (PI) is used, the number given is the acceleration factor. PI is typically performed with generalized auto-calibrating partially parallel acquisition.
e Scan time (in minutes): The time given in parenthesis is the total scan times for performing the secretin-enhanced MRCP series and the 3 postgadolinium series.

Table 2
Parameters for pancreatic imaging on 3.0 T MR imaging scanners

Parameter	3D SPGR DIXON	T2 2D SSFSE	T2 2D SSFSE	MRCP 2D Slab	MRCP 3D	MRCP Secretin	3D SPGR FS
Plane of acquisition	Axial	Axial	Coronal	Coronal	Coronal	Coronal	Axial
TR/TE (msec)	5.45/2.45 (in), 3.68 (out)	2000/96	2000/97	4500/622	2400/719	4500/746	4.19/1.47
Flip angle (°)	9	150	150	160	Variable	180	9
ST/SG	4.0/-	5/5.2	4/4.4	40/-	1.2/-	40/-	2.6/-
NEX	1	1	1	1	2	1	1
RBW	500 or 780	780	780	383	318	161	350
Phase direction	A to P	A to P	R to L	R to L	R to L	R to L	A to P
Echo train length	1	168	256	307	101	288	1
Matrix	320 × 224	320 × 224	320 × 256	384 × 306	380 × 380	384 × 306	308 × 210
Field of view	400	380	350	300	380	300	400
Respiration	BH	BH	Navigator	BH	Navigator	BH	BH
Fat saturation	No	SPAIR	No	Fat sat	SPAIR	Fat sat	SPAIR
Concatenation	1	4	1	8	1	1	1
Parallel imaging	2	2	3	2	2	2	2
Scan time (min:sec)	0:16	1:08	1:50	0:36	3:54	0:04 (9:56)	0:19 (3:19)

See legend for Table 1.

contrast is helpful in reducing the signal from the overlying stomach and duodenum. Pineapple or blueberry juice has also been used as oral contrast agents.[1–3] The manganese content of these juices results in an increased signal on T1-weighted images and a reduced signal on T2-weighted images. The authors prefer the use of 300 mL of proprietary silicone-coated superparamagnetic iron oxide particle suspension (ferumoxsil, Gastromark, Covidien Pharmaceuticals, Hazelwood, MO, USA) (Fig. 1) taken orally a few minutes before the MR imaging examination. Alternatively, diluted gadolinium (eg, 5 mL in 75 mL of saline) can also null the signal in the upper gastrointestinal tract on T2-weighted images.

T1-Weighted Sequences

Because of the presence of proteins and manganese, the normal pancreas has one of the highest signal intensities of the abdominal viscera on fat-suppressed T1-weighted images. T1-weighted sequences are useful for assessing hemorrhage, such as those that occur within inflammatory collections in acute pancreatitis (Fig. 2), and can help identify the presence of pancreatic fat (Fig. 3). Traditionally, 2-dimensional gradient-echo sequences with 2 echo times (TE) have been used. This sequence yields images in which water and fat protons have the same or opposing phases. The fat content may be estimated by assessing the signal loss on opposed-phase images. Three-dimensional, 2-point Dixon techniques (see Fig. 3), which acquire thinner, contiguous slices within a breath-hold, are preferable to 2-dimensional gradient-echo sequences because they are less affected by field inhomogeneities and can assess fat content of more than 50%. Three-point Dixon techniques may be able to correct for T2* decay by using the data from a third echo.

T2-Weighted Sequences

Normal pancreatic parenchyma has a shorter T2 than most abdominal organs and, therefore, exhibits a low to intermediate signal on T2-weighted images. T2-weighted sequences are useful to assess the nature of peripancreatic inflammatory collections and determine their internal solid versus fluid content. These sequences are also useful in the assessment of cystic pancreatic masses. Depending on the scanner, TSE, single-shot fast spin echo (SSFSE), or steady-state free precession (SSFP) sequences are used. SSFP, such as fast imaging employing steady-state acquisition (FIESTA), true fast imaging with steady-state precession (FISP), or balanced fast-field echo (FFE), have a high signal-to-noise ratio (SNR). In these sequences, contrast is determined by a ratio of T2/T1. By keeping the repetition time (TR) and TE short, T1 remains constant and the principal component of image contrast is T2. Balanced SSFP techniques are insensitive to flow voids and do not show the artificial filling defects in bile ducts because of the flow that may sometimes be seen on SSFSE images (Fig. 4). Pancreatic vessels are bright on SSFE sequences, making them advantageous in surgical planning for tumor resectability. However, small cystic lesions adjacent to splenic vessels may be difficult to discern on this sequence. Balanced SSFP sequences are prone to susceptibility artifact. Off-resonance effects may produce alternating dark and light bands. Shimming and maintaining a short TR help to reduce this artifact. Studies on liver lesions have not found a significant difference in diagnostic ability between balanced SSFP and SSFSE sequences.[4,5]

In general, the image quality of SSFSE sequence is superior to TSE sequences. SSFSE is used to obtain T2-weighted sequence, with a TE of about 100 milliseconds, and MRCP, with a TE of about 600 milliseconds (see Tables 1 and 2). Fat is bright

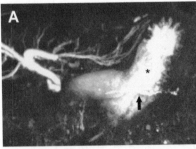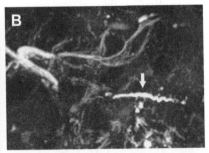

Fig. 1. A 65-year-old man with history of intraductal papillary mucinous neoplasm, status post-Whipple operation. (A) Coronal MRCP image shows the bright signal from the fluid within the stomach (asterisk), which overlies the body and tail of pancreas, obscuring the main pancreatic duct and a cystic mass (black arrow) in pancreatic body. (B) Same patient was reexamined after ingestion of negative oral contrast. Repeat study shows good visualization of cystic mass and main pancreatic duct (arrow).

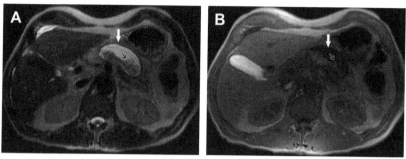

Fig. 2. A 44-year-old male patient with acute pancreatitis and sudden drop in hematocrit level. (*A*) Axial T2-weighted image shows a fluid collection (*white arrow*) with low signal debris (*black arrow*) in dependent aspect. (*B*) Axial T1-weighted opposed-phase image shows high signal (*black arrow*) in dependent aspect of cyst indicating presence of blood products. Simple fluid has low signal on T1-weighted images (*white arrow*). Patient was diagnosed to have hemorrhagic pseudocyst.

on these sequences, thus, fat suppression may be required. In addition, T2-weighted sequences are too long to be acquired within one breath-hold. They may be obtained over 2 or 3 breath-holds. Alternatively, the sequences may be performed during free breathing with the motion correction techniques explained later.

Fat suppression

Two different approaches are traditionally used to suppress fat. Chemical shift fat suppression is based on the difference of resonance frequency between fat and water. Before the main sequence, a spectrally selective radiofrequency pulse tuned to the fat frequency is applied, followed by spoiler

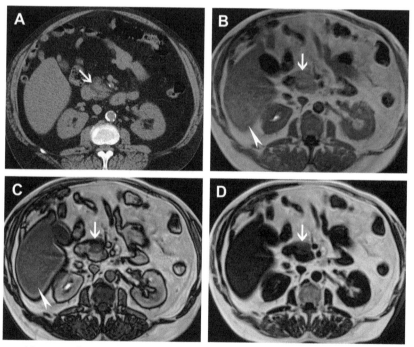

Fig. 3. A 64-year-old man underwent an unenhanced chest computed tomography (CT) and was found to have a pancreatic head mass worrisome for malignancy. Further evaluation with MR imaging was recommended. (*A*) Axial CT image shows inhomogeneous hypodensity in the head of the pancreas (*arrow*). In-phase (*B*) and opposed-phase (*C*) images of 3-dimensional T1-weighted MR imaging show focal area of signal loss on opposed-phase within the pancreatic head (*arrow*) corresponding to the CT finding. Liver shows diffuse loss of signal consistent with hepatic steatosis (*arrowhead*). (*D*) Using the Dixon technique, it is possible to derive fat-only or water-only images. On fat-only image (*D*), pancreatic head shows focal increased signal (*arrow*). Appearances are consistent with fatty deposition in pancreatic head, simulating tumor.

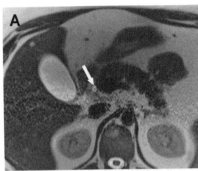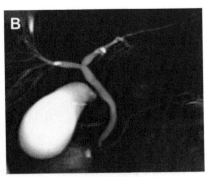

Fig. 4. A 33-year-old woman with right upper-quadrant pain. (*A*) Axial SSFSE T2-weighted image shows apparent filling defect (*arrow*) in distal common bile duct (CBD). (*B*) Coronal MRCP image on the same study shows no obvious CBD stone. The apparent calculus on axial SSFSE image is artifactual and caused by flow of bile. Endoscopic retrograde cholangiopancreatography (*not shown*) did not reveal choledocholithiasis.

gradient pulses. The frequency of precession of fat protons depends on the magnetic field. Therefore, this technique is adversely affected by magnetic field inhomogeneity. Another approach is inversion-recovery (IR) fat suppression, such as short tau inversion recovery (STIR), which is based on the difference in T1 relaxation times between fat and water. By using an inversion time (TI) of 150 to 170 milliseconds at 1.5 T MR imaging, the fat signal can be selectively suppressed. In general, IR techniques have more homogenous fat suppression and a better contrast-to-noise ratio compared with spectral fat saturation techniques. On the other hand, they have lower spatial resolution, with other MR parameters being the same, or longer acquisition times.

In the conventional implementation of IR fat suppression, the inversion pulse has a wide frequency bandwidth to invert both fat and water spins. Therefore, the water signal is also partially suppressed at the TI of fat. This suppression results in a lower SNR that may affect lesion conspicuity. Spectral adiabatic inversion recovery (SPAIR) is a newer IR fat-suppression technique. In this sequence, the inversion pulse is spectrally selective and affects only the fat protons. The adiabatic inversion is also insensitive to B1 inhomogeneity. The benefits of adiabatic inversion recovery over conventional IR include better SNR (**Fig. 5**) and reduced susceptibility artifact, especially at 3.0 T.[6] However, the specific absorption rate (SAR) is higher with adiabatic inversion recovery compared with conventional IR sequences.

In addition to the 2 techniques of fat suppression discussed previously (ie, chemical shift selective saturation and inversion recovery), T2-weighted Dixon techniques are being evaluated. Three-point Dixon techniques with iterative decomposition of water and fat may be used with TSE sequences but require a long acquisition time.[7] A prototype 3-point Dixon technique in which each TSE readout gradient is replaced with 3 readout gradient pulses with different fat/water phase shifts may, in the future, provide high-quality, fat-suppressed, breath-hold T2-weighted images.[8,9]

Motion suppression

Techniques of motion suppression during free breathing include the use of respiratory triggering, respiratory monitoring with navigator pulse, and rotatory k-space sampling. Most T2-weighted SSFSE and 3-dimensional MRCP sequences are too long to be performed within a single breath-hold and require respiratory triggering. Traditionally, this is accomplished by placing pneumatic bellows around the lower chest to detect respiratory motion. A more recent development is the use of 2-dimensional navigator pulses. The most commonly used navigator technique is 2-dimensional prospective acquisition correction encoding (2D PACE) (**Fig. 6**). This method is further discussed in the "MRCP" section.

Rotatory filling of the k-space allows for inherent motion-correction capabilities. With these techniques, named periodically rotated overlapping parallel lines with enhancement reconstruction (PROPELLER) or BLADE (not an acronym), the k-space is covered by multiple rectangle regions shaped like blades rotated around the center.[10,11] Each blade consists of a small number of phase-encoding lines that can be filled with a multiple echo acquisition after a single excitation. Any in-plane motion that occurs between the acquisitions of the 2 blades can be determined by comparing the k-space data in the overlapping part of 2 blades and may be corrected. After repeating such process for all the blades, the full k-space can be created from motion-corrected blades to reconstruct an image with reduced motion artifacts (**Fig. 7**). These techniques require longer

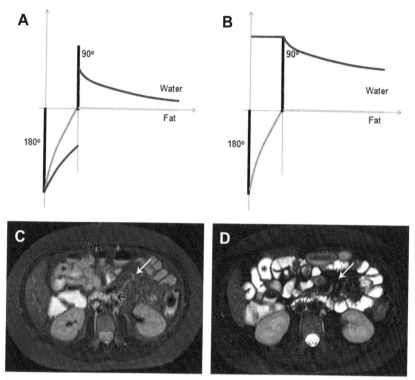

Fig. 5. (A, B) Line diagrams of conventional IR (A) and SPAIR (B) sequences. The vertical axis shows signal and time is given in the horizontal axis. The orange lines show signal from fat and the red lines show the signal from water. Note that the water signal from SPAIR is higher than that from IR. (C, D) A 31-year-old man with abdominal pain underwent evaluation with 3.0 T MR imaging. Axial images of conventional IR (C) and SPAIR (D) are compared. Mesenteric vessels within the fat (arrow) are better depicted with SPAIR. Motion artifacts in midline abdomen distorting the image (C) (black arrows) is not present on the image (D) with SPAIR sequence. There is reduced water signal (asterisk) in conventional IR sequence. Bowel wall is more conspicuous on SPAIR image.

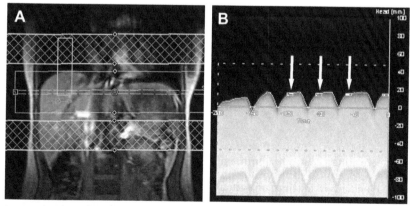

Fig. 6. Navigator monitoring of respiratory motion. (A) In this technique, coronal 2-dimensional, low-resolution gradient-echo images with small flip angle (to prevent magnetization saturation) are acquired in about 100 milliseconds. Technique traces the motion of the right hemi-diaphragm in real time. (B) This respiratory trace allows synchronization of data acquisition with patient's respiratory cycle. On initial respiratory cycles, range of motion is determined. On subsequent respiratory cycles, data acquisition is triggered when diaphragm is stationary (arrows).

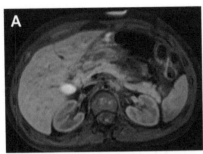 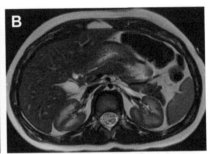

Fig. 7. Motion-related artifact reduction using motion correction (BLADE) sequence in a 5-year-old male pediatric patient. (*A*) Axial, T1-weighted, fat-saturated images obtained free breathing without motion correction shows motion-related artifacts significantly degrading the image quality in the midline abdomen. (*B*) During the same study, an axial, T2-weighted image with BLADE was also obtained; these motion-corrected images show substantially reduced artifacts in this difficult-to-scan patient.

scan times than conventional rectilinear data acquisition because of the redundancy in k-space data. However, the oversampling in the center of the k-space also improves the SNR. These techniques are based on the assumption of rigid body motion and are not as effective in correcting elastic motion for organs, such as the liver and pancreas. In addition, they do not correct in-plane motion. With rotatory k-space filling techniques, image quality is best with wider blades, longer echo train lengths, and oversampling of the k-space.[12] Inadequate k-space sampling may result in streak artifacts (Fig. 8). Increasing echo train length improves flow suppression. Studies have shown the improved diagnostic quality of upper abdominal organs with rotatory k-space filling technique sequences compared

with conventional breath-hold and navigator-corrected T2-weighted SSFSE sequences.[10,13]

Flip-angle modulation techniques

A limitation of 3-dimensional, constant, flip-angle, T2-weighted sequences at 3.0 T is the high radio-frequency energy deposition. Newer 3-dimensional TSE techniques use variable flip angles. Such techniques are termed SPACE (sampling perfection with application optimized contrasts using different flip angle evolutions), XETA (extended echo train acquisition), or CUBE (not an acronym). Variable refocusing flip-angle techniques can maintain higher signal intensity in a long echo train to produce higher SNR.[14] SAR may be reduced by about 70% at 3.0 T by using varying flip angles.[15] A study comparing traditional constant flip-angle, 3-dimensional MRCP with variable refocused flip-angle MRCP in healthy volunteers imaged on a 3.0 T MR scanner found significantly better image quality of intrahepatic bile ducts with the latter sequence.[14] In addition, the improved image quality, with the variable, refocused flip-angle technique, has been found in healthy subjects scanned at 1.5 T,[16] when energy deposition is not a major factor. This result may be caused by the shorter echo spacing and the resultant lesser image blurring that is possible with variable refocusing flip angles. The advantages and disadvantages of flip-angle modulation techniques over constant flip-angle techniques are given in Table 3.[17]

Fig. 8. BLADE sequence artifact caused by insufficient sampling of k-space. A 46-year-old patient with right upper-quadrant pain underwent MR imaging evaluation. T2-weighted, fat-saturated, axial image obtained with BLADE shows streaky artifacts (*arrows*) that obscure the structures in and around the gastric wall within the lesser sac. These artifacts arise in the process of gridding data acquired from an oblique trajectory in k-space and may be improved by oversampling of the k-space.

MRCP

MRCP refers to the acquisition of heavily T2-weighted images, with variants of TSE sequences. These sequences consist of a single 90° pulse followed by multiple, constant refocusing pulses. The refocusing pulses were typically 180° pulses, although pulses of 130° to 160° are often used to

Table 3
Advantages and disadvantages of flip-angle modulation techniques, such as SPACE, with constant flip-angle TSE T2-weighted sequences

Advantages	Disadvantages
Reduced SAR, especially at 3.0 T Reduced echo space, less blurring Reduced N/2 ghosting artifacts	Longer acquisition times
Isotropic acquisition, allowing multiplanar reconstructions	Altered contrast, with partial T1-weighting
Improved flow suppression	Increased B1 inhomogeneity artifact

Variable flip-angle techniques may fill the k-space partition in a respiratory cycle. Constant flip-angle, 3-dimensional techniques may fill the k-space partition in 2 breathing cycles. If the diaphragmatic position in the 2 cycles is different, N/2 ghosting artifacts may occur. Ghost signal is shifted by one half length of field of view (FOV) in phase-encoding direction (or FOV/4 if parallel imaging with acceleration factor of 2 is used).
   Data from Haystead CM, Dale BM, Merkle EM. N/2 ghosting artifacts: elimination at 3.0-T MR cholangiography with SPACE pulse sequence. Radiology 2008;246:589–95.

reduce energy deposition, especial at 3.0 T. Very long echo trains may be required to acquire all data in a slice within a single TR, which can result in blurring of the images. The commonly used sequences use a partial Fourier technique in which 50% to 60% of the k-space is filled by data. The remainder of the k-space is filled by extrapolation using the symmetry of the k-space. Sequences that acquire the dataset within one TR and use partial Fourier technique are called SSFSE or half

Fourier acquisition single-shot turbo spin echo (HASTE). Two-dimensional MRCP has traditionally been used with coronal SSFSE slabs. The 40-mm slabs in multiple coronal oblique planes can be acquired to image the pancreatic ductal system (Fig. 9).

Three-dimensional MRCP
A 3-dimensional TSE sequence can produce high-spatial-resolution MRCP images (Fig. 10). Thin

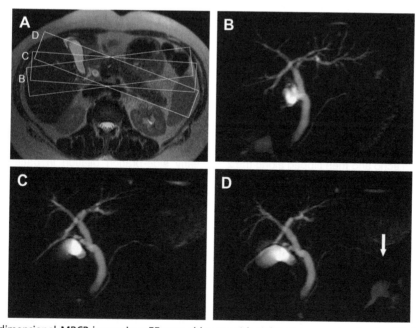

Fig. 9. Two-dimensional MRCP image in a 55-year-old man with right upper-quadrant pain. (*A*) Positioning of MRCP slabs. Three slabs were placed for demonstration purposes on axial SSFSE image and correspond to images (*B–D*). In the authors' practice, 6 coronal oblique slabs (40 mm thick) are used to ensure that the pancreaticobiliary ductal system is included. (*B–D*) Two-dimensional MRCP coronal images, corresponding to slab selections on image (*A*), demonstrate different portions of the pancreatic duct. Note that pancreatic tail is only seen on image (*D*) (*arrow*) and not visualized on (*B*) or (*C*).

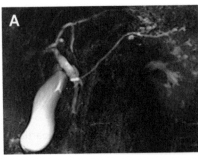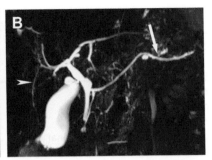

Fig. 10. A 74-year-old woman with cystic pancreatic lesions. Coronal image of 2-dimensional MRCP (*A*) and coronal maximum intensity projection image of 3-dimensional MRCP (*B*) demonstrate that the posterior branch of right hepatic duct (*arrowhead*) is better visualized on 3-dimensional sequence. In addition, the 3-dimensional sequence shows the ductal connection of the cystic lesion (*arrow*) better than the 2-dimensional sequence. This was a critical finding highly suggestive of a side-branch intraductal papillary mucinous neoplasm. In the authors' practice, both 2- and 3-dimensional MRCP are routinely performed because the former may have better image quality in patients with irregular or rapid respiratory cycles.

sections without slice gap allow for better assessment of small stones, side branches of main pancreatic duct, and the intrahepatic biliary system.[18,19] Three-dimensional MRCP may be performed as a series of breath-holds or during free breathing. In the authors' practice, 1- to 2-mm contiguous slices during free breathing are acquired and navigator-echo techniques reduce motion artifact. The main disadvantage of this technique is the long acquisition time. In addition, navigator-based triggering requires uniform and regular breathing cycles for optimal image quality. If patients have rapid or irregular breathing, the image quality may be impaired. An alternative method of producing 3-dimensional MRCP images is to use a TSE sequence with a 90° flip-back pulse. Such sequences are called fast recovery fast spin echo (FRFSE), DRIVE, or RESTORE (not acronyms). The unique feature of these sequences is that after a long echo train, the residual transverse magnetization is refocused into a final spin echo and then flipped along the z-axis by a 90° fast-recovery pulse.[18,20] This action accelerates the relaxation of the longitudinal magnetization, leading to a reduction in TR without loss of SNR. It is possible to perform a breath-hold 3-dimensional MRCP with this sequence. However, the number of slices that may be obtained is substantially less than with respiratory-triggered versions of 3-dimensional MRCP.

S-MRCP

Secretin is a polypeptide hormone secreted by duodenal mucosa in response to increased luminal acidity.[21] It induces pancreatic secretion of water and bicarbonate. In the first 3 to 5 minutes after administration, the tone of sphincter of Oddi is increased. These effects result in the temporary distention of the pancreatic ducts. Synthetic human secretin (ChiRhoStim, ChiRhoClin, Inc, Burtonsville, Maryland) is given intravenously over 1 minute to avoid potential abdominal pain that may occur with a bolus injection. An adult dose of 16 μg (0.2 μg/kg body weight) is used. At the commencement of injection, a baseline scan is obtained, followed by an oblique coronal SSFSE image (2-second scan time) every 30 seconds for 10 minutes. In average patients, the maximal effect of intravenous secretin is between 7 to 10 minutes (Fig. 11).

S-MRCP is used routinely in all patients undergoing MRCP at the authors' institution. Secretin is valuable in the assessment of complex pancreatic ductal anomalies, such as annular pancreas (Fig. 12) and anomalous pancreaticobiliary junction.[22] S-MRCP increases the confidence of the diagnosis of pancreas divisum, although in many instances the diagnosis may be suspected on nonsecretin MRCP. S-MRCP helps in assessing early side-branch dilation in patients with mild changes of chronic pancreatitis because the sensitivity of conventional MRCP is not adequate to detect side-branch dilation (Fig. 13).[23–26] In addition, the exocrine functional reserve can be quantitatively or semiquantitatively assessed with S-MRCP (see Fig. 13; Fig. 14). Quantitative measurements of exocrine response to secretin have been calculated using volumetric or signal intensity measurements of fluid released into duodenum following secretin injection.[27–30] The authors routinely use a semiquantitative description of exocrine function.[31] If the maximum output fills only the duodenal bulb, pancreatic exocrine function is considered to be poor. Filling of the bulb and the second part of the duodenum is considered suboptimal function. Filling of the

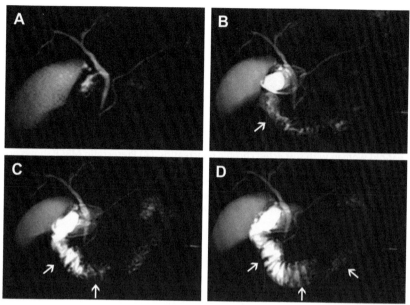

Fig. 11. A 47-year-old man with abdominal pain evaluated with MRCP. These images are obtained before injection of secretin (*A*) and at 3 minutes (*B*), 7 minutes (*C*), and 10 minutes (*D*) after intravenous administration of secretin. Note progressive filling of first through fourth portions of the duodenum, which become distended with excreted pancreatic fluid (*arrows*). On the 7-minute image, fluid has reached the duodenojejunal junction.

duodenum or loops of jejunum is considered normal function. In addition, S-MRCP is also useful in the evaluation of patients with pancreatic duct leak following severe pancreatitis, pancreatic surgery, or blunt trauma.[32,33]

The authors have performed more than 6000 S-MRCP since 2003 and are aware of only 3 cases of acute pancreatitis that resulted shortly after secretin administration. In the authors' practice, secretin is used even in patients with mild acute pancreatitis but its use is avoided in patients with severe pancreatitis in the acute setting. The major

drawbacks of S-MRCP are the 10 minutes of acquisition time and the cost of secretin (estimated to be $300 per adult dose).

Contrast-Enhanced Sequences

Contrast administration is not necessary in the evaluation of patients with suspected choledocholithiasis or follow-up of cystic pancreatic lesions. For most other indications, the acquisition of gadolinium-enhanced sequences is advisable. The sequence of choice for pregadolinium and

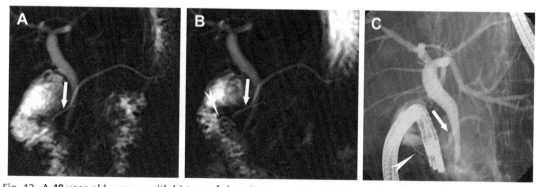

Fig. 12. A 48-year-old woman with history of chronic pancreatitis. (*A*) Conventional MRCP shows incomplete divisum anatomy with a prominent Santorini duct (*arrow*) connected to the main duct in the body and tail. However, there was no obvious evidence of annular pancreas. (*B*) Postsecretin MRCP shows the divisum anatomy (*arrow*) and a thin duct (*arrowhead*) overlying the duodenum. This finding was considered to be consistent with annular pancreas. (*C*) The diagnosis of divisum (*arrow*) and annular pancreas (*arrowhead*) were proven on ERCP.

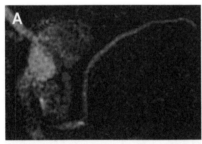
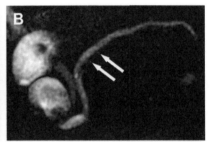

Fig. 13. A 52-year-old woman with suspected chronic pancreatitis. (*A*) Presecretin MRCP shows an unremarkable pancreatogram. (*B*) Image obtained 8 minutes after intravenous secretin shows early side-branch dilation (*arrows*), indicating mild chronic pancreatitis (diagnosed by dilation of 3 or more side branches). Exocrine response to secretin is poor, with fluid only filling duodenal bulb. In the authors' experience, exocrine functional deficiencies may be substantially worse than anatomic abnormalities of the pancreatic duct.

postgadolinium series is the 3-dimensional, fat-suppressed, spoiled gradient echo. This sequence has many names, such as volume interpolated breath-hold (VIBE), fast gradient echo (F-GRE), liver acquisition with volume acceleration (LAVA), and T1-weighted, high-resolution, isotropic volume examination (THRIVE), and allows the acquisition of 2- to 5-mm contiguous slices within a 20-second breath-hold. Typically, gadolinium is injected at 2 mL/sec using a power injector and followed with a 20 mL of saline flush administered at the same rate. It is usual to acquire images of the liver (and pancreas) in multiple phases. Timing of the scan may be performed using fixed time delays, real-time bolus tracking, or with a test bolus. Traditionally, scans are obtained in the arterial, venous, and delayed phases acquired 25, 60, and 180 seconds, respectively, after the start of contrast infusion. Bolus tracking has been primarily used in MR angiography but is increasingly used in abdominal imaging. The delay from the onset of infusion to

the arrival of contrast in the distal aorta varies from 12 to 30 seconds, with a mean of 17 to 18 seconds.[34,35] Thus, it may be expected that bolus tracking would be superior to using fixed delays. In patients without cardiovascular comorbidity, fixed time delays may be adequate.[36] However, patients with cirrhosis or hypertension, bolus tracking gives a more reliable arterial phase.[35] There is no consensus on the optimal bolus tracking technique. The authors prefer to monitor the distal aorta at the diaphragmatic hiatus with bolus tracking sequence and real-time reconstructions. As soon as contrast appears, the bolus-tracking scan ends and patients are given breathing instructions. The arterial phase is started 8 seconds later. For an acceptable arterial phase, there should be good contrast in the aorta, superior mesenteric artery, and portal vein and no contrast in the hepatic veins. Lack of contrast in the portal vein suggests that the phase was acquired too early. To obtain an arterial phase without motion artifact, it is

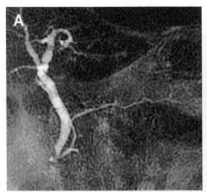
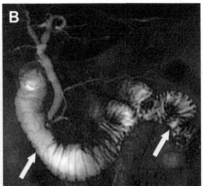

Fig. 14. A 37-year-old woman being investigated for unexplained abdominal pain, possibly biliopancreatic origin. (*A*) Presecretin image shows low signal in the duodenum since the patient ingested iron oxide suspension before the MR imaging examination. (*B*) Postsecretin image shows high signal fluid throughout the duodenum and some loops of jejunum (*arrows*). This fluid was discharged into the duodenum because of secretin-induced stimulation of the pancreas. The exocrine response to secretin is good because it fills the duodenal lumen (compare with Fig. 13).

important that the technologist coaches patients about breath-hold and gives clear instructions before intravenous contrast injection. Timing of the venous and delayed phases is less stringent compared with the arterial phase.

The contraindications to the use of gadolinium are severe allergy, pregnancy, and end-stage renal dysfunction. When the estimated glomerular filtration rate (eGFR) is more than 60 mL/min/1.73 m^2, the authors use the standard dose of gadolinium (0.1 mmol/kg). With an eGFR of 30- to 60-mL/min/1.73 m^2, a reduced dose is used, typically half the standard dose. At the authors' institution, gadolinium is not administered when the eGFR is less than 30 mL/min/1.73 m^2.

1.5 T Versus 3.0 T MR Imaging

The main advantage of scanning at 3.0 T is the higher SNR. Parallel imaging is a technique used more often in 3.0 T MR imaging than at 1.5 T. It allows the creation of images with ample field of view and spatial resolution using fewer k-space lines. This outcome is possible because the spatial sensitivity information from independent receiver coils may be used to overcome the aliasing effect of acquiring a reduced number of phase encoding lines.[37,38] As a result, the scan time is reduced, allowing the acquisition of breath-hold images or multiphasic studies in a shorter period. In addition, parallel-imaging techniques can be used to reduce T2 blurring in TSE techniques and reduce SAR and susceptibility effects by allowing shorter echo trains.[39] The main limitation of parallel imaging is the associated reduction in SNR, which is usually not an issue at 3.0 T whereby the overall SNR is higher than at 1.5 T. Parallel imaging may produce artifacts with lines or bands in the center of the images. Image domain–based techniques, such as sensitivity encoding (SENSE), and k-space–based techniques, such as generalized autocalibrating partially parallel acquisition (GRAPPA), are the 2 main types of parallel imaging. Details of these techniques have been discussed elsewhere.[37,40,41]

The improved availability of radiofrequency coils that are optimal for 3.0 T has reduced many of the limitations of 3.0 T, with a decrease in chemical shift and susceptibility artifacts and artifacts caused by interference of radiofrequency waves. Studies comparing 1.5 T and 3.0 T abdominal MR imaging suggest that 3.0 T does not offer substantial improvement in image quality for precontrast images.[42–49] However, the SNR of contrast-enhanced images is thought to be superior at 3.0 T compared with 1.5 T.[50,51] Continuing improvements in hardware and imaging sequences may allow 3.0 T MR imaging to become the system of choice for imaging the pancreas.

SUMMARY (OBJECTIVES FOR RECALL)

As a result of recent technological advances, there has been a substantial change in the pancreatic MR imaging protocol. The 3-dimensional, 2-point Dixon technique acquires thinner slices and is preferable to 2-dimensional, gradient-echo sequences. T1-weighted sequences are useful for assessing hemorrhage and the presence of pancreatic fat. Improved fat and motion suppression allows for better contrast resolution and image quality. The diagnostic potential of MRCP is close to that of endoscopic retrograde cholangiopancreatography (ERCP), obviating most diagnostic ERCP studies. Three-dimensional MRCP sequences with thin, contiguous slices offer good spatial resolution and better depiction of the pancreatic duct compared with 2-dimensional, thick-slab MRCP images. Secretin stimulation results in temporary distention of the pancreatic ducts and is, therefore, valuable in the assessment of patients with complex pancreatic ductal anomalies and chronic pancreatitis. The parallel-imaging technique reduces the scan time and improves image quality, particularly in 3.0 T scanners. Negative oral contrast can be used to reduce the signal from the overlying stomach and duodenum.

The future direction of pancreatic MR imaging will likely include more functional assessment of the pancreas with S-MRCP, diffusion-weighted MR imaging, MR imaging perfusion, and MR elastography. These tools may become part of the MR protocol for specific indications, such as assessing the malignant potential of cystic pancreatic tumor, or evaluating the severity of chronic pancreatitis. The future of pancreas MR imaging seems to be exciting.

REFERENCES

1. Coppens E, Metens T, Winant C, et al. Pineapple juice labeled with gadolinium: a convenient oral contrast for magnetic resonance cholangiopancreatography. Eur Radiol 2005;15:2122–9.
2. Papanikolaou N, Karantanas A, Maris T, et al. MR cholangiopancreatography before and after oral blueberry juice administration. J Comput Assist Tomogr 2000;24:229–34.
3. Riordan RD, Khonsari M, Jeffries J, et al. Pineapple juice as a negative oral contrast agent in magnetic resonance cholangiopancreatography: a preliminary evaluation. Br J Radiol 2004;77:991–9.

4. Herborn CU, Vogt F, Lauenstein TC, et al. MRI of the liver: can true FISP replace HASTE? J Magn Reson Imaging 2003;17:190–6.

5. Numminen K, Halavaara J, Isoniemi H, et al. Magnetic resonance imaging of the liver: true fast imaging with steady state free precession sequence facilitates rapid and reliable distinction between hepatic hemangiomas and liver malignancies. J Comput Assist Tomogr 2003;27:571–6.

6. Lauenstein TC, Sharma P, Hughes T, et al. Evaluation of optimized inversion-recovery fat-suppression techniques for T2-weighted abdominal MR imaging. J Magn Reson Imaging 2008;27:1448–54.

7. Reeder SB, Yu H, Johnson JW, et al. T1- and T2-weighted fast spin-echo imaging of the brachial plexus and cervical spine with IDEAL water-fat separation. J Magn Reson Imaging 2006;24:825–32.

8. Low RN, Ma J, Panchal N. Fast spin-echo triple-echo Dixon: initial clinical experience with a novel pulse sequence for fat-suppressed T2-weighted abdominal MR imaging. J Magn Reson Imaging 2009;30:569–77.

9. Ma J, Son JB, Zhou Y, et al. Fast spin-echo triple-echo Dixon (fTED) technique for efficient T2-weighted water and fat imaging. Magn Reson Med 2007;58:103–9.

10. Bayramoglu S, Kilickesmez O, Cimilli T, et al. T2-weighted MRI of the upper abdomen: comparison of four fat-suppressed T2-weighted sequences including PROPELLER (BLADE) technique. Acad Radiol 2010;17(3):368–74. [Epub 2009 Dec 30].

11. Nanko S, Oshima H, Watanabe T, et al. Usefulness of the application of the BLADE technique to reduce motion artifacts on navigation-triggered prospective acquisition correction (PACE) T2-weighted MRI (T2WI) of the liver. J Magn Reson Imaging 2009;30:321–6.

12. Hirokawa Y, Isoda H, Maetani YS, et al. Evaluation of motion correction effect and image quality with the periodically rotated overlapping parallel lines with enhanced reconstruction (PROPELLER) (BLADE) and parallel imaging acquisition technique in the upper abdomen. J Magn Reson Imaging 2008;28:957–62.

13. Michaely HJ, Kramer H, Weckbach S, et al. Renal T2-weighted turbo-spin-echo imaging with BLADE at 3.0 tesla: initial experience. J Magn Reson Imaging 2008;27:148–53.

14. Arizono S, Isoda H, Maetani YS, et al. High-spatial-resolution three-dimensional MR cholangiography using a high-sampling-efficiency technique (SPACE) at 3T: comparison with the conventional constant flip angle sequence in healthy volunteers. J Magn Reson Imaging 2008;28:685–90.

15. Weigel M, Hennig J. Contrast behavior and relaxation effects of conventional and hyperecho-turbo spin echo sequences at 1.5 and 3 T. Magn Reson Med 2006;55:826–35.

16. Morita S, Ueno E, Masukawa A, et al. Comparison of SPACE and 3D TSE MRCP at 1.5T focusing on difference in echo spacing. Magn Reson Med Sci 2009;8:101–5.

17. Haystead CM, Dale BM, Merkle EM. N/2 ghosting artifacts: elimination at 3.0-T MR cholangiography with SPACE pulse sequence. Radiology 2008;246:589–95.

18. Sodickson A, Mortele KJ, Barish MA, et al. Three-dimensional fast-recovery fast spin-echo MRCP: comparison with two-dimensional single-shot fast spin-echo techniques. Radiology 2006;238:549–59.

19. Yoon LS, Catalano OA, Fritz S, et al. Another dimension in magnetic resonance cholangiopancreatography: comparison of 2- and 3-dimensional magnetic resonance cholangiopancreatography for the evaluation of intraductal papillary mucinous neoplasm of the pancreas. J Comput Assist Tomogr 2009;33:363–8.

20. Busse RF, Riederer SJ, Fletcher JG, et al. Interactive fast spin-echo imaging. Magn Reson Med 2000;44:339–48.

21. Chey WY, Chang TM. Secretin, 100 years later. J Gastroenterol 2003;38:1025–35.

22. Motosugi U, Ichikawa T, Araki T, et al. Secretin-stimulating MRCP in patients with pancreatobiliary maljunction and occult pancreatobiliary reflux: direct demonstration of pancreatobiliary reflux. Eur Radiol 2007;17:2262–7.

23. Balci NC, Alkaade S, Magas L, et al. Suspected chronic pancreatitis with normal MRCP: findings on MRI in correlation with secretin MRCP. J Magn Reson Imaging 2008;27:125–31.

24. Czako L. Diagnosis of early-stage chronic pancreatitis by secretin-enhanced magnetic resonance cholangiopancreatography. J Gastroenterol 2007;42(Suppl 17):113–7.

25. Sai JK, Suyama M, Kubokawa Y, et al. Diagnosis of mild chronic pancreatitis (Cambridge classification): comparative study using secretin injection-magnetic resonance cholangiopancreatography and endoscopic retrograde pancreatography. World J Gastroenterol 2008;14:1218–21.

26. Sugiyama M, Haradome H, Atomi Y. Magnetic resonance imaging for diagnosing chronic pancreatitis. J.Gastroenterol 2007;42(Suppl 17):108–12.

27. Bali MA, Sztantics A, Metens T, et al. Quantification of pancreatic exocrine function with secretin-enhanced magnetic resonance cholangiopancreatography: normal values and short-term effects of pancreatic duct drainage procedures in chronic pancreatitis. Initial results. Eur Radiol 2005;15:2110–21.

28. Czako L, Endes J, Takacs T, et al. Evaluation of pancreatic exocrine function by secretin-enhanced magnetic resonance cholangiopancreatography. Pancreas 2001;23:323–8.

29. Lee NJ, Kim KW, Kim TK, et al. Secretin-stimulated MRCP. Abdom Imaging 2006;31:575–81.

30. Punwani S, Gillams AR, Lees WR. Non-invasive quantification of pancreatic exocrine function using secretin-stimulated MRCP. Eur Radiol 2003;13:273–6.

31. Cappeliez O, Delhaye M, Deviere J, et al. Chronic pancreatitis: evaluation of pancreatic exocrine function with MR pancreatography after secretin stimulation. Radiology 2000;215:358–64.

32. Hellund JC, Skattum J, Buanes T, et al. Secretin-stimulated magnetic resonance cholangiopancreatography of patients with unclear disease in the pancreaticobiliary tract. Acta Radiol 2007;48:135–41.

33. Ragozzino A, Manfredi R, Scaglione M, et al. The use of MRCP in the detection of pancreatic injuries after blunt trauma. Emerg Radiol 2003;10:14–8.

34. Earls JP, Rofsky NM, Decorato DR, et al. Hepatic arterial-phase dynamic gadolinium-enhanced MR imaging: optimization with a test examination and a power injector. Radiology 1997;202:268–73.

35. Sharma P, Kitajima HD, Kalb B, et al. Gadolinium-enhanced imaging of liver tumors and manifestations of hepatitis: pharmacodynamic and technical considerations. Top Magn Reson Imaging 2009;20:71–8.

36. Materne R, Horsmans Y, Jamart J, et al. Gadolinium-enhanced arterial-phase MR imaging of hypervascular liver tumors: comparison between tailored and fixed scanning delays in the same patients. J Magn Reson Imaging 2000;11:244–9.

37. Glockner JF, Hu HH, Stanley DW, et al. Parallel MR imaging: a user's guide. Radiographics 2005;25:1279–97.

38. Pruessmann KP. Encoding and reconstruction in parallel MRI. NMR Biomed 2006;19:288–99.

39. Hussain SM, Wielopolski PA, Martin DR. Abdominal magnetic resonance imaging at 3.0 T: problem or a promise for the future? Top Magn Reson Imaging 2005;16:325–35.

40. Akisik FM, Sandrasegaran K, Aisen AM, et al. Abdominal MR imaging at 3.0 T. Radiographics 2007;27:1433–44.

41. Bammer R, Schoenberg SO. Current concepts and advances in clinical parallel magnetic resonance imaging. Top Magn Reson Imaging 2004;15:129–58.

42. Edelman RR, Salanitri G, Brand R, et al. Magnetic resonance imaging of the pancreas at 3.0 tesla: qualitative and quantitative comparison with 1.5 tesla. Invest Radiol 2006;41:175–80.

43. Isoda H, Kataoka M, Maetani Y, et al. MRCP imaging at 3.0 T vs. 1.5 T: preliminary experience in healthy volunteers. J Magn Reson Imaging 2007;25:1000–6.

44. Kim SY, Byun JH, Lee SS, et al. Biliary tract depiction in living potential liver donors: intraindividual comparison of MR cholangiography at 3.0 and 1.5 T. Radiology 2010;254:469–78.

45. Koelblinger C, Schima W, Weber M, et al. Gadoxate-enhanced T 1-weighted MR cholangiography: comparison of 1.5 T and 3.0 T. Rofo 2009;181:587–92.

46. Onishi H, Kim T, Hori M, et al. MR cholangiopancreatography at 3.0 T: intraindividual comparative study with MR cholangiopancreatography at 1.5 T for clinical patients. Invest Radiol 2009;44:559–65.

47. Ramalho M, Heredia V, Tsurusaki M, et al. Quantitative and qualitative comparison of 1.5 and 3.0 tesla MRI in patients with chronic liver diseases. J Magn Reson Imaging 2009;29:869–79.

48. Schmidt GP, Wintersperger B, Graser A, et al. High-resolution whole-body magnetic resonance imaging applications at 1.5 and 3 Tesla: a comparative study. Invest Radiol 2007;42:449–59.

49. von Falkenhausen MM, Lutterbey G, Morakkabati-Spitz N, et al. High-field-strength MR imaging of the liver at 3.0 T: intraindividual comparative study with MR imaging at 1.5 T. Radiology 2006;241:156–66.

50. Goncalves Neto JA, Altun E, Elazzazi M, et al. Enhancement of abdominal organs on hepatic arterial phase: quantitative comparison between 1.5- and 3.0-T magnetic resonance imaging. Magn Reson Imaging 2010;28:47–55.

51. Lee VS, Hecht EM, Taouli B, et al. Body and cardiovascular MR imaging at 3.0 T. Radiology 2007;244:692–705.

Ultrasonography of the Pancreas

Giulia A. Zamboni, MD*, Maria Chiara Ambrosetti, MD,
Mirko D'Onofrio, MD, Roberto Pozzi Mucelli, MD

KEYWORDS

- Ultrasonography • Pancreatic ultrasound
- Pancreatic diseases • Contrast-enhanced ultrasonography

Although the pancreas is often thought of as an organ that is difficult to explore using ultrasound (US), due to its deep retroperitoneal location, with the appropriate technique it can be studied successfully in most patients. US can provide information that is useful for diagnosis of pathologic conditions, especially with the use of harmonic imaging, color-Doppler, and contrast agent administration.

EXAMINATION TECHNIQUES

To improve visualization of the pancreas, the ultrasound (US) examination is usually performed after at least 6 hours of fasting. In this way, the presence of bowel gas is limited, the stomach is empty of food, and the entire organ can be visualized. Nevertheless, technical success is also dependent on the skill and persistence of the examiner.[1]

US should be performed routinely along multiple scan planes, including transverse, longitudinal, and angled oblique, to visualize the entire organ: the head with the uncinate process, the body, and the tail. These multiple scan planes should allow examination of the entire pancreas in at least 2 views. When needed, the spleen can be used as an acoustic window to visualize the pancreatic tail.

When visualization of the pancreas is limited, it is possible to use other scanning techniques, such as moving the transducer and applying compression to displace bowel gas, filling the stomach with water, examining the patient in suspended inspiration or expiration, and changing the patient to a decubitus position.

Conventional gray-scale US with multifrequency transducers is usually the first step when examining the pancreas, selecting the best frequency for each depth. Usually, convex probes are used, with frequencies ranging between 3 and 5 MHz. Doppler frequency must be set to record flows from deep abdominal vessels (1–4 MHz). Lower Doppler frequencies allow better penetration and are used to evaluate the peripancreatic vessels, whereas higher Doppler frequencies are useful for evaluating slower flows in thin patients whose pancreas is more superficial.[2]

Tissue Harmonic Imaging

The routine examination technique should include the use of tissue harmonic imaging (THI), which can improve visualization of the pancreas by increasing the signal-to-noise ratio and reducing the reverberation artifacts from the body wall, especially when studying large patients or deep structures. Shapiro and colleagues[3] demonstrated that harmonic imaging had better penetration detail and overall image quality than conventional US. In a prospective study on 107 patients, Hohl and colleagues[4] demonstrated that sensitivity for the detection of pancreatic lesions with THI using the phase inversion technique was higher than for conventional B-mode US.

Color-Doppler and Power-Doppler Ultrasound

Doppler ultrasound is another fundamental part of the conventional US examination for evaluating the peripancreatic vessels (portal vein, superior

Disclosures: G.A.Z., M.C.A., and R.P.M. have no disclosures. M.D. was an Advisory Board member, Siemens Healthcare (2010).
Istituto di Radiologia, Policlinico GB Rossi, Azienda Ospedaliera Universitaria Integrata Verona, P.le LA Scuro 10, 37134 Verona, Italy
* Corresponding author.
E-mail address: gzamboni@hotmail.com

Radiol Clin N Am 50 (2012) 395–406
doi:10.1016/j.rcl.2012.03.010
0033-8389/12/$ – see front matter © 2012 Elsevier Inc. All rights reserved.

mesenteric artery and vein, splenic artery and vein, aorta and inferior vena cava). Doppler imaging allows the visualization of smaller peripancreatic and intrapancreatic vessels, and at the same time the assessment of patency and characteristics of blood flow.[2]

The normal color-Doppler and pulsed-Doppler features of peripancreatic vessels in healthy subjects are well known[5]: the mean flow velocity is about 103 ± 18 cm/s in the celiac trunk, 78 ± 16 cm/s in the hepatic artery, 85 ± 18 cm/s in the splenic artery, 100 ± 22 cm/s in the superior mesenteric artery,[2] and 12 to 20 cm/s in the portal vein.[2] The resistance index in the superior mesenteric artery is general higher than in the other arterial vessels.[2]

Contrast-Enhanced Ultrasound

Contrast-enhanced ultrasound (CEUS) with second-generation contrast agents is not currently approved by the Food and Drug Administration for the study of solid abdominal organs in the United States, but is used in many other countries for the study of the pancreas and other abdominal organs.

CEUS with second-generation contrast agents (Sonovue, Bracco, Milan, Italy; Sonazoid, GE Health care, Oslo, Norway; Optison, GE Health care, NJ, USA; Definity, Lantheus Medical Imaging, MA, USA) and the use of contrast-specific US techniques allows a continuous dynamic observation of pancreatic parenchymography. CEUS can, therefore, be used for a better identification of pancreatic lesions as compared with conventional US and for characterization and staging of focal lesions already identified at US.[6]

The technique of CEUS of the pancreas should vary according to the clinical indication.[6] The patient should be in the position that provides the best visualization of the area of interest in the pancreas, most commonly the supine position. Harmonic microbubble (MB)-specific imaging with a low acoustic US pressure (mechanical index <0.2) is required for a dynamic CEUS examination: with specific US software, the background tissue signals are canceled and only the signals related the responses of the MBs are visualized. In our institution, we routinely administer a 2.4-mL intravenous bolus of second-generation contrast agent, constituted of sulfur hexafluoride–filled MBs with a phospholipid peripheral shell (SonoVue, Bracco) followed by a 5-mL saline flush. The enhancement is evaluated in real time, maintaining the same scanning frame rate as in the previous conventional gray-scale examination. The dynamic continuous observation of the contrast-enhanced phases

(arterial, portal/venous, and late phases) starts immediately after the contrast agent injection.[7] Still images or clips are saved according to the radiologist's preferences; however, most often still images are saved for the baseline and delayed parts of the examination, whereas clips are saved for the early arterial and parenchymographic phases (starting from the arrival of the contrast in the aorta).

In our institution, the most common indication is characterization and staging of focal lesions: the lesion must be examined in the arterial, pancreatic, and venous contrast-enhanced phases. The relationship with the peripancreatic vessels must be assessed. With second-generation agents, after the study of the pancreas, the liver can be studied in the delayed "sinusoidal" phase to exclude the presence of liver metastases[8]; for the study of the liver, the left lateral decubitus position may be useful.

When the objective is detection or study of a small pancreatic lesion, often the case for endocrine tumors, 2 boluses of contrast agent can be used, each of 2.4 mL, to be able to explore all the portions of the pancreas in the arterial phase.[6] Also, the use of a high–acoustic pressure flash, which almost completely eliminates saturation of the area immediately adjacent to the parenchyma already studied by disrupting the MBs, can provide another pure arterial phase.

The complete examination of the pancreas (Box 1) should include the evaluation of size, contour, and texture of the gland, and the echo pattern of the head, body, and tail (Fig. 1). The main pancreatic duct and the common bile duct must be identified, as well as the major peripancreatic vessels, such as the portal vein, superior mesenteric artery and vein, splenic artery and vein, and aorta and inferior vena cava.

NORMAL ANATOMY

The pancreas is located at the level of the first or second lumbar vertebra in the retroperitoneal

---

Box 1
What to look for in pancreatic US

- Size
- Contour
- Texture
- Echogenicity
- Main pancreatic duct
- Common bile duct
- Major peripancreatic vessels (portal vein, superior mesenteric artery and vein, splenic artery and vein, aorta and inferior vena cava)

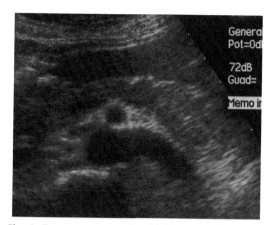

Fig. 1. Tranverse conventional US image of a normal pancreas in a young adult: the pancreas appears isoechoic to the normal liver parenchyma.

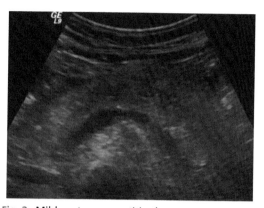

Fig. 2. Mild acute pancreatitis: the transverse conventional US image depicts the pancreas slightly enlarged, with a heterogeneous texture.

space, and its position can vary with respiration. The pancreas is usually divided into the head, with the uncinate process posteriorly and inferiorly, neck, body, and tail. The normal pancreatic parenchyma usually has a homogeneous texture and is isoechoic or hyperechoic to the normal liver parenchyma. With age, fatty replacement of the pancreas (pancreatic lipomatosis) is common, and the parenchyma may appear as echogenic as the adjacent retroperitoneal fat in up to 35% of cases.[9]

The main pancreatic duct normally measures between 95 and 250 mm in length. The diameter is greatest in the head (3–4 mm), and tapers in the body (2–3 mm) and tail (1–2 mm).[10]

INFLAMMATORY DISEASE
Acute Pancreatitis

Acute pancreatitis is an acute inflammatory process of the pancreas; the diagnosis is usually based on elevated serum amylase and lipase levels and clinical findings. Although computed tomography (CT) is the imaging modality of choice in patients with suspicion of acute pancreatitis, US is often the first examination performed in patients with acute abdominal pain. US can also help in identifying the presence of biliary stones; therefore, allowing a diagnosis of biliary pancreatitis.

Most commonly, patients with mild acute pancreatitis will show normal findings at US. When the disease is more severe, the pancreas becomes enlarged and hypoechoic to the normal liver, with a heterogeneous texture as a result of edema (**Fig. 2**).

Pancreatitis can involve the entire gland or only a portion. Diffuse acute pancreatitis is usually easily recognized, without problems in differential diagnosis. Focal acute pancreatitis, appearing as a homogeneously hypoechoic segmental enlargement of the pancreas, can be difficult to differentiate from a neoplasm. Color-Doppler can aid in the differential diagnosis, showing increased signal owing to hyperemia. CEUS can also be useful in the differential diagnosis between focal pancreatitis and pancreatic cancer: the inflamed parenchyma shows increased parenchymography, different from a neoplastic lesion (**Box 2**).[6]

US can also detect the complications of acute pancreatitis, and guide treatment. Complications include acute fluid collections, abscesses, pseudocysts, infected necrosis, and hemorrhage. The most common complications are acute fluid collections, seen in up to 50% of patients, and are most commonly localized within the anterior pararenal space and in the lesser sac.[11]

Pseudocysts are delayed complications of acute pancreatitis (typically after 4 weeks of symptom onset).[12] Pseudocysts can contain inclusions that can hinder the sonographic distinction from cystic tumors, especially mucinous cystadenoma. CEUS can aid in this differential diagnosis because the endoluminal debris is not vascularized and will appear completely and homogeneously anechoic at CEUS (**Box 3, Fig. 3**).[6]

Box 2
Focal acute pancreatitis

- Homogeneously hypoechoic segmental enlargement of the pancreas (differential diagnosis with neoplasms).

- Color-Doppler: increased signal owing to hyperemia.

- CEUS: the inflamed parenchyma shows increased parenchymography, as opposed to ductal adenocarcinoma, which appears hypovascular.

Other delayed complications that can develop weeks after the onset of pancreatitis are infected pseudocysts (abscesses) (ie, collections of purulent material in or around the pancreas). Infected pseudocysts at US are anechoic or heterogeneously isoechoic or hypoechoic because of bright echoes from pus, debris, or gas bubbles.[13] Pancreatic abscesses require drainage, either percutaneous drainage, often US guided, or surgical or endoscopic intervention.

Chronic Pancreatitis

Chronic pancreatitis is an inflammatory process in which the pancreatic parenchyma is replaced by fibrous tissue. The diagnosis is based on clinical findings, laboratory evaluation, and imaging findings: these imaging findings are readily recognized in the advanced phases of the disease, but are often subtle in the early phases.[1] US is able to identify the fine alterations in the parenchyma echotexture that can present in the early stages of the disease, which can be important for the diagnosis (Box 4); however, especially in the early stages of the disease, the texture of the parenchyma can be normal in up to 40% of cases.[14–16]

With advanced disease, atrophy and alterations in size occur, which are the most easily identified findings. The organ has irregular contour and the parenchyma becomes hyperechoic owing to fatty infiltration and fibrosis[1,10]: this sign is sensitive but nonspecific.

The most typical imaging findings for the diagnosis of chronic pancreatitis are intraductal calcifications and pancreatic duct dilation (Fig. 4).

According to the Japan Pancreas Society, the presence of calcifications is the most important and pathognomonic diagnostic criterion for chronic pancreatitis.[17] At US, calcifications appear as hyperechoic foci with posterior shadowing, a feature that smaller calcifications may lack. Calcifications are better demonstrated with harmonic imaging.

Dilatation of the main pancreatic duct (ie, caliber >3 mm) can be easily identified at US in patients with chronic pancreatitis and has 60% to 70% sensitivity and 80% to 90% specificity for the diagnosis.[1,18] Main pancreatic duct dilatation is a specific but not sensitive sign for the diagnosis of chronic pancreatitis: Bolondi and colleagues[18] reported that the main pancreatic duct was dilated in 52.3% of patients with chronic pancreatitis. Although identifying alterations of the contour of the main pancreatic duct may be difficult, the presence of irregularly dilated portions of the duct is typical of the more advanced stages of chronic pancreatitis.

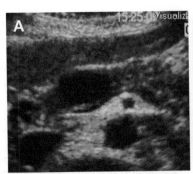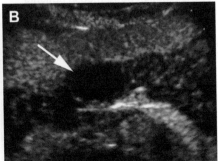

Fig. 3. Pseudocyst: small cystic lesion in the pancreatic head with anechoic content and well-defined wall (*A*). CEUS shows the absence of enhancing septations or nodules (*arrow* in *B*).

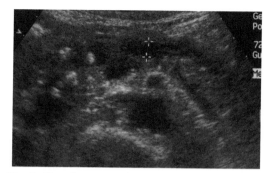

Fig. 4. Chronic pancreatitis: Conventional US shows the pancreatic head, heterogeneously hypoechoic with a multiple hyperechoic parenchymal calcifications. The main pancreatic duct is dilated (between calipers).

Mass-forming pancreatitis is usually observed in patients with a history of chronic pancreatitis.[19] The differential diagnosis with adenocarcinoma may be challenging because the lesions can present with very similar US features, as well as similar symptoms and signs (Table 1). In most cases, mass-forming pancreatitis appears as a hypoechoic mass with enlargement of a limited portion of the organ, most commonly the head. The presence of small calcifications may suggest the diagnosis,[10] but contrast-enhanced examinations and biopsy are necessary for the diagnosis. CEUS can aid in the differential diagnosis, because although ductal adenocarcinoma is hypoechoic in all contrastographic phases, mass-forming pancreatitis shows "parenchymographic" enhancement similar to the surrounding parenchyma in all the phases (Fig. 5). This enhancement has an intensity that is inversely correlated with the length of the inflammatory process: the longer the inflammatory process, the less intense the enhancement.[20]

Autoimmune chronic pancreatitis is characterized by periductal fibrosis, with lymphocytic infiltration and evolution to fibrosis.[21] The process can be diffuse or focal, depending on extension of the disease. US findings are characteristic in the diffuse form: the pancreas is enlarged with the typical "sausage"-like morphology, with markedly hypoechoic parenchyma, and the main pancreatic duct is compressed by the surrounding parenchyma.[21] At CEUS, the parenchyma involved by autoimmune pancreatitis shows a moderate to marked enhancement in the early contrast-enhanced phases,[22] followed by washout.

SOLID TUMORS
Ductal Adenocarcinoma

The aims of imaging in pancreatic neoplasms are detection and staging to ensure proper management for the patient. US is often the first examination for the initial evaluation of the pancreas.[1] Ductal adenocarcinoma represents up to 90% of all tumors of the exocrine pancreas. At US, adenocarcinoma typically appears as a solid hypoechoic lesion with ill-defined margins that alter the gland contours or, when the mass is small, is completely surrounded by parenchyma.

Masses in the pancreatic head cause ductal obstruction, with secondary dilatation of the common bile duct and the pancreatic duct, the so-called "double-duct sign"; however, these features can also be frequently seen in chronic pancreatitis. In the more aggressive tumors, the imbalance between growth rate and angiogenesis may cause necrosis.[6]

As observed at contrast-enhanced CT and magnetic resonance (MR) imaging, during CEUS, ductal adenocarcinoma shows poor enhancement in all contrast-enhancement phases and appears hypoechoic compared with the adjacent normal parenchyma. Contrast medium administration enables better evaluation of the margins and size of the lesion and its relationship with peripancreatic arterial and venous vessels for local staging (Box 5, Fig. 6).[6] By using second-generation contrast agents, after studying the pancreas in the first dynamic phases, it is possible to scan the liver in the delayed phase to detect the presence of metastases.

Table 1
US differential diagnosis between mass-forming pancreatitis and adenocarcinoma

	Mass-Forming Pancreatitis	Adenocarcinoma
US	Hypoechoic mass	Hypoechoic mass
Calcifications	Pathognomonic	Absent
Ductal dilatation	Present	Present
CEUS	Enhancement similar to adjacent normal parenchyma	Hypovascular compared with adjacent normal parenchyma

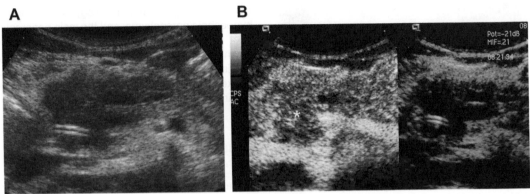

Fig. 5. Mass-forming pancreatitis. (*A*) Transverse conventional US shows the pancreatic head, enlarged and hypoechoic. (*B*) After contrast-agent administration, the parenchyma in the head (*asterisk*) shows "parenchymographic" enhancement, appearing isoechoic to the rest of the organ.

Endocrine Tumors

Pancreatic endocrine tumors arise from the neuroendocrine cells of the pancreas; these tumors are classified as functional or hyperfunctioning versus nonfunctional or nonhyperfunctioning based on the presence of clinical symptoms related to hormone overproduction by the tumor. Usually, hyperfunctioning endocrine tumors, the most common of which are insulinomas and gastrinomas, are small at the time of diagnosis, whereas nonhyperfunctioning tumors are frequently large at detection and more often malignant.[23] Endocrine tumors are hypervascular, which influences the imaging features (**Box 6**).[12] Color- and power-Doppler US can show a "spot pattern" within endocrine tumors, from small vessels that have flow visible at Doppler: this feature, however, can be absent in small tumors or in tumors with a poorly developed vascular network.[24]

CEUS features are dependent on the size and vascularity of the tumor. Most often these lesions enhance rapidly and intensely in the early contrast-enhanced phases and retain the MBs in the late phase.[24]

In a minority of cases, however, the presence of dense and hyalinized stroma inside the lesion can cause hypovascularity of endocrine tumors.[24] Nevertheless, it has been reported that a clear enhancement during CEUS can be seen in some pancreatic endocrine tumors that appear hypodense on multidetector CT[24]: this is probably because of the high resolution power of state-of-the-art US imaging, combined with the size and blood-pool distribution of MB contrast agents, along with the advantage of continuous observation of the arrival of the contrast agent. CEUS can, therefore, improve the identification and characterization of endocrine tumors,[24,25] and further aid in their locoregional and hepatic staging (**Fig. 7**).[24]

CYSTIC PANCREATIC TUMORS

Cystic tumors represent 10% to 15% of all pancreatic tumors; serous and mucinous subtypes are the most common cystic neoplasms of the pancreas (**Table 2**).

Serous Cystadenoma

Serous cystadenoma (SCA) is a benign lesion with a strong female predilection, usually seen in patients older than 60 years. SCA is generally characterized by tiny cysts (smaller than 2 cm in diameter) and is most commonly located in the head of the pancreas.[12]

The content of the cysts appears anechoic at US; however, when the cysts are extremely small, the lesion may appear solid on US and CT. A central scar may be present in up to 15% of the cases, appearing as a central solid hyperechoic portion of the tumor, sometimes with calcifications. US can show the microcystic appearance of the tumor. US features of SCA that are typical and often diagnostic include sharp lobulated

---

Box 5
US features of pancreatic adenocarcinoma

- Solid hypoechoic mass with ill-defined margins
- Possible areas of necrosis (rare)
- CEUS: hypoenhancing mass; better evaluation of margins and relationship with vessels for local staging.

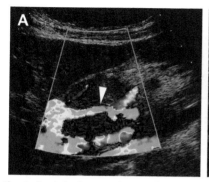
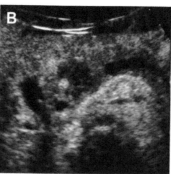
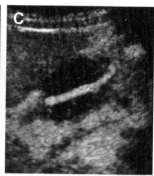

Fig. 6. Ductal adenocarcinoma. (A) Sagittal US image shows a large hypoechoic solid mass in the pancreatic head encasing the gastroduodenal artery (*arrowhead*). Axial (B) and sagittal (C) CEUS shows that the mass is hypovascular and confirms vascular encasement.

margins, thin wall, and internal septations that are radially arranged and converge to a central scar (Fig. 8). CEUS can demonstrate the enhancement of intralesional septations revealing the microcystic nature of the lesion even in lesions that might appear solid at baseline US.[6]

Mucin-Producing Tumors

Mucin-producing tumors of the pancreas arise from the peripheral ducts (mucinous cystic tumors) or from the main pancreatic duct and its side branches (intraductal papillary mucinous neoplasms [IPMNs]).[26]

Mucinous cystic tumors are most common in women 40 to 60 years of age, are malignant or potentially malignant lesions, and most commonly are observed in the body or tail of the pancreas.[27]

Mucinous cystic tumors are located peripherally in the parenchyma and show cysts that are fewer in number and larger in size than those observed in SCA. At US, mucinous cystic neoplasms appear round or ovoid-shaped, and are made up of unilocular or multilocular cysts with thick walls. Mucinous cystadenoma may have calcifications in the wall and/or septations, parietal nodules, and papillary vegetations. The visualization of the wall and inclusions may be impaired because of the mucinous content of

the cysts, which demonstrates fine echoes at US. For these reasons, harmonic imaging is used to allow better evaluation of the walls, septations, nodules, and papillary vegetations.[28] Also, contrast administration may significantly improve the US identification of the parietal nodules and septa, and can aid in differentiating these lesions from pseudocysts (Fig. 9).[6]

IPMNs are tumors that induce dilation of the main pancreatic duct and/or side branches, or result in formation of cysts because of proliferation of ductal epithelium and excessive mucin production. IPMNs are classified on the basis of their site of involvement into main duct type, branch duct type, or a combination of the two.[29] In the main duct type, dilatation of the main pancreatic duct is visible at US (Fig. 10).

Especially for the ductectatic mucin-hypersecreting type of the branch duct IPMNs, it can be difficult to differentiate mucin from solid portions of the tumor. Therefore, harmonic imaging may be used to better identify the fluid components.

With CEUS, intraductal papillary tumoral vegetations may be more visible because they enhance in the dynamic phase, especially in the papillary-villous variant[20]; however, US may not easily demonstrate the communication between side branch lesions and the main pancreatic duct.[30]

ACOUSTIC RADIATION FORCE IMPULSE

The assessment of the viscoelastic properties of tissues with US has gained increasing interest in recent years. Many types of software have been proposed for US tissue-strain analysis performed under compression, such as Hitachi Real-time Tissue Elastography (HI-RTE, Hitachi Medical Systems Europe, Zurich, Switzerland), eSie Touch (Siemens, Erlangen, Germany), or Elasticity Imaging (Siemens), or without compression, such as

---

Box 6
US features of endocrine tumors

- US: solid hypoechoic/isoechoic, well-defined mass
- Color- and power-Doppler US: "spot" pattern
- CEUS: rapid and intense enhancement in the arterial phase with retention of MBs in the late phase

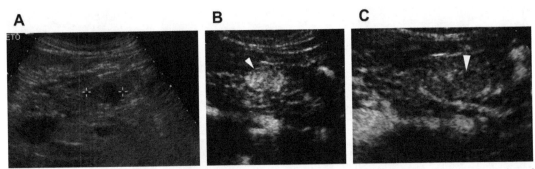

Fig. 7. Pancreatic endocrine tumor: small hypoechoic solid mass in the pancreatic body (*A*, between calipers). CEUS shows strong enhancement in the arterial phase (*B*, *arrowhead*) and MB retention in the delayed phase (*C*, *arrowhead*).

acoustic radiation force impulse (ARFI) imaging and its new implementations, Virtual Touch tissue imaging (Siemens) and Virtual Touch tissue quantification (Siemens).

ARFI imaging is a new US imaging modality that evaluates the stiffness of deep tissues by short-duration acoustic radiation forces that produce localized displacements in a "pushed" region of interest (ROI). Through the use of acoustic push pulses to generate shear waves on a fixed target, ROI qualitative visual and quantitative value measurements can be obtained (**Fig. 11**). Virtual Touch tissue quantification provides numerical measurements (wave-velocity values) of tissue stiffness at a precise image-based anatomic location. The normal values of shear-wave speed for normal liver, gallbladder, pancreas, spleen, and kidneys have been defined.[31] A recent study assessed the role of ARFI in the characterization of pancreatic cystic lesions, suggesting a potential

Table 2
Clinical and US features of cystic lesions of the pancreas

	SCA	MCN	IPMN
Location	Head	Body, tail	Ubiquitous
Age	Older than 60 years	40–60 years	Older
Sex	Female	Female	Indifferent
b-mode	Microcystic appearance Lobulated margins Internal septa arranged radially and converging on the central scar	Round or ovoid-shaped Unilocular or multilocular cysts	Dilatation of the main pancreatic duct and/or its side branches or formation of cysts
THI	—	Better evaluation of the walls, septa, nodules, and papillary vegetations	Identify the fluid portions of IPMN
Duct dilation	Absent	Absent	Present in the main duct type
Cyst features	Small and multiple Anechoic content	Larger and fewer Content with fine echoes Thick walls Calcifications on the wall or the septa Parietal nodules and papillary vegetations	—
CEUS	Enhancement of thin intralesional septa	Enhancement of parietal nodules and thick septa	Enhancement of vegetations

Abbreviations: CEUS, contrast-enhanced ultrasound; IPMN, intraductal papillary mucinous neoplasm; MCN, mucinous cystic neoplasm; SCA, serous cystadenoma; THI, tissue harmonic imaging.

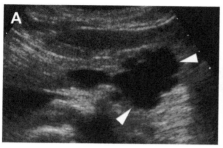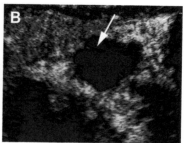

Fig. 8. Serous cystadenoma: conventional US shows a cystic lesion with sharp lobulated margins and internal septations that converge radially (*arrowheads* in *A*). CEUS demonstrates enhancement of thin intralesional septations (*arrow* in *B*).

new approach for a noninvasive analysis of the fluid content.[32]

INTRAOPERATIVE ULTRASOUND

Intraoperative ultrasound (IOUS) can guarantee high-resolution B-mode imaging of the pancreas and liver. Image quality is improved by placing the probe either directly on the surface of the organ or with a minimal fluid interface, avoiding any interference by the abdominal wall or the gas-filled bowel.

Several investigators have reported that sensitivity of IOUS in the detection of carcinomas is 92.3% to 100.0% and that its use can modify the surgical treatment in up to 67.0% of cases.[33–36] This imaging technique is especially useful for selected cases when preoperative studies indicate possible vascular invasion by the pancreatic mass or possible hepatic involvement.

Pancreatic IOUS can have a clinical role in lesion identification and/or in lesion staging. In the first scenario, IOUS is used for lesion detection; for example, a hyperfunctioning endocrine tumor not identified at preoperative imaging. For lesion staging and operative guidance, the examination requires an evaluation of the relationship of the lesion with the main pancreatic duct and the assessment of resectability from the major peripancreatic vessels.

INTERVENTIONAL ULTRASOUND

The use of Interventional ultrasound for the diagnosis and therapy of some pancreatic pathologies has definitely modified diagnostic and therapeutic management. Percutaneous US-guided procedures are widely used because of the possibility for continuous monitoring, the high spatial resolution, availability, and the low cost of this technique. For US-guided procedures, the entry points to the pancreas can be selected freely because of the possibility of scanning along oblique planes.[37]

Percutaneous Diagnostic Procedures

The accuracy of US-guided percutaneous diagnostic biopsy procedures can vary according to the site of the lesion. Brandt and colleagues[38] reported a 93% to 94% accuracy for body-tail lesions and a slightly lower accuracy for head lesions (83%–84%).[39] In a more recent series of 545 diagnostic fine-needle aspirations (FNAs) of pancreatic lesions, 63% of which were located in

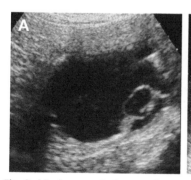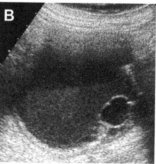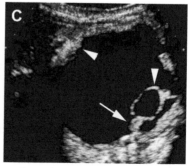

Fig. 9. Mucinous cystadenoma: large cystic lesion with thick walls and septations, the content shows fine echoes at conventional US (*A*). Harmonic imaging allows better visualization of the posterior wall of the cyst (*B*). CEUS shows enhancement of the thick wall and septations (*arrowheads* in *C*) and of parietal nodule (*arrow* in *C*).

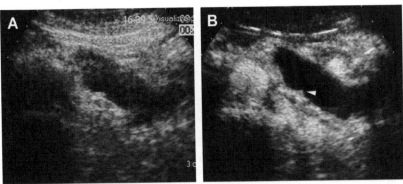

Fig. 10. Main duct IPMN: segmental dilatation of the main pancreatic duct in the body-tail (*A*), the duct content shows fine echoes owing to the presence of mucin. CEUS reveals enhancement of papillary parietal vegetations (*arrowhead* in *B*).

the head or uncinate process, we obtained a 99.4% sensitivity, 100.0% specificity, 99.4% accuracy, and a 1.5% incidence of minor complications.[40] Indeed, US guidance for percutaneous diagnostic procedures has a low reported incidence of complications, ranging from 1.5% to 5.0%.[40,41]

The safest and most commonly used entry point for FNA and biopsy is the left upper quadrant, left of the midline, which allows avoidance of major vessels. The angle of the needle track will vary depending on the location of the lesion in the pancreas.[40] The safest entry point and track are selected to avoid passage into hollow organs. Although transgastric passage is not absolutely contraindicated, transcolonic passage always should be avoided.

For interventional procedures, 2 types of probes are commonly used: probes with lateral support, and probes with noncontinuous crystals and central support. The use of a lateral-support probe will allow only oblique needle tracks, whereas a central support probe will allow both vertical and oblique tracks. In our institution, we routinely use probes ranging in frequency from 2.5 to 5.0 MHz with a laterally mounted guide kit (**Fig. 12**). Color-Doppler images are fundamental for identifying major blood vessels and excluding them from the needle track.

Percutaneous Therapeutic Procedures

The other major use of US-guidance is for the positioning of percutaneous drainage catheters. US guidance can guarantee a direct access route to the pancreas, avoiding involvement of the neighboring structures, such as vessels, and allows efficient treatment of infected pancreatic necrosis or

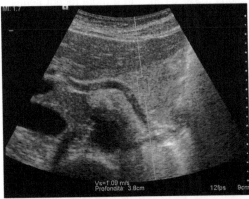

Fig. 11. Acoustic radiation force impulse (ARFI) imaging of the normal pancreatic body, with Virtual Touch tissue quantification providing a numerical measurement (wave-velocity value) of the stiffness of the parenchyma.

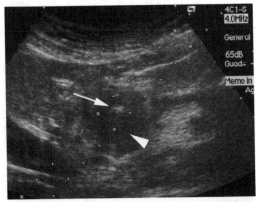

Fig. 12. Transverse US image shows a hypoechoic mass in the pancreatic head (*arrowhead*). A probe with lateral support is used, providing the oblique needle track shown. The needle tip (*arrow*) can be seen inside the lesion.

pseudocysts. During the procedure, a fluid sample can be obtained to assess the presence of amylase, which proves a communication with the main pancreatic duct.

SUMMARY

With the appropriate technique, US can provide useful information on the pancreas and its diseases in most patients. US can also be used to guide diagnostic and therapeutic procedures and for intraoperative guidance.

REFERENCES

1. Martinez-Noguera A, D'Onofrio M. Ultrasonography of the pancreas. 1. Conventional imaging. Abdom Imaging 2007;32(2):136–49.
2. Bertolotto M, D'Onofrio M, Martone E, et al. Ultrasonography of the pancreas. 3. Doppler imaging. Abdom Imaging 2007;32(2):161–70.
3. Shapiro RS, Wagreich J, Parsons RB, et al. Tissue harmonic imaging sonography: evaluation of image quality compared with conventional sonography. AJR Am J Roentgenol 1998;171(5):1203–6.
4. Hohl C, Schmidt T, Haage P, et al. Phase-inversion tissue harmonic imaging compared with conventional B-mode ultrasound in the evaluation of pancreatic lesions. Eur Radiol 2004;14(6):1109–17.
5. Taylor KJ, Burns PN, Woodcock JP, et al. Blood flow in deep abdominal and pelvic vessels: ultrasonic pulsed-Doppler analysis. Radiology 1985; 154(2):487–93.
6. D'Onofrio M, Zamboni G, Faccioli N, et al. Ultrasonography of the pancreas. 4. Contrast-enhanced imaging. Abdom Imaging 2007;32(2):171–81.
7. D'Onofrio M, Gallotti A, Principe F, et al. Contrast-enhanced ultrasound of the pancreas. World J Radiol 2010;2(3):97–102.
8. D'Onofrio M, Martone E, Faccioli N, et al. Focal liver lesions: sinusoidal phase of CEUS. Abdom Imaging 2006;31(5):529–36.
9. Rumack C, Wilson S, Charboneau J. Diagnostic ultrasound. New York: Mosby Year Book; 1991.
10. Remer EM, Baker ME. Imaging of chronic pancreatitis. Radiol Clin North Am 2002;40(6):1229–42, v.
11. Baron TH, Morgan DE. The diagnosis and management of fluid collections associated with pancreatitis. Am J Med 1997;102(6):555–63.
12. Procacci C, Biasiutti C, Carbognin G, et al. Pancreatic neoplasms and tumor-like conditions. Eur Radiol Suppl 2001;11(Suppl 2):S167–92.
13. Procacci C, Mansueto G, D'Onofrio M, et al. Nontraumatic abdominal emergencies: imaging and intervention in acute pancreatic conditions. Eur Radiol 2002;12(10):2407–34.
14. Alpern MB, Sandler MA, Kellman GM, et al. Chronic pancreatitis: ultrasonic features. Radiology 1985; 155(1):215–9.
15. Grant TH, Efrusy ME. Ultrasound in the evaluation of chronic pancreatitis. J Am Osteopath Assoc 1981; 81(3):183–8.
16. Lees WR, Vallon AG, Denyer ME, et al. Prospective study of ultrasonography in chronic pancreatic disease. Br Med J 1979;1(6157):162–4.
17. Homma T, Harada H, Koizumi M. Diagnostic criteria for chronic pancreatitis by the Japan Pancreas Society. Pancreas 1997;15(1):14–5.
18. Bolondi L, Priori P, Gullo L, et al. Relationship between morphological changes detected by ultrasonography and pancreatic exocrine function in chronic pancreatitis. Pancreas 1987;2(2):222–9.
19. Kim T, Murakami T, Takamura M, et al. Pancreatic mass due to chronic pancreatitis: correlation of CT and MR imaging features with pathologic findings. AJR Am J Roentgenol 2001;177(2):367–71.
20. D'Onofrio M, Zamboni G, Malago R, et al. Pancreatic pathology. In: Quaia E, editor. Contrast media in ultrasonography. Berlin: Springer-Verlag; 2005. p. 335–47.
21. Furukawa N, Muranaka T, Yasumori K, et al. Autoimmune pancreatitis: radiologic findings in three histologically proven cases. J Comput Assist Tomogr 1998;22(6):880–3.
22. Numata K, Ozawa Y, Kobayashi N, et al. Contrast-enhanced sonography of autoimmune pancreatitis: comparison with pathologic findings. J Ultrasound Med 2004;23(2):199–206.
23. Buetow PC, Miller DL, Parrino TV, et al. Islet cell tumors of the pancreas: clinical, radiologic, and pathologic correlation in diagnosis and localization. Radiographics 1997;17(2):453–72 [quiz: 472A–B].
24. D'Onofrio M, Mansueto G, Falconi M, et al. Neuroendocrine pancreatic tumor: value of contrast enhanced ultrasonography. Abdom Imaging 2004; 29(2):246–58.
25. D'Onofrio M, Mansueto G, Vasori S, et al. Contrast-enhanced ultrasonographic detection of small pancreatic insulinoma. J Ultrasound Med 2003; 22(4):413–7.
26. Procacci C, Graziani R, Bicego E, et al. Intraductal mucin-producing tumors of the pancreas: imaging findings. Radiology 1996;198(1):249–57.
27. Procacci C, Biasiutti C, Carbognin G, et al. Characterization of cystic tumors of the pancreas: CT accuracy. J Comput Assist Tomogr 1999;23(6):906–12.
28. Hammond N, Miller FH, Sica GT, et al. Imaging of cystic diseases of the pancreas. Radiol Clin North Am 2002;40(6):1243–62.
29. Procacci C, Megibow AJ, Carbognin G, et al. Intraductal papillary mucinous tumor of the pancreas: a pictorial essay. Radiographics 1999;19(6): 1447–63.

30. Procacci C, Schenal G, Dalla Chiara E, et al. Intraductal papillary mucinous tumors: imaging. In: Procacci C, Megibow A, editors. Imaging of the pancreas. Cystic and rare tumors. Berlin: Springer-Verlag; 2003. p. 97–137.

31. Gallotti A, D'Onofrio M, Pozzi Mucelli R. Acoustic Radiation Force Impulse (ARFI) technique in ultrasound with Virtual Touch tissue quantification of the upper abdomen. Radiol Med 2010;115(6):889–97.

32. D'Onofrio M, Gallotti A, Mucelli RP. Pancreatic mucinous cystadenoma at ultrasound acoustic radiation force impulse (ARFI) imaging. Pancreas 2010;39(5):684–5.

33. D'Onofrio M, Vecchiato F, Faccioli N, et al. Ultrasonography of the pancreas. 7. Intraoperative imaging. Abdom Imaging 2007;32(2):200–6.

34. Sun MR, Brennan DD, Kruskal JB, et al. Intraoperative ultrasonography of the pancreas. Radiographics 2010;30(7):1935–53.

35. Sugiyama M, Hagi H, Atomi Y. Reappraisal of intraoperative ultrasonography for pancreatobiliary carcinomas: assessment of malignant portal venous invasion. Surgery 1999;125(2):160–5.

36. Sahani DV, Kalva SP, Tanabe KK, et al. Intraoperative US in patients undergoing surgery for liver neoplasms: comparison with MR imaging. Radiology 2004;232(3):810–4.

37. D'Onofrio M, Malago R, Zamboni G, et al. Ultrasonography of the pancreas. 5. Interventional procedures. Abdom Imaging 2007;32(2):182–90.

38. Brandt KR, Charboneau JW, Stephens DH, et al. CT- and US-guided biopsy of the pancreas. Radiology 1993;187(1):99–104.

39. Mallery JS, Centeno BA, Hahn PF, et al. Pancreatic tissue sampling guided by EUS, CT/US, and surgery: a comparison of sensitivity and specificity. Gastrointest Endosc 2002;56(2):218–24.

40. Zamboni GA, D'Onofrio M, Idili A, et al. Ultrasound-guided percutaneous fine-needle aspiration of 545 focal pancreatic lesions. AJR Am J Roentgenol 2009;193(6):1691–5.

41. Di Stasi M, Lencioni R, Solmi L, et al. Ultrasound-guided fine needle biopsy of pancreatic masses: results of a multicenter study. Am J Gastroenterol 1998;93(8):1329–33.

Imaging of Pancreatic Adenocarcinoma: Update on Staging/Resectability

Eric P. Tamm, MD[a],*, Aparna Balachandran, MD[a],
Priya R. Bhosale, MD[a], Matthew H. Katz, MD[b],
Jason B. Fleming, MD[b], Jeffrey H. Lee, MD[c],
Gauri R. Varadhachary, MD[d]

KEYWORDS

- Pancreatic cancer • Staging • Resectability • Imaging
- Treatment • Pancreatic adenocarcinoma

Pancreatic cancer remains one of the most challenging tumors to treat. The tumor is seated deep in the retroperitoneum and typically infiltrates a network of crucial arteries, veins, and nerves that supply or drain the liver, spleen, stomach, pancreas, and large and small bowel. Most patients present with metastatic disease that obviates potentially curative surgical intervention. Through the close cooperation of a variety of specialists, including oncologists, radiation oncologists, and surgeons, there has been an ongoing effort to improve treatment regimens and surgical techniques to maximize tumor control while minimizing potentially devastating effects. As a consequence, the criteria for resectable disease have been evolving, increasing the demands for accurate staging.

Imaging has simultaneously assumed a crucial role in helping to stratify patients to stage-appropriate therapies and clinical trials, which has also highlighted the need for consistency in radiology reporting.

This article reviews recent surgical advances and general treatment approaches that have led to a change in the understanding of resectable disease and staging, the current criteria for staging, current classifications of resectable disease, imaging techniques, imaging, and imaging criteria for staging. It also includes a brief discussion of current efforts to standardize radiology reporting for this disease.

RECENT ADVANCES LEADING TO CHANGES IN STAGING

The only option for cure remains multimodality treatment strategies that include surgical resection. For the 15% to 20% of patients who can undergo surgery, the overall survival rate is approximately 15% to 27%,[1–3] which has led to the push to develop techniques and therapies to increase the percentage of patients who can undergo surgery. These techniques include venous interposition

[a] Department of Diagnostic Radiology, The University of Texas MD Anderson Cancer Center, 1515 Holcombe Boulevard, Unit 1473, Houston, TX 77030, USA; [b] Department of Surgical Oncology, The University of Texas MD Anderson Cancer Center, 1515 Holcombe Boulevard, Unit 0444, Houston, TX 77030, USA; [c] Department of Gastroenterology, Hepatology & Nutrition, The University of Texas MD Anderson Cancer Center, 1515 Holcombe Boulevard, Unit 1466, Houston, TX 77030, USA; [d] Department of GI Medical Oncology, The University of Texas MD Anderson Cancer Center, 1515 Holcombe Boulevard, Unit 0426, Houston, TX 77030, USA
* Corresponding author. Department of Diagnostic Radiology, The University of Texas MD Anderson Cancer Center, PO Box 301402, Unit 1473, Houston, TX 77230-1402.
E-mail address: etamm@mdanderson.org

Radiol Clin N Am 50 (2012) 407–428
doi:10.1016/j.rcl.2012.03.008
0033-8389/12/$ – see front matter © 2012 Elsevier Inc. All rights reserved.

grafts, hepatic arterial interposition grafts, and the use of chemotherapy and/or radiation before surgery (neoadjuvant). Knowledge of vascular anatomy is important to understand these procedures and is described in **Fig. 1.**

VENOUS RESECTION AND RECONSTRUCTION

Venous resection with reconstruction is typically performed to allow removal of tumor involving sections of the superior mesenteric vein, portal vein, and/or splenoportal confluence in a manner to reconstitute flow. This approach can include a variety of techniques (**Figs. 2** and **3**) such as saphenous venous patches, interposition grafts (such as with the internal jugular vein), primary anastomosis (if there remains sufficient length of native venous structures following resection), as well as splenic vein ligation when necessary.[4] Key to this procedure is that the 2 venous ends

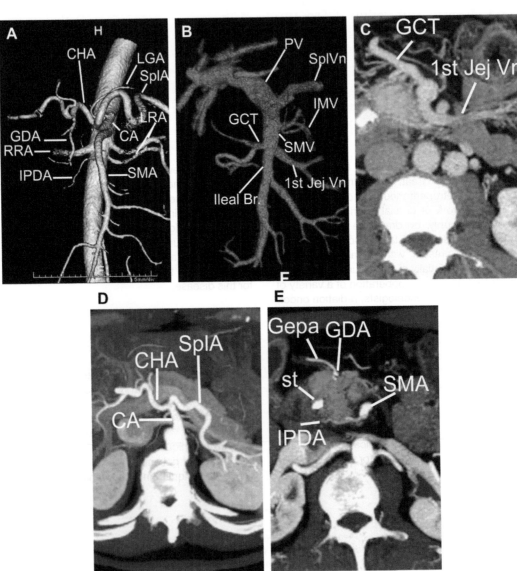

Fig. 1. Regional arterial and venous anatomy of the pancreas. Volume-rendered coronal image segmented to show (*A*) arterial anatomy and (*B*) venous anatomy. Axial 15-mm maximum-intensity projection (MIP) images show (*C*) the gastrocolic trunk (GCT) and first jejunal vein (1st Jej Vn), (*D*) celiac axis (CA), common hepatic artery (CHA) and splenic artery (Spl A), and (*E*) superior mesenteric artery (SMA), inferior pancreaticoduodenal artery (IPDA) proceeding posterior to pancreatic head, gastroduodenal artery (GDA) forming the right anterior boundary, and the right gastroepiploic artery (Gepa) originating from the gastroduodenal artery. Stent (st) is noted. Ileal Br., ileal branch of the SMV; IMV, inferior mesenteric vein; LGA, left gastric artery; LRA, left renal artery; PV, portal vein; RRA, right renal artery; SMV, superior mesenteric vein; SplVn, splenic vein.

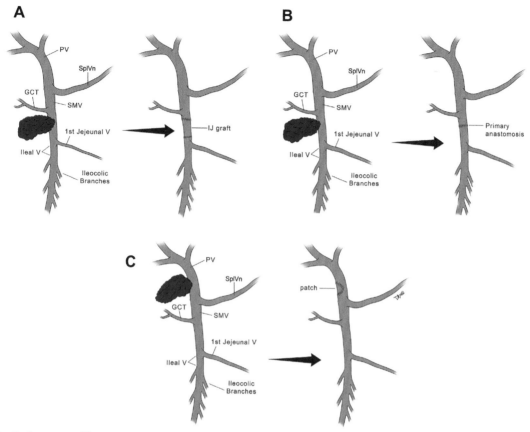

Fig. 2. Summary of basic types of venous reconstruction including (*A*) interposition internal jugular venous graft for when a segment of vein is resected, (*B*) primary anastomosis for short-segment resection, and (*C*) placement of a patch, for minimal venous involvement.

to be joined have only a single lumen. It is currently not possible to anastomose a single lumen (ie, patent portal vein) to multiple lumens (ie, ileocolic branches, Fig. 4). Although it is possible to do venous reconstruction in situations of venous involvement, including even short-segment occlusion, extension of tumor into branches such as the ileocolic branches precludes graft placement, even if the vessels involved are not occluded. Involvement of the jejunal vein has been considered

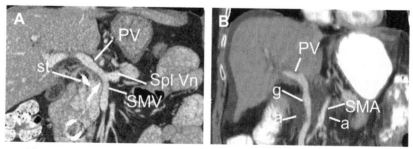

Fig. 3. A 62-year-old woman with pancreatic head/neck ductal adenocarcinoma. Coronal raysum reconstruction, portal venous phase of the baseline pancreatic CT study shows (*A*) tumor (*white arrow*) abutting the SMV. Portal vein (PV), splenic vein (Spl Vn) and stent (st) are also noted. (*B*) Postoperative coronal raysum shows the internal jugular graft (g), restoring continuity of flow back to the PV. Also noted is the SMA, and the presence of ascites (a) that resolved on subsequent scans.

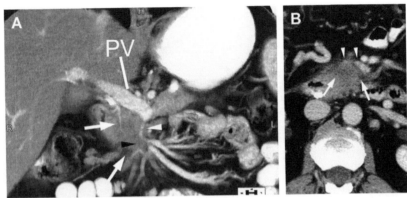

Fig. 4. A 49-year-old man with pancreatic head cancer with tumor (*white arrows*) shown (*A*) on coronal volume-rendered image to markedly narrow the SMV (*white arrowhead*) and inferiorly to occlude it focally (*black arrowhead*) and on the axial image (*B*) to infiltrate the ileocolic branches (*white arrowheads*).

at some, but not all, institutions to be a contraindication to resection.[5,6] It has been noted that reconstruction of the ileal branch of the superior mesenteric vein is preferred to reconstruction of the jejunal branch, given the latter's thin wall, as well as its posterior location.[6]

Tseng and colleagues,[4] in a study of 141 patients at our institution who underwent vascular resection (mostly venous reconstructions), showed similar survival between those who underwent resection with reconstruction (23.4 months) compared with those who underwent resection without reconstruction (26.5 months, *P* = .177). The American Hepato-Pancreatico-Biliary Association and Society of Surgical Oncology published a consensus statement in 2009 concluding that pancreaticoduodenectomy with vein resection and reconstruction is a viable option for treatment of some pancreatic adenocarcinomas.[7] Christians and colleagues[6] reported on the operation's safety, and also noted that detailed knowledge of the anatomy of the root of the mesentery is needed to optimize success.

HEPATIC ARTERY SEGMENTAL RESECTION AND/OR RECONSTRUCTION

Given that 60% of pancreatic cancers occur in the pancreatic head,[8] it is common for them to involve the gastroduodenal artery. The common hepatic artery is therefore a common site for involvement secondary to cephalad growth along the gastroduodenal artery. Another concern is for involvement of accessory or replaced right hepatic arteries, or even common hepatic arteries, originating from the superior mesenteric artery (SMA) because these vessels typically course in close proximity to the posterior pancreatic head and, therefore, are at high risk for involvement by pancreatic head tumors.[9,10] Tseng and colleagues[4] also

reported on 17 hepatic arterial segmental resections with or without reconstructions. They performed a primary anastomosis for short-segment involvement of the common and/or proper hepatic arteries if the common/hepatic artery was sufficiently redundant, or interposed a reversed saphenous vein graft if it was not (**Figs. 5** and **6**). Replaced and/or accessory right hepatic arteries inseparable from tumor were resected without reconstruction when such resection was feasible. Because of the small number of patients involved, it was not possible to calculate survival statistics for this group of patients.

APPROACHES TO CHEMOTHERAPY AND/OR RADIATION THERAPY

Because survival of patients status post resection with surgery alone has been limited (median survival 11–20 months), and includes high local recurrence rates (up to 60%),[11] supplemental approaches using chemotherapy and radiation therapy have been used. These approaches are typically in 1 of 2 groups: adjuvant (postoperative) or neoadjuvant (preoperative) therapy.

ADJUVANT (POSTOPERATIVE) THERAPY

This approach treats possible residual tumor with chemotherapy or chemotherapy and radiation therapy. The European Organization for Research and Treatment of Cancer evaluated 218 patients with periampullary tumors who were randomized to either observation or treatment with radiation and 5-fluorouracil (5FU).[12] The median survival for the treated group was 17.1 months versus 12.6 for those who were observed, but the difference was not statistically significant. A subsequent long-term follow-up study of these patients also

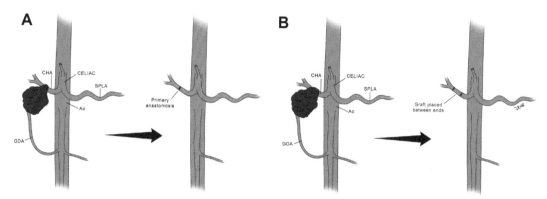

Fig. 5. Types of CHA reconstructions. Pancreatic head tumors typically ascend the gastroduodenal artery (GDA) to involve the CHA. If tumor involvement is minimal (*A*), then a primary anastomosis of the existing CHA ends can be done. However, if the involved CHA segment is longer (*B*), then a vascular graft is needed. For an anastomosis to be possible, tumor must not involve the proximal 1 cm of the common hepatic artery as it originates from the celiac trunk.

showed no statistically significant difference in survival.[13] The European Study Group for Pancreatic Cancer (ESPAC-1) trial subsequently stratified 541 patients to multiple categories including postoperative chemotherapy alone, postoperative chemoradiation, postoperative chemoradiation plus subsequent additional chemotherapy, and postoperative observation alone. That study showed a statistically significant improvement in survival from chemotherapy versus no chemotherapy (19.7 months vs 14 months, *P* = .0005) but not for chemoradiation,[14] A follow-up analysis showed a slight decrease in survival for those undergoing chemoradiation (15.9 months) compared with those without chemoradiation (17.9 months, *P* = .05).[15] Another study, the Radiation Therapy Oncology Group trial 97-04, showed a trend to increased overall survival for gemcitabine-based chemotherapy followed by 5FU chemoradiation, although results were not statistically significant (both arms in this study had

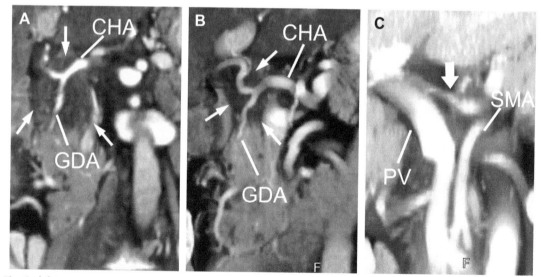

Fig. 6. (*A*) Pancreatic head tumor (*white arrows*) seen at baseline coronal raysum reconstruction to encase (involve more than 180°) the gastroduodenal artery (GDA) and the common hepatic (CHA). The patient then underwent preoperative chemotherapy and radiation therapy. (*B*) Coronal raysum reconstruction from follow-up scan shows the primary mass to have decreased (*white arrows*) but to still encase the gastroduodenal and common hepatic arteries. The patient underwent surgery, which showed no viable tumor involving the CHA. Arterial graft was placed and is shown with an arrow on the postoperative MIP image (*C*). The lower quality of postoperative reconstructions is because of thicker axial source images.

chemoradiation).[16] Further studies are underway to clarify the roles of chemotherapy and radiation therapy in the adjuvant setting. Guidelines from the National Comprehensive Cancer Network (NCCN) support the use of postoperative chemotherapy or chemoradiation therapy.[11] One of the limitations noted for the adjuvant approach has been that up to 33% cannot undergo adjuvant therapy, or it is delayed, because of illness.[12,17,18] It has been advocated that restaging imaging evaluations be performed immediately before starting adjuvant therapy to exclude residual tumor or early progression.[11]

PREOPERATIVE THERAPY

Preoperative therapy was developed as an alternative approach to adjuvant therapy for the following reasons. Preoperative therapy avoids the problem of postoperative morbidity delaying or excluding patients from undergoing adjuvant therapy. Preoperative therapy treats presumed micrometastases likely present at the time of presentation given that most patients who undergo potentially curative resection still die of recurrent pancreatic cancer. Preoperative therapy also provides a time interval before surgery in which indeterminate lesions that may be metastases can be better characterized by imaging follow-up (Fig. 7). It has also been suggested that patients who develop overt metastases during this period of intense preoperative therapy likely have an aggressive tumor biology and therefore would have done poorly even if they had proceeded directly to surgery. Potentially needless surgery may therefore be avoided. In addition, preoperative chemoradiation may allow for tumor downstaging (Fig. 8) and, in single-institution studies, has been shown to result in lower rates of surgical margin positivity.[19–23] Studies at our institution have shown median survival of up to 34 months for those who undergo preoperative therapy and surgery, but survival for those who did not proceed to surgery has been only 7 to 11 months.[24,25] Up to 30% of patients who undergo neoadjuvant therapy do not undergo surgery because of development of metastases; in contrast, isolated locoregional progression in the preoperative phase has been rare (ie, loss of a window of opportunity for surgical resection).[24,26] To our knowledge, there have been no prospective trials comparing preoperative therapy followed by surgery with upfront surgery followed by adjuvant treatment.

STAGING OF PANCREATIC CANCER: AMERICAN JOINT COMMITTEE ON CANCER GUIDELINES

The most commonly used staging system is that from the American Joint Committee on Cancer (AJCC).[27] This system assesses the status of the primary tumor (T), lymph nodes (N), and metastases (M). Stages are defined based on TNM grades.

The T status can be summarized as follows (Fig. 9): the T0, TX, and Tis classifications refer to lack of evidence for a primary tumor, inability to evaluate the primary tumor, or carcinoma in situ, respectively. T1 tumors are those less than

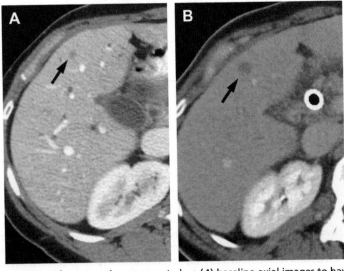

Fig. 7. A 39-year-old woman with pancreatic cancer, noted on (A) baseline axial images to have indeterminate liver lesion (black arrow), too small to characterize. Patient was therefore considered borderline for resectability, and underwent preoperative chemotherapy and radiation therapy. Follow-up axial portal venous phase imaging (B) shows lesion (black arrow) to have increased in size, consistent with a liver metastasis.

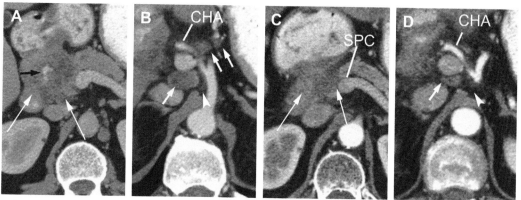

Fig. 8. A 61-year-old man with cancer of the pancreatic head. Baseline portal venous phase imaging (*A*) shows tumor (*long white arrows*) measuring nearly 5 cm, with central ulceration (*black arrow*) opacifying with gastrointestinal contrast from communication with duodenum. More superiorly obtained axial image (*B*) shows adenopathy (*white arrows*) near the CHA and in the portacaval region. Soft tissue stranding (*white arrowhead*) is seen to abut (meaning ≤180° of involvement) the celiac trunk. Follow-up imaging after chemoradiation (*C*) shows that tumor (*long white arrows*) has decreased, but still abuts the splenoportal confluence (SPC). On a more superiorly obtained image (*D*) adenopathy (*white arrow*) has decreased or resolved. Soft tissue stranding (*white arrowhead*) near the celiac trunk is similar or slightly increased. Patient went on to surgery, with successful tumor resection, only 1% viable tumor, and no positive regional lymph nodes for cancer.

or equal to 2 cm and bounded by the pancreas. T2 tumors are larger than 2 cm but still bounded by pancreas. T3 tumors are those that extend beyond the pancreas, but do not involve the celiac or superior mesenteric arteries. T4 tumors involve either the celiac or the superior mesenteric arteries and, in most institutions, represent unresectable tumor. With the advent of vascular resections and reconstructions, there has been a shift in staging to emphasize arterial involvement, and references to venous involvement for the T grades have been eliminated.[28] The N term can be summarized as follows: NX (unable to evaluate nodal status), N0 (no metastases to regional nodes), and N1 (presence of metastases to regional nodes). The M term is either M0 (no metastases) or M1 (distant metastases are present).

Staging can be summarized as follows (**Fig. 10**): the presence of any metastases classifies a patient as stage IV. The presence of T4 disease (celiac or SMA involvement) without metastases renders any patient as stage III. Stage IIA is T3 disease in the absence of nodal or distant metastases, and stage IIB is T1 to T3 disease in the setting of regional

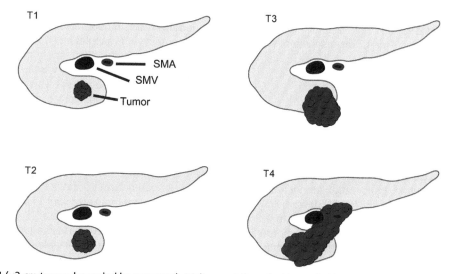

Fig. 9. T1 (<2-cm tumor, bounded by pancreas), T2 (tumor ≥2 cm, but bounded by pancreas), T3 (tumor extending beyond pancreas but not involving the celiac or superior mesenteric arteries), and T4 disease (tumor involving the celiac or superior mesenteric arteries). SMV, superior mesenteric vein; SMA, superior mesenteric artery.

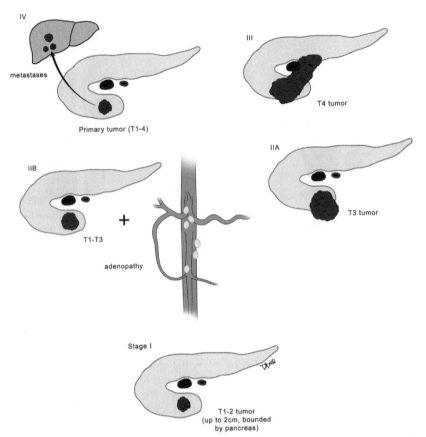

Fig. 10. Current staging of pancreatic cancer. Stage IV disease is the presence of distant metastases. Stage III disease is any other disease in which tumor involves the celiac or superior mesenteric arteries. Stage IIB disease is any other disease with adenopathy, and T1 to T3. Stage IIA is T3 disease (extending beyond the pancreas but without superior mesenteric or celiac artery involvement) without adenopathy or distant metastases. Stage I disease is any other disease (no metastases, no adenopathy) with primary tumor confined to the pancreas (T1–T2).

nodal metastases but not distant metastases. Stage I disease is T1 or T2 disease without nodal or distant metastases.[28]

CLASSIFICATION OF RESECTABLE, BORDERLINE, AND UNRESECTABLE DISEASE

Although the AJCC criteria provide classifications for staging, other efforts have been made to group patients for purposes of clinical management. Recently published pancreatic adenocarcinoma oncology guidelines by the NCCN describe grouping patients based on radiographic criteria into those with clearly resectable disease, borderline resectable disease, or clearly unresectable disease,[29,30] which supports other publications using such groupings.[7,19,31,32]

Clearly resectable disease (AJCC stages I and II) is defined as no overt metastatic disease, no overt

adenopathy, and, importantly, no evidence of any tumor contact with vasculature (**Fig. 11**) other than perhaps the gastroduodenal artery in the case of pancreatic head tumors (this vessel is resected as part of a Whipple procedure). This classification means that an intact, uninvolved, so-called clean fat plane surrounds vessels such as the SMA, the celiac trunk, and the common hepatic artery. For other vessels that are in contact with the pancreas, such as the superior mesenteric vein, vessels only have contact with clearly normal pancreatic parenchyma or fat and show no deformity or narrowing that is thought to be secondary to tumor involvement.

Clearly unresectable disease (stages III and IV) is represented by clearly identifiable distant metastases (stage IV), overt adenopathy outside the surgical field, or tumor encasement (>180° of circumferential involvement, **Fig. 12**) of such arteries (**Fig. 13**) as the SMA, celiac trunk, or origin

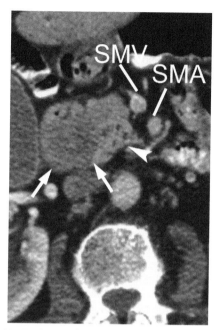

Fig. 11. A 52-year-old woman with pancreatic ductal adenocarcinoma of the pancreatic head (*white arrows*) involving the duodenum, which is effaced. Tumor is resectable, because the SMV and SMA are separated from the tumor by either an intact fat plane or normal-appearing pancreatic parenchyma (*white arrowhead*).

borderline or marginal resectable disease. According to the current NCCN definitions, borderline resectable patients have no distant metastases, venous involvement that is at most short-segment occlusion with suitable vessel above and below the point of obstruction for resection and reconstruction (Fig. 14), superior mesenteric and celiac arterial involvement limited to abutment (no >180° of the circumference of involvement) of these vessels (Fig. 15), and common hepatic artery involvement limited to at most short-segment encasement (up to 360 involvement) with sparing of the origin from the celiac of sufficient length to allow for placement of an arterial bypass graft (see Fig. 6).[30] These terms are similar to those outlined by our institution for borderline resectable patients in the article by Varadhachary and colleagues,[19] although in the NCCN guidelines any degree of venous abutment is considered borderline disease. More recently, our institution defined these patients as having anatomically borderline disease (type A), and added 2 other categories, B and C.[11] Type B borderline resectable patients are those with possible extrapancreatic disease, namely computed tomography (CT) findings suspicious but not definite for metastatic disease (see Fig. 7) and/or N1 disease confirmed by prereferral laparotomy or endoscopic ultrasound (EUS) with fine-needle aspiration (FNA). Type C patients are those with preexisting comorbidities (including those with potentially prohibitive comorbidities thought not to have been sufficiently evaluated) or reversible degradation of performance status (even if marginal performance status).[11]

of the common hepatic artery (which would preclude placement of an arterial jump graft).

The more difficult group to classify, given the evolution of treatment techniques (surgery, radiation therapy, and chemotherapy), is that of

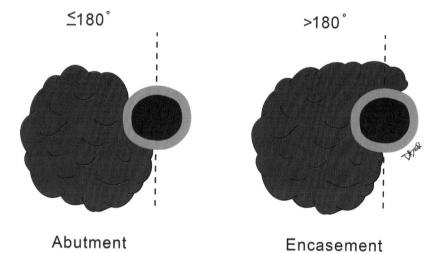

Fig. 12. The terms abutment (defined as ≤180° of tumor involvement of a vessel's circumference) and encasement (>180° of tumor involvement of a vessel's circumference). Either the terms abutment/encasement or degrees of circumferential involvement should be used to describe vascular involvement to facilitate communication with specialties outside radiology.

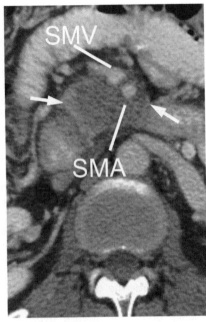

Fig. 13. A 66-year-old man with unresectable (stage III) cancer of the pancreatic head. Axial portal venous phase images show tumor (*white arrows*) encasing greater than 180° of circumferential involvement of the SMV, with 360° of circumferential involvement of the SMA.

IMAGING: TECHNIQUE

The characteristics used to define resectable, borderline resectable, and unresectable disease are based on the use of cross-sectional imaging and require the use of imaging techniques that optimize the visualization of tumor, its relationship to adjacent anatomic structures and its possible spread to nodes outside the surgical field, and distant sites such as the liver, peritoneum, lung, and bone.[11,19,30] The NCCN guidelines recommend pancreas-specific CT or MR imaging.[30]

Before discussing techniques, it is important to consider the timing for using specific imaging techniques. In our experience, the work-up for patients with abdominal pain and/or jaundice usually began with transabdominal ultrasound to evaluate the possibility of cholecystitis or simply the presence of gallstones. If ultrasound showed extrahepatic biliary dilatation, patients then typically underwent endoscopic retrograde cholangiopancreatography (ERCP) for diagnostic work-up and for treatment. However, the subsequent immediate placement of a biliary stent often eliminated visualization of the point of biliary obstruction, eliminating a useful diagnostic imaging feature for subsequent imaging with CT, MR imaging, or EUS (and for guiding biopsy for subtle lesions). More importantly, ERCP, brushings, and/or biopsy procedures can all cause postprocedure pancreatitis (**Fig. 16**), which can markedly limit the ability to visualize the tumor and the interface between tumor and vessel, limiting subsequent biopsy attempts and preventing accurate staging, and delaying or precluding enrollment in clinical trials. For this reason, at our institution, patients who present with suspicion of pancreatic cancer undergo cross-sectional imaging for staging (CT or MR imaging) before any intervention.

CT

Multidetector-row CT (MDCT) is probably the most widely used cross-sectional modality for the staging of pancreatic cancer. Thin-section (3 mm

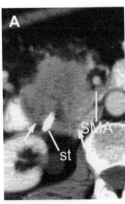
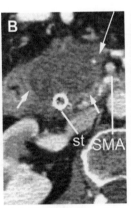
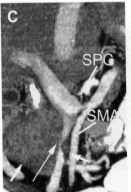
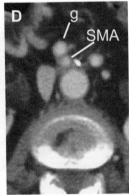

Fig. 14. Borderline venous occlusion in a 60-year-old woman. Baseline axial portal venous phase image (*A*) shows pancreatic head mass (*white arrows*) that occludes the SMV. Only the SMA is visualized. Stent (st) is present. Following a course of chemoradiation, follow-up study (*B*) axial image and (*C*) coronal reconstruction image show new minimal patency of the SMV (*long white arrow*). SMA and SPC are noted. Postoperative (*D*) axial image shows graft (g) that was successfully placed. SMA is noted.

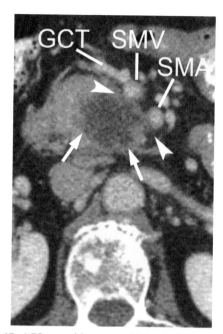

Fig. 15. A 76-year-old woman with borderline stage II to III pancreatic ductal adenocarcinoma of the pancreatic head. Axial portal venous phase imaging shows tumor (*white arrows*) with abutment (here <180° of circumferential involvement) of the SMA and SMV (*white arrowheads*). Gastrocolic trunk (GCT) is also noted.

or thinner), biphasic technique is crucial to identify the primary tumor, determine its local extent, as well as to identify distant metastases. Usually, injection rates of 3 to 5 mL/s are used with a sufficient volume of contrast for a 30-second injection duration.[33–35] The first postcontrast phase of imaging is obtained during the phase of peak pancreatic parenchymal enhancement to maximize the conspicuity of the tumor (Fig. 17). This phase is approximately 40 to 50 seconds after the start of contrast injection.[36] The later portal venous phase, which maximizes enhancement of the liver parenchyma (approximately 60–70 seconds after injection), is useful for identification of liver metastases and also results in excellent opacification of the mesenteric, splenic, and portal veins, which is useful for evaluation for tumor involvement of these structures.[36] We typically reconstruct axial images to 2 slice thicknesses, 2.5 mm for primary review, and 0.625 to 1.25 mm (depending on the MDCT platform) to allow for postprocessing. For example, we create coronal and sagittal 2.5-mm thick contiguous multiplanar reconstructions (see Fig. 17), but these thinner axial images are also useful for creating curved planar reformations, maximum-intensity projection (MIP), minimum-intensity projection, as well as volume-rendered and segmented volume rendered images.

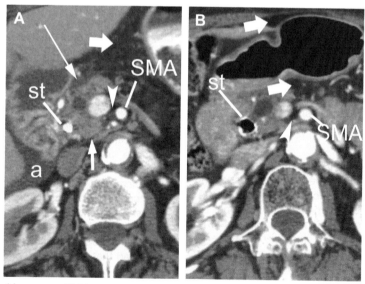

Fig. 16. A 72-year-old woman with biopsy-proven stage I pancreatic adenocarcinoma. Baseline axial CT image at our institution (*A*) shows stent (st) placed by outside institution. Large white arrow shows edematous changes in mesenteric fat, ascites (a), and fluid near the pancreatic head (*long white arrow*) consistent with post–stent placement pancreatitis. In this setting, it is not clear whether stranding (*white arrowhead*) near the SMA represents tumor or inflammation. Tumor (*medium white arrow*) involves the pancreatic head and uncinate process. (*B*) Posttreatment scan shows resolution of pancreatitis, with resolution of ascites, and fat (*big white arrows*) anterior and posterior to the stomach no longer appearing edematous. Fat interface (*white arrowhead*) near SMA now appears intact with previously seen stranding having resolved. Plastic stent was replaced with a metallic stent (st).

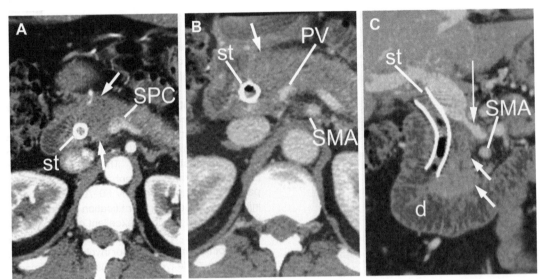

Fig. 17. A 53-year-old man with stage II-III borderline pancreatic head ductal adenocarcinoma on baseline multi-phasic examination. (*A*) Axial pancreatic parenchymal phase image shows tumor (*white arrows*) abutting the SPC and surrounding stent (*st*). (*B*) On portal venous phase image, tumor (*white arrow*) is less conspicuous. Tumor narrows the well-opacified portal vein (PV) superior to the SPC. Nonspecific stranding abuts the right border of the SMA. Coronal reconstruction of the portal venous phase (*C*) shows that the tumor (*white arrows*) causes marked narrowing of the portal vein (*long white arrow*). d, duodenum.

Pancreatic adenocarcinoma has a typically hypodense appearance on the pancreatic parenchymal phase (see Fig. 17) but can be isodense, and either remains hypodense on the portal venous phase or may become isodense. Axial images and coronal and sagittal reformations are useful for providing a comprehensive review of the celiac, superior mesenteric, common hepatic, and splenic arteries as well as the main portal, splenic, and superior mesenteric veins and their major branches (gastrocolic trunk, first jejunal vein, and ileocolic tributaries).

MR IMAGING

MR imaging offers the advantage of multiple sequences that can provide information regarding the primary tumor, its local extent, vascular involvement, and distant metastases. Multiple recent technical developments include platforms with higher field strength, increasingly powerful multichannel coils, new contrast agents, and new sequences. An example of a typical imaging examination (Figs. 18 and 19) includes T2-weighted fat-suppressed, T1-weighted, in and out of phase, diffusion-weighted, and T1-weighted dynamically obtained postcontrast multiplanar imaging (such as three-dimensional [3D] gradient recalled echo volumes obtained with parallel imaging). Dynamically obtained images can be obtained as single breath holds at 20, 60, 120, and 180 seconds after the start of contrast injection.[37,38] Such sequences as Fast Imaging Employing Steady-State Acquisition (FIESTA; GE Medical Systems, Milwaukee, WI) with fat suppression (see Fig. 19) can help to differentiate fat, vessels, tumor, and uninvolved pancreas. Images are most commonly obtained directly in the axial plane. However, other planes can be obtained directly. Coronal-plane FIESTA images are useful for evaluating the relationship of tumor to vessels, particularly the origin of the celiac and superior mesenteric arteries in cross section, and to visualize the extent of common hepatic artery involvement.

Pancreatic adenocarcinoma has a variable appearance on MR imaging depending on the sequence being examined. On dynamic images, its appearance is similar to that on contrast-enhanced CT, being hypointense to adjacent pancreatic parenchyma, but at times also appearing isointense, in which case identification of primary tumor can be difficult. A recent article suggested that MR imaging may be able to visualize up to 79% of tumors that appear isodense to normal pancreatic parenchyma on multiphasic CT studies.[39]

EUS

Using a combination of radial and curvilinear arrays, EUS has developed a significant role in the ability to image lesions and provide tissue

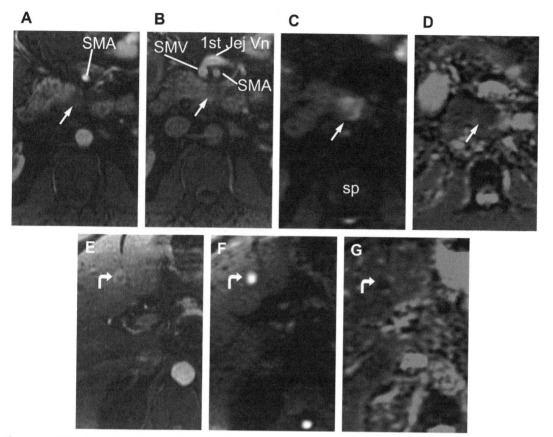

Fig. 18. MR imaging of a 56-year-old man with history of stage IV pancreatic cancer. Pancreatic tumor (*white arrow*) appears hypointense on (*A*) pancreatic parenchymal phase and (*B*) portal venous phase. Venous structures such as the SMV and first jejunal vein (1st Jej Vn) are well opacified on the portal venous phase, optimizing evaluation for venous involvement. On diffusion weighted imaging (*C*), tumor appears bright, and on apparent diffusion coefficient (ADC) map (*D*), tumor appears dark, indicating restricted water movement. Liver metastasis (*curved white arrow*) on dynamic three-dimensional (3D) spoiled gradient echo late arterial phase (*E*) shows ring enhancement; on (*F*) diffusion weighted imaging appears bright and shows low signal on ADC (*G*) consistent with restricted water movement, supporting that this is a metastasis.

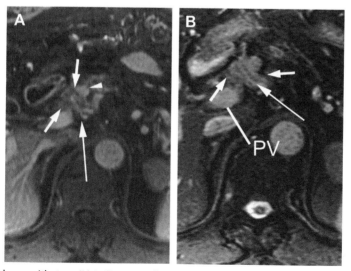

Fig. 19. A 61-year-old man with stage IIA to B pancreatic cancer. Portal venous phase 3D spoiled gradient T1-weighted fat-suppressed image (*A*) shows tumor (*white arrows*) abutting enlarged common hepatic artery node (*white arrowhead*) and encasing the CHA (*long white arrow*). (*B*) Fat-suppressed Fast Imaging Employing Steady-State Acquisition (FIESTA) image similarly shows CHA encasement.

diagnoses via EUS-guided FNA for pancreatic cancer through real-time imaging without the need for administration of a contrast agent.[40,41] Future directions include the possibility of contrast enhancement, as well as potentially the use of elastography.[42] This ability to visualize and obtain tissue specimens in real time is also useful for the evaluation of suspicious lymph nodes. However, the role of EUS for staging is likely more limited than CT or MR imaging, given its limited view of abdominal anatomy (discussed later).

POSITRON EMISSION TOMOGRAPHY/CT

Positron emission tomography (PET)/CT is usually performed without intravenous contrast, and therefore has had a limited role in the local staging of pancreatic cancer given its poor depiction of tumor and its relationship to adjacent vasculature. However, a study comparing PET, unenhanced PET/CT, and intravenous contrast-enhanced PET/CT showed, as expected, improved accuracy for intravenous contrast-enhanced PET/CT (88% vs 76% for unenhanced PET/CT) for staging, and was suggested as a possible single technique for the staging of pancreatic cancer.[43] The role of unenhanced PET/CT has primarily been to detect metastatic disease and has been useful especially for unexpected sites because it is a whole-body imaging modality (**Figs. 20** and **21**).[44]

IMAGING AND STAGING
Local Staging

Staging on cross-sectional imaging currently involves determining in cross section the degrees of circumferential involvement of regional arteries and veins (see **Figs. 11–13** and **15**) by tumor and narrowing/occlusion of veins (see **Fig. 14**). As described originally by Lu and colleagues[45] in 1997, using a threshold of greater than 180° of circumferential vessel involvement as indicating unresectable disease on contrast-enhanced CT imaging yielded a sensitivity of 84% and specificity of 98% for unresectable disease, which maximized the sending of all those with resectable disease to surgery, at the expense of undercalling unresectable disease. This was in the setting of older staging criteria in which venous involvement meant unresectable disease, and likely did not include the use of preoperative therapy.[45] Determining the accuracy of CT and MR imaging for staging has currently become more complex given the variability of therapy and surgical approaches between institutions. As noted previously, institutions vary in their use of neoadjuvant and/or adjuvant therapy. Nevertheless, more recent staging studies have shown sensitivities for unresectable disease between 52% and 91%, and specificities of 92% to 100%, but there were likely differences between institutions in what was considered surgically resectable disease.[46–50] In addition, in these

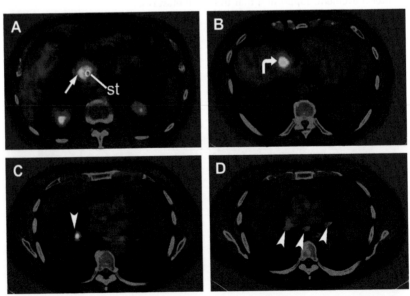

Fig. 20. A 78-year-old man with biopsy-proven stage IV pancreatic cancer. Axial fused images from PET/CT study shows (*A*) fluorodeoxyglucose (FDG) avid pancreatic head mass (*white arrow*) surrounding stent (st), (*B*) liver metastasis (*curved white arrow*), (*C*) right hilar nodal metastasis (*curved white arrowhead*), and (*D*) other, slightly less FDG avid, hilar and mediastinal nodes (*curved white arrowheads*).

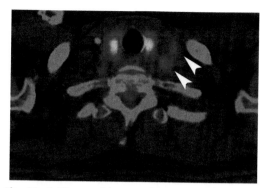

Fig. 21. A 59-year-old man with stage IV pancreatic adenocarcinoma. Axial fused PET/CT image shows FDG-avid left supraclavicular adenopathy (*curved white arrowheads*) consistent with metastatic disease.

studies, small-volume metastases to the liver or peritoneum were as common, or more common, than vascular invasion as causes for patients being identified as unresectable at surgery who were identified as resectable on cross-sectional imaging. A study that compared different generations of MDCT equipment in the same institution did not show a significant difference in performance between generations.[48] Another question is that of MR versus CT for staging. MR offers inherently better soft tissue contrast (see **Figs. 18** and **19**), whereas CT offers higher spatial resolution and the ability to freeze bowel motion. Although it is difficult to compare 2 modalities

that are evolving so rapidly, several studies have shown comparable performance between MR and CT for local staging.[46,51] It is therefore probably best to use the strengths of a given institution (CT vs MR imaging) in terms of equipment, experience, and skill when choosing which modality to use for determining local staging.

Another confounding factor is that of preoperative chemoradiation (**Fig. 22**). To date, it is not possible to distinguish on imaging between nonviable tumor and remaining viable tumor following therapy. Another issue is that of posttreatment changes. Radiation therapy can cause changes around vessels that we have found to primarily manifest as soft tissue stranding. We have found baseline studies useful for identifying the extent of tumor before radiation therapy; in our experience, patients undergoing preoperative therapy who develop, or show stable, minimal stranding without significant soft tissue thickening adjacent to vessels should not be prevented from undergoing surgery.[49] Overall, we found the accuracy of determining vascular involvement to be similar to that reported in the absence of preoperative therapy.[49]

The role of EUS for local staging and determining vascular invasion is not clear, because results have been mixed. A study by Dewitt and colleagues of 120 patients showed EUS to be superior to CT for tumor staging (67% vs 41%), but equivalent for nodal staging (44% vs 47%), and similar or slightly inferior to CT for judging

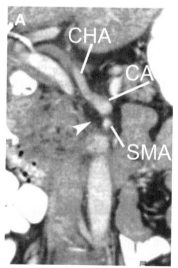

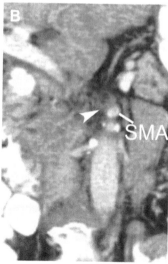

Fig. 22. A 53-year-old woman with borderline stage II to III pancreatic cancer, with imaging before, and following, chemoradiation. (*A*) Coronal gray scale reformation shows, at presentation, subtle stranding (*white arrowhead*) near the SMA origin. CA, celiac axis. (*B*) Follow-up coronal reconstruction at the same level following chemoradiation, before surgery. Soft tissue thickening has become more prominent (*white arrowhead*) but does not have the appearance of definite solid tissue. The patient underwent surgery, with negative resection margin on microscopy, and no positive regional lymph nodes.

resectability (88 vs 92%). However, in another study, the EUS feature of loss of the integrity of the echoplane surrounding a vessel indicated tumor adherence to vasculature in only 29% of cases, and in none was there histologic evidence of invasion.[52] A prospective blinded study of 62 patients evaluating accuracy of locoregional staging using surgical confirmation compared EUS, MR imaging, and CT and showed accuracies of 62%, 68%, and 74% respectively.[53] In the same study, CT had an accuracy of 83% for vascular invasion versus 75% for EUS. These investigators concluded that EUS may be best used as a potentially confirmatory test following CT for resectable tumors.[53] A systematic review of the literature by Dewitt and colleagues[54] concluded that heterogeneous study design, study quality, and differing results prevented a clear determination of whether CT or EUS was better for evaluation of patients before surgery and that well-controlled prospective studies were necessary.

Unenhanced PET/CT, as already noted, does not have a role for local staging of pancreatic cancer. However, as also already noted, when performed with intravenous contrast, it seems to perform comparably with contrast-enhanced CT. Attention to technique, including thin-section imaging and the timing of phases of image acquisition, likely remain important for accurate staging.

Nodal Disease

The accuracy for assessing nodal disease is limited regardless of the modality used. Nodal size of greater than 1 cm in the short axis has most commonly been used on MR imaging and CT as a threshold for identifying metastatic nodes, but is nonspecific. In a study using a size criterion of 1.5 cm or larger on CT as a sign of metastatic nodal disease, only 16.7% of patients with nodal involvement were identified as having nodal disease on preoperative CT.[50] Nevertheless, it is important to identify nodes outside the conventional surgical field, such as nodes to the left of the SMA (Fig. 23). PET/CT has been reported to have sensitivities of 46% to 71% and specificities of 63% to 100%[55–57] for nodal disease (see Figs. 20 and 21). PET/CT is probably useful in the setting of identifying nodes most suspicious for biopsy, but is limited for small-volume disease, and cannot differentiate between inflammatory adenopathy versus metastatic adenopathy. The limited field of visibility of EUS prevents a comprehensive evaluation of the abdomen for adenopathy, particularly for nodes outside the surgical field.[58] As with other modalities, its sensitivity is also limited because of the inability to detect nodal micrometastases. The

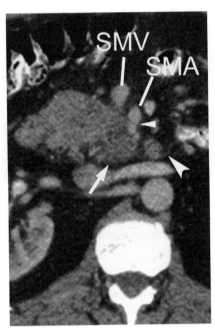

Fig. 23. A 54-year-old man with biopsy-proven borderline stage II to III pancreatic cancer and regional nodal disease. Axial image from baseline CT study shows tumor in the uncinate (*white arrow*) abutting by more than 90° the SMA, by extension along the IPDA (*white arrowhead*). To the left of the SMA is adenopathy (*curved white arrowhead*).

combination of EUS with FNA has been shown to greatly increase the specificity of diagnosis for pancreatic cancer,[59] and although information in the literature is limited, it is expected that EUS-FNA would have high specificity, and therefore usefulness, in the evaluation of suspicious lymph nodes, making it a useful problem solver when such determinations need to be made, although its ability to evaluate such nodes is again limited by the range of visualization of the abdomen by EUS, the range of safe access for FNA biopsy, and the problems of sampling error inherent with nodal micrometastases. Early work suggests that EUS paired with elastography may have promise in improving its sensitivity and specificity for nodal involvement.[60]

Metastases

Pancreatic cancer most commonly metastasizes to liver, peritoneum, lungs, and bone, although bone metastases typically occur late in the course of this disease. CT, MR imaging, and PET/CT play complementary roles in the evaluation for metastatic disease.

Liver metastases are most commonly assessed by either CT or MR imaging. Although older studies have reported CT (see Fig. 7; Fig. 24) having

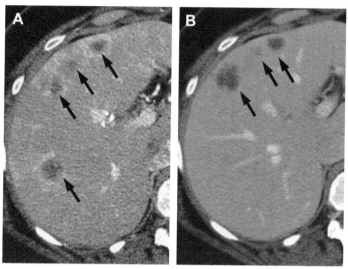

Fig. 24. A 54-year-old woman with multiple liver metastases from pancreatic cancer. (*A*) Pancreatic parenchymal phase shows multiple metastases (*black arrows*) that show peripheral hyperdense enhancement and central hypodensity. (*B*) Portal venous phase image shows only a hypodense appearance of metastases (*black arrows*).

a sensitivity of 75% to 87%,[61–63] a recent study comparing MDCT with CT arterial portography and CT-assisted hepatic arteriography showed MDCT to have a sensitivity of 48.4% and specificity of 97.9% for liver metastases.[64] Small-volume metastases to liver, particularly peritoneal implants to the liver surface, have been a difficulty for cross-sectional imaging, as is also the lack of

specificity of very small lesions.[47–49] MR imaging has often served as a problem solver for liver metastases (**Fig. 25**), and recent developments such as diffusion-weighted imaging (**Fig. 26**) and the use of liver-specific contrast agents are promising. In a study of 15 patients with 62 liver metastases, comparing gadoxetic acid MR imaging (a liver-specific agent that can also be used for

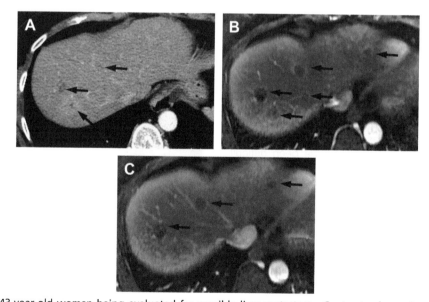

Fig. 25. A 43-year-old woman being evaluated for possible liver metastases. Contrast-enhanced portal venous phase CT image (*A*) shows lesions suspicious for metastases (*black arrows*) appearing slightly hypodense or showing unusual, slightly prominent, enhancement. Subsequent MR imaging examination (*B*) shows late arterial phase ring enhancement for several lesions with (*C*) washout on portal venous phase, appearing more prominent on the MR imaging than on CT and confirming that several of these lesions are liver metastases.

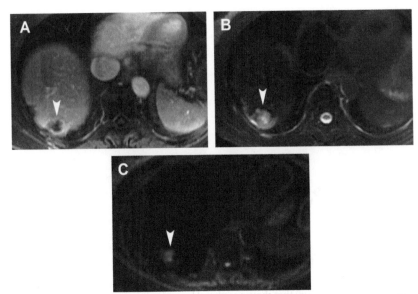

Fig. 26. A 71-year-old woman with pancreatic cancer status post Whipple procedure 2 years earlier. Lesion (*white arrowhead*) in liver on (*A*) portal venous phase shows low-intensity center and peripheral enhancement. (*B*) On fat-suppressed T2-weighted imaging, the lesion shows bright central focus likely representing necrosis. On diffusion (*C*), the lesion appears bright. Note that the rim of enhancement of liver metastases is a variable finding between patients on MR imaging.

dynamic imaging) with MDCT, MR imaging had greater sensitivity than CT (85% vs 69%).[65] MR imaging assessment of the primary tumor was thought to be similar to that of MDCT for the purposes of local staging.[65] Limited information is available on the role of PET/CT in the diagnosis of liver metastases (see **Fig. 20**). Studies that evaluated whole-body fluorodeoxyglucose (FDG) PET showed sensitivities of approximately 67% to 70%.[66–68] A more recent study comparing intravenous contrast-enhanced PET/CT, unenhanced PET/CT, and PET alone showed sensitivities for liver metastases of 82%, 46%, and 46%, respectively.[43]

Pancreatic metastases to the peritoneum are usually of small volume and have been difficult to detect by any modality (Fig. 27). This difficulty has led to the suggestion of using laparoscopy to screen patients for peritoneal disease. This approach has the limitation that sites identified on laparoscopy may not be identifiable on cross-sectional imaging, and therefore would not be amenable to imaging follow-up. In addition, a meta-analysis suggested that, in the setting of dual-phase thin-section CT, the use of additional exploratory laparoscopy would alter management in, at most, 4% to 15% of patients.[69]

PET/CT has been advocated as a means for identifying unexpected distant sites of metastatic disease (see **Figs. 20** and **21**) because it is a whole-body modality, as opposed to conventional MDCT and MR imaging, which are typically used in a narrow range of anatomic regions (abdomen, abdomen/pelvis, or, in the case of CT, chest, abdomen, and pelvis). A study of 103 patients in which the FDG-PET data were reviewed and compared with MDCT, the detection rate for liver metastases was less than that of CT, but better than CT for detection of remote

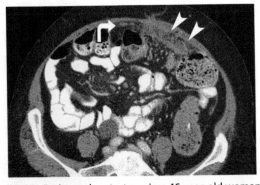

Fig. 27. Peritoneal metastases in a 46-year-old woman with pancreatic cancer. Axial contrast-enhanced portal venous phase CT image shows peritoneal disease manifesting as small nodule (*curved white arrow*) and as broad soft tissue thickening (*white arrowheads*).

lymph node and bone metastases.[70] However, the same study also noted that MDCT "indicated other noncurative factors in these patients." All patients who were not resectable could be identified as such without FDG-PET. Additional information is needed to identify whether there is added benefit for PET/CT compared with MDCT. Another consideration is the use of contrast-enhanced PET/CT, which could allow for this modality to become a single technique for whole-body staging of pancreatic cancer, providing information on the full gamut from local vascular involvement to distant liver, lung, bone, and far distant nodal metastases.[43]

REPORTING OF IMAGING FINDINGS

Following imaging and its accurate interpretation, probably the next most important issue is that findings be described in a clear, consistent manner, understandable by all physicians who are involved in a patient's care. Unclear reports can create confusion that can potentially result in patients being assigned incorrectly to treatment trials. For patients traveling between institutions, unclear reports could result in the repeating of imaging studies.

For this reason, attempts have been made to standardize reporting of imaging findings for pancreatic cancer. An article from our institution regarding multidisciplinary care of patients with pancreatic cancer proposed a template for dictation of CT findings for patients with pancreatic cancer, including descriptions of the primary tumor's size, location, relationship to vessels (using the terms abutment, ≤180° of contact, and encasement, >180° of contact), vessel occlusion, variant vascular anatomy, a grade regarding local tumor resectability (resectable, borderline resectable, or locally advanced), and extent and location of extrapancreatic disease.[71] A template published by the Radiologic Society of North America (RSNA), and available on the Internet, similarly characterizes the primary lesion but also includes descriptive features for cystic lesions, suggested descriptors for vascular involvement (degrees of enhancement, abutment/encasement, or contiguous/noncontiguous), as well as providing additional descriptors of the adjacent parenchyma, nodes, and whether distant metastases are present.[72] It is our understanding that other organizations, such as the American Pancreatic Association (APA), are developing similar suggested reporting standards. It is our opinion that these templates serve 2 important functions: a checklist of features to be reported, and a standardized vocabulary (most importantly for vascular involvement) understood by multiple specialties.

REFERENCES

1. Wolff RA, Abbruzzese JL, Evans DB. Neoplasms of the exocrine pancreas. In: Bast RC Jr, Kufe DW, Pollock RE, editors. Cancer medicine. 6th edition. Hamilton (Ontario): American Cancer Society and BC Decker; 2003. p. 1585–614.
2. Sener SF, Fremgen A, Menck HR, et al. Pancreatic cancer: a report of treatment and survival trends for 100,313 patients diagnosed from 1985-1995, using the National Cancer Database. J Am Coll Surg 1999;189(1):1–7.
3. Katz MH, Wang H, Fleming JB, et al. Long-term survival after multidisciplinary management of resected pancreatic adenocarcinoma. Ann Surg Oncol 2009;16(4):836–47.
4. Tseng JF, Raut CP, Lee JE, et al. Pancreaticoduodenectomy with vascular resection: margin status and survival duration. J Gastrointest Surg 2004;8(8):935–49 [discussion: 949–50].
5. Lall CG, Howard TJ, Skandarajah A, et al. New concepts in staging and treatment of locally advanced pancreatic head cancer. AJR Am J Roentgenol 2007;189(5):1044–50.
6. Christians KK, Lal A, Pappas S, et al. Portal vein resection. Surg Clin North Am 2010;90(2):309–22.
7. Evans DB, Farnell MB, Lillemoe KD, et al. Surgical treatment of resectable and borderline resectable pancreas cancer: expert consensus statement. Ann Surg Oncol 2009;16(7):1736–44.
8. Clark LR, Jaffe MH, Choyke PL, et al. Pancreatic imaging. Radiol Clin North Am 1985;23(3):489–501.
9. Balachandran A, Darden DL, Tamm EP, et al. Arterial variants in pancreatic adenocarcinoma. Abdom Imaging 2008;33(2):214–21.
10. Okahara M, Mori H, Kiyosue H, et al. Arterial supply to the pancreas; variations and cross-sectional anatomy. Abdom Imaging 2010;35(2):134–42.
11. Katz MH, Fleming JB, Lee JE, et al. Current status of adjuvant therapy for pancreatic cancer. Oncologist 2010;15(11):1205–13.
12. Klinkenbijl JH, Jeekel J, Sahmoud T, et al. Adjuvant radiotherapy and 5-fluorouracil after curative resection of cancer of the pancreas and periampullary region: phase III trial of the EORTC gastrointestinal tract cancer cooperative group. Ann Surg 1999;230(6):776–82 [discussion: 782–4].
13. Smeenk HG, van Eijck CH, Hop WC, et al. Long-term survival and metastatic pattern of pancreatic and periampullary cancer after adjuvant chemoradiation or observation: long-term results of EORTC trial 40891. Ann Surg 2007;246(5):734–40.

14. Neoptolemos JP, Dunn JA, Stocken DD, et al. Adjuvant chemoradiotherapy and chemotherapy in resectable pancreatic cancer: a randomised controlled trial. Lancet 2001;358(9293):1576–85.

15. Neoptolemos JP, Stocken DD, Friess H, et al. A randomized trial of chemoradiotherapy and chemotherapy after resection of pancreatic cancer. N Engl J Med 2004;350(12):1200–10.

16. Regine WF, Winter KA, Abrams RA, et al. Fluorouracil vs gemcitabine chemotherapy before and after fluorouracil-based chemoradiation following resection of pancreatic adenocarcinoma: a randomized controlled trial. JAMA 2008;299(9):1019–26.

17. Kalser MH, Ellenberg SS. Pancreatic cancer. Adjuvant combined radiation and chemotherapy following curative resection. Arch Surg 1985;120(8):899–903.

18. Aloia TA, Lee JE, Vauthey JN, et al. Delayed recovery after pancreaticoduodenectomy: a major factor impairing the delivery of adjuvant therapy? J Am Coll Surg 2007;204(3):347–55.

19. Varadhachary GR, Tamm EP, Abbruzzese JL, et al. Borderline resectable pancreatic cancer: definitions, management, and role of preoperative therapy. Ann Surg Oncol 2006;13(8):1035–46.

20. Sasson AR, Wetherington RW, Hoffman JP, et al. Neoadjuvant chemoradiotherapy for adenocarcinoma of the pancreas: analysis of histopathology and outcome. Int J Gastrointest Cancer 2003;34(2–3):121–8.

21. White RR, Xie HB, Gottfried MR, et al. Significance of histological response to preoperative chemoradiotherapy for pancreatic cancer. Ann Surg Oncol 2005;12(3):214–21.

22. Pingpank JF, Hoffman JP, Ross EA, et al. Effect of preoperative chemoradiotherapy on surgical margin status of resected adenocarcinoma of the head of the pancreas. J Gastrointest Surg 2001;5(2):121–30.

23. Heinrich S, Schafer M, Weber A, et al. Neoadjuvant chemotherapy generates a significant tumor response in resectable pancreatic cancer without increasing morbidity: results of a prospective phase II trial. Ann Surg 2008;248(6):1014–22.

24. Evans DB, Varadhachary GR, Crane CH, et al. Preoperative gemcitabine-based chemoradiation for patients with resectable adenocarcinoma of the pancreatic head. J Clin Oncol 2008;26(21):3496–502.

25. Varadhachary GR, Wolff RA, Crane CH, et al. Preoperative gemcitabine and cisplatin followed by gemcitabine-based chemoradiation for resectable adenocarcinoma of the pancreatic head. J Clin Oncol 2008;26(21):3487–95.

26. Heinrich S, Pestalozzi BC, Schafer M, et al. Prospective phase II trial of neoadjuvant chemotherapy with gemcitabine and cisplatin for resectable adenocarcinoma of the pancreatic head. J Clin Oncol 2008;26(15):2526–31.

27. Exocrine and endocrine pancreas. In: Edge SB, Byrd DR, Compton CC, et al, editors. AJCC cancer staging manual. 7th edition. New York: Springer; 2010. p. 241–50.

28. Fuhrman GM, Leach SD, Staley CA, et al. Rationale for en bloc vein resection in the treatment of pancreatic adenocarcinoma adherent to the superior mesenteric-portal vein confluence. Pancreatic Tumor Study Group. Ann Surg 1996;223(2):154–62.

29. Tempero MA, Arnoletti JP, Behrman S, et al. Pancreatic adenocarcinoma. J Natl Compr Canc Netw 2010;8(9):972–1017.

30. National Comprehensive Cancer Network I. Clinical practice guidelines in oncology: pancreatic adenocarcinoma. [pdf file]. 2011. 1.2012. Available at: http://www.nccn.org/professionals/physician_gls/PDF/pancreatic.pdf. Accessed November 7, 2011.

31. Katz MH, Pisters PW, Lee JE, et al. Borderline resectable pancreatic cancer: what have we learned and where do we go from here? Ann Surg Oncol 2011;18(3):608–10.

32. Abrams RA, Lowy AM, O'Reilly EM, et al. Combined modality treatment of resectable and borderline resectable pancreas cancer: expert consensus statement. Ann Surg Oncol 2009;16(7):1751–6.

33. Kim T, Murakami T, Takahashi S, et al. Pancreatic CT imaging: effects of different injection rates and doses of contrast material. Radiology 1999;212(1):219–25.

34. Schueller G, Schima W, Schueller-Weidekamm C, et al. Multidetector CT of pancreas: effects of contrast material flow rate and individualized scan delay on enhancement of pancreas and tumor contrast. Radiology 2006;241(2):441–8.

35. Tublin ME, Tessler FN, Cheng SL, et al. Effect of injection rate of contrast medium on pancreatic and hepatic helical CT. Radiology 1999;210(1):97–101.

36. Fletcher JG, Wiersema MJ, Farrell MA, et al. Pancreatic malignancy: value of arterial, pancreatic, and hepatic phase imaging with multi-detector row CT. Radiology 2003;229(1):81–90.

37. Fayad LM, Mitchell DG. Magnetic resonance imaging of pancreatic adenocarcinoma. Int J Gastrointest Cancer 2001;30(1–2):19–25.

38. Pamuklar E, Semelka RC. MR imaging of the pancreas. Magn Reson Imaging Clin North Am 2005;13(2):313–30.

39. Kim JH, Park SH, Yu ES, et al. Visually isoattenuating pancreatic adenocarcinoma at dynamic-enhanced CT: frequency, clinical and pathologic characteristics, and diagnosis at imaging examinations. Radiology 2010;257(1):87–96.

40. Tamm EP, Loyer EM, Faria SC, et al. Retrospective analysis of dual-phase MDCT and follow-up EUS/EUS-FNA in the diagnosis of pancreatic cancer. Abdom Imaging 2007;32(5):660–7.

41. Wiersema MJ, Vilmann P, Giovannini M, et al. Endosonography-guided fine-needle aspiration biopsy: diagnostic accuracy and complication assessment. Gastroenterology 1997;112(4):1087–95.

42. Giovannini M. The place of endoscopic ultrasound in bilio-pancreatic pathology. Gastroenterol Clin Biol 2010;34(8–9):436–45.

43. Strobel K, Heinrich S, Bhure U, et al. Contrast-enhanced 18F-FDG PET/CT: 1-stop-shop imaging for assessing the resectability of pancreatic cancer. J Nucl Med 2008;49(9):1408–13.

44. Delbeke D, Martin WH. PET and PET/CT for pancreatic malignancies. Surg Oncol Clin North Am 2010; 19(2):235–54.

45. Lu DS, Reber HA, Krasny RM, et al. Local staging of pancreatic cancer: criteria for unresectability of major vessels as revealed by pancreatic-phase, thin-section helical CT. AJR Am J Roentgenol 1997;168(6):1439–43.

46. Lee JK, Kim AY, Kim PN, et al. Prediction of vascular involvement and resectability by multidetector-row CT versus MR imaging with MR angiography in patients who underwent surgery for resection of pancreatic ductal adenocarcinoma. Eur J Radiol 2010;73(2):310–6.

47. Kaneko OF, Lee DM, Wong J, et al. Performance of multidetector computed tomographic angiography in determining surgical resectability of pancreatic head adenocarcinoma. J Comput Assist Tomogr 2010;34(5):732–8.

48. Zamboni GA, Kruskal JB, Vollmer CM, et al. Pancreatic adenocarcinoma: value of multidetector CT angiography in preoperative evaluation. Radiology 2007;245(3):770–8.

49. Tamm EP, Loyer EM, Faria S, et al. Staging of pancreatic cancer with multidetector CT in the setting of preoperative chemoradiation therapy. Abdom Imaging 2006;31(5):568–74.

50. Valls C, Andia E, Sanchez A, et al. Dual-phase helical CT of pancreatic adenocarcinoma: assessment of resectability before surgery. AJR Am J Roentgenol 2002;178(4):821–6.

51. Arslan A, Buanes T, Geitung JT. Pancreatic carcinoma: MR, MR angiography and dynamic helical CT in the evaluation of vascular invasion. Eur J Radiol 2001;38(2):151–9.

52. Aslanian H, Salem R, Lee J, et al. EUS diagnosis of vascular invasion in pancreatic cancer: surgical and histologic correlates. Am J Gastroenterol 2005; 100(6):1381–5.

53. Soriano A, Castells A, Ayuso C, et al. Preoperative staging and tumor resectability assessment of pancreatic cancer: prospective study comparing endoscopic ultrasonography, helical computed tomography, magnetic resonance imaging, and angiography. Am J Gastroenterol 2004;99(3): 492–501.

54. Dewitt J, Devereaux BM, Lehman GA, et al. Comparison of endoscopic ultrasound and computed tomography for the preoperative evaluation of pancreatic cancer: a systematic review. Clin Gastroenterol Hepatol 2006;4(6):717–25 [quiz: 664].

55. Pakzad F, Groves AM, Ell PJ. The role of positron emission tomography in the management of pancreatic cancer. Semin Nucl Med 2006;36(3): 248–56.

56. Bares R, Dohmen BM, Cremerius U, et al. Results of positron emission tomography with fluorine-18 labeled fluorodeoxyglucose in differential diagnosis and staging of pancreatic carcinoma. Radiologe 1996;36(5):435–40 [in German].

57. Bares R, Klever P, Hauptmann S, et al. F-18 fluoro-deoxyglucose PET in vivo evaluation of pancreatic glucose metabolism for detection of pancreatic cancer. Radiology 1994;192(1):79–86.

58. Kala Z, Valek V, Hlavsa J, et al. The role of CT and endoscopic ultrasound in pre-operative staging of pancreatic cancer. Eur J Radiol 2007;62(2): 166–9.

59. Mitsuhashi T, Ghafari S, Chang CY, et al. Endoscopic ultrasound-guided fine needle aspiration of the pancreas: cytomorphological evaluation with emphasis on adequacy assessment, diagnostic criteria and contamination from the gastrointestinal tract. Cytopathology 2006;17(1):34–41.

60. Giovannini M, Thomas B, Erwan B, et al. Endoscopic ultrasound elastography for evaluation of lymph nodes and pancreatic masses: a multicenter study. World J Gastroenterol 2009;15(13): 1587–93.

61. Richter GM, Simon C, Hoffmann V, et al. Hydrospiral CT of the pancreas in thin section technique. Radiologe 1996;36(5):397–405 [in German].

62. Trede M, Rumstadt B, Wendl K, et al. Ultrafast magnetic resonance imaging improves the staging of pancreatic tumors. Ann Surg 1997;226(4): 393–405 [discussion: 405–7].

63. Calculli L, Casadei R, Diacono D, et al. Role of spiral computerized tomography in the staging of pancreatic carcinoma. Radiol Med 1998;95(4):344–8 [in Italian].

64. Ikuta Y, Takamori H, Ikeda O, et al. Detection of liver metastases secondary to pancreatic cancer: utility of combined helical computed tomography during arterial portography with biphasic computed tomography-assisted hepatic arteriography. J Gastroenterol 2010;45(12):1241–6.

65. Motosugi U, Ichikawa T, Morisaka H, et al. Detection of pancreatic carcinoma and liver metastases with gadoxetic acid-enhanced MR imaging: comparison

with contrast-enhanced multi-detector row CT. Radiology 2011;260(2):446–53.

66. Sahani DV, Kalva SP, Fischman AJ, et al. Detection of liver metastases from adenocarcinoma of the colon and pancreas: comparison of mangafodipir trisodium-enhanced liver MRI and whole-body FDG PET. AJR Am J Roentgenol 2005;185(1): 239–46.

67. Frohlich A, Diederichs CG, Staib L, et al. Detection of liver metastases from pancreatic cancer using FDG PET. J Nucl Med 1999;40(2):250–5.

68. Diederichs CG. Pancreatic cancer. In: Ruhlmann J, Oehr P, Biersack HJ, editors. PET in oncology. Berlin: Springer-Verlag; 1999. p. 128–34.

69. Pisters PW, Lee JE, Vauthey JN, et al. Laparoscopy in the staging of pancreatic cancer. Br J Surg 2001; 88(3):325–37.

70. Izuishi K, Yamamoto Y, Sano T, et al. Impact of 18-fluorodeoxyglucose positron emission tomography on the management of pancreatic cancer. J Gastrointest Surg 2010;14(7):1151–8.

71. Evans DB, Crane CH, Charnsangavej C, et al. The added value of multidisciplinary care for patients with pancreatic cancer. Ann Surg Oncol 2008; 15(8):2078–80.

72. Gottlieb R, et al. CT onco primary pancreas mass template. 2011. Available at: http://www.radreport. org/txt/0000018. Accessed November 14, 2011.

Imaging of Acute Pancreatitis: Update of the Revised Atlanta Classification

Thomas L. Bollen, MD

KEYWORDS

• Acute pancreatitis • Classification • Severity
• Pancreatic necrosis • Peripancreatic collections

INTRODUCTION

Acute pancreatitis (AP) is defined as an acute inflammatory state of the pancreas and is conventionally categorized as either mild or severe disease. Approximately 80% to 85% of patients with AP will have the mild form with an uncomplicated clinical course, whereas 15% to 20% develop a complicated clinical course characterized by organ failure and/or local complications.[1]

Worldwide the incidence of AP is increasing, probably related to the rising incidence of gallstones, obesity, and aging of the population; all are well-known risk factors for AP.[2] Besides gallstones, alcohol abuse is the second most common cause of AP.[1] Although the pathophysiology of AP is incompletely understood, it is believed that in gallstone and alcoholic pancreatitis a chain of events is triggered by a temporary or permanent pancreatic duct obstruction. Locally this leads to activation and release of pancreatic enzymes into the pancreatic interstitium and peripancreatic tissues. When severe, autodigestion and necrosis occur.[1] Systemically, this results in release of inflammatory mediators termed cytokines, such as tumor necrosis factor, which is toxic to acinar cells. Cytokines activate and intensify the inflammatory cascade that may ultimately culminate in (multi)organ failure. Alternatively, the ischemia-reperfusion theory has been proposed as a unifying mechanism for AP; microcirculatory disturbances are the cause of local tissue injury and cytokine-mediated inflammatory response that may lead to the systemic inflammatory response syndrome (SIRS) and the development of organ failure.[3,4] There are evolving data that the magnitude of the inflammatory response, mediated by the immune system, is responsible for most of the morbidity and mortality in AP rather than the degree and extent of local pancreatic damage.[5,6]

Clinically, severe AP is characterized by an early toxic phase with variable organ dysfunction lasting 1 to 2 weeks and a later phase dominated by the effects of local complications (primarily infected necrosis).[5,7,8] Mortality from AP closely follows this biphasic pattern; in the first weeks, patients with severe AP die from sustained (multiple) organ failure, whereas in the later phase mortality can largely be attributed to infection of necrotic pancreatic and peripancreatic tissues, often superimposed by organ failure.[5,8]

Over the past decades, several classification systems for AP have emerged, with the 1992 Atlanta Classification (AC) being the latest.[9] The International Symposium on Acute Pancreatitis (Atlanta, Georgia, September 11–13, 1992) proposed a clinically based classification system that provided definitions for the disease, its severity, organ failure, and the local complications of AP.[9] Better understanding of the pathophysiology of AP, improved diagnostic imaging of AP, and the development of minimally invasive radiologic, endoscopic, and operative techniques for the management of local complications have made it necessary to revise the AC.

The author declares no competing interests.
Department of Radiology, St Antonius Hospital, PO Box 2500, Koekoekslaan 1, 3430 EM Nieuwegein, The Netherlands
E-mail address: t.bollen@antoniusziekenhuis.nl

Radiol Clin N Am 50 (2012) 429–445
doi:10.1016/j.rcl.2012.03.015

Important topics to be incorporated in a new state-of-the-art classification are assessment of clinical and morphologic severity, and recognition that there is no direct correlation between clinical severity and morphologic manifestations of AP. In addition, such a classification should make appropriate use of terms relating to peripancreatic collections; should include recognition of distinct entities, such as peripancreatic or extrapancreatic necrosis alone and walled-off necrosis; and should outline other important findings to be evaluated by contrast-enhanced computed tomography (CECT). Computed tomography (CT) is the most widely available imaging modality and is the standard for evaluation of AP. Magnetic resonance (MR) imaging and transabdominal or endoscopic ultrasonography (EUS) may also be used in specific situations. Both latter techniques depict more precisely the heterogeneity of peripancreatic collections and are superior to CECT in detecting the presence of nonliquid tissue components within collections[10]; however, because these techniques may not be readily available, the revised classification principally concentrates on CECT. The working group that revised the AC is composed of internationally renowned pancreatologists of different disciplines. These experts first convened in 2006, and many drafts of the revised AC have been circulating on the World Wide Web since then, some of which have been referred to in review articles in the radiologic[11,12] and nonradiologic literature.[13,14] The working document of the revised AC is, however, still in progress and probably will be published in its final form in 2012. Therefore, slight changes must be anticipated, in particular regarding definitions of clinical severity. This article reviews the CT features of AP and presents terms found in the latest version of the document describing the revised AC, with emphasis on the radiologic evaluation of AP.

DEFINITION OF ACUTE PANCREATITIS

The clinical diagnosis of AP requires 2 of the following 3 features:

1. Abdominal pain strongly suggestive of AP (epigastric, radiating to the back)
2. Serum amylase and/or lipase activity at least 3 times the upper limit of normal
3. Characteristic findings of AP on imaging, with CT the best, most universally available imaging modality.

If abdominal pain is strongly suggestive of AP but the serum amylase and/or lipase activity is less than 3 times the upper limit of normal, characteristic findings of AP on a CECT or MR imaging are required to confirm the diagnosis.

CT FINDINGS OF ACUTE PANCREATITIS

Most cases of AP are diagnosed clinically and do not require imaging for diagnosis. Sometimes, however, the clinical history and presentation of a patient are not straightforward, and a reliable imaging modality is needed to ascertain the diagnosis. Of all imaging techniques available, CT is the preferred imaging modality in the initial evaluation and in follow-up of AP. The sensitivity of CT for the diagnosis of AP is not known, particularly in mild cases, but a good-quality CECT demonstrates distinct pancreatic and peripancreatic abnormalities in most patients with moderate to severe AP.[15]

AP is a dynamic disease with continuously altering appearances on imaging. CECT findings of AP are time dependent. The development of morphologic and clinical complications approximately run along a well-described timetable, as observed in previous studies: parenchymal necrosis is infrequently found within the first day after onset of symptoms[15,16]; infection of pancreatic and extrapancreatic necrosis needs several weeks to develop, with a peak incidence between the second and fourth weeks[17]; and full encapsulation of peripancreatic collections takes approximately 3 to 4 weeks.[9,16]

On CT the mild, moderate, and severe morphologic forms of AP are staged by the CT Severity Index (CTSI) (Table 1), a radiologic grading system on a 10-point severity scale developed by Balthazar and colleagues[18] that combines quantification of pancreatic/extrapancreatic inflammatory changes (0–4 points) with the extent of pancreatic parenchymal necrosis (0–6 points), both of which can be assessed by CECT. Besides prognostic information on patient morbidity and mortality, the CTSI depicts

Table 1
CT severity index

Characteristics	Points
Pancreatic inflammation	
Normal pancreas	0
Focal or diffuse enlargement of the pancreas	1
Peripancreatic inflammation	2
Single acute peripancreatic fluid collection	3
Two or more acute peripancreatic fluid collections	4
Pancreatic parenchymal necrosis	
None	0
Less than 30%	2
Between 30% and 50%	4
More than 50%	6

the order in which morphologic manifestations in AP appear on CT.

In its mildest forms, AP is characterized by a normal (CTSI 0) or minimal increase in size of the pancreas caused by interstitial edema that might be focal or diffuse (CTSI 1) (Fig. 1). This feature is often not appreciated, however, when comparison with prior imaging is not available. Release of pancreatic enzymes in the interstitial space results in peripancreatic fat planes becoming blurred and thickened (CTSI 2) (Fig. 2). Peripancreatic extension of the inflammatory process is common because the pancreas does not have a capsule. At this stage, pancreatic and peripancreatic alterations generally resolve over time, leaving no residual findings.

As AP progresses, peripancreatic collections accumulate in and around the pancreas (CTSI 3 and 4) (Fig. 3). The most common sites of peripancreatic collections are the lesser sac, a potential space located directly anterior to the pancreas and posterior to the stomach, and the left anterior pararenal space. Early peripancreatic collections lack a well-defined capsule and are confined by the anatomic space in which they arise. The natural course of these early collections is variable: they can persist or enlarge and evolve into encapsulated collections, or they can resolve spontaneously. The significance of peripancreatic collections in AP is their susceptibility to undergo secondary infection or hemorrhage or to cause symptoms attributable to mass effect.

The most severe morphologic forms of AP are denoted by the formation of pancreatic parenchymal necrosis, the extent of which is often classified in terms of less than 30%, between 30% and

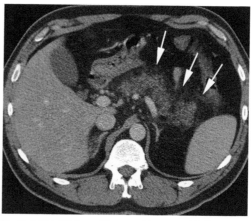

Fig. 2. Mild AP in a 45-year-old man with history of cholelithiasis. CT reveals an edematous pancreas, which is enlarged and heterogeneous. The peripancreatic fat planes are blurred and show increased attenuation, also called fat stranding (arrows). Grade C, no parenchymal necrosis; CTSI 2.

50%, and more than 50% (CTSI 5–6, 7–8, and 9–10, depending on the number of accompanying fluid collections, respectively) (Fig. 4). Parenchymal necrosis, defined as diffuse or focal areas of nonviable pancreatic parenchyma, tends to occur early in the course of the disease (within 4 days after onset of disease).[16,19]

On CECT, the diagnosis of parenchymal necrosis is based on demonstrating a focal or diffuse area of parenchymal nonenhancement. Excellent correlation between the lack of pancreatic enhancement on CT and parenchymal necrosis is observed when the affected region is at least 3 cm or larger in diameter or involves more than one-third of the gland.[16,20]

Although it is not necessary to perform CT imaging for all patients presenting with AP, it is generally recommended in the following circumstances:

1. When the clinical diagnosis is in doubt
2. For patients with organ failure or other reliable clinical or biochemical predictors of severe AP
3. For patients who are suspected to have a severe local complication (ie, intestinal ischemia or perforation)

Follow-up CT studies are reserved for patients who have severe morphologic findings on the index CT (such as parenchymal necrosis and peripancreatic fluid collections) together with clinical suspicion of complications, mainly infection of necrosis or hemorrhage, or when there is failure of clinical response to treatment.[15,16] Finally, CT is helpful if intervention is contemplated because the information provided by the scan helps guide percutaneous, endoscopic, and surgical aspiration or drainage.

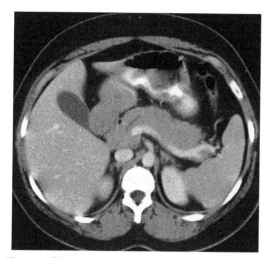

Fig. 1. Mild AP (ethanol-induced) in a 40-year-old man. Diagnosis was made on clinical grounds and elevated serum amylase and lipase. CT shows a slightly enlarged pancreatic gland. Grade B, no parenchymal necrosis; CTSI 1.

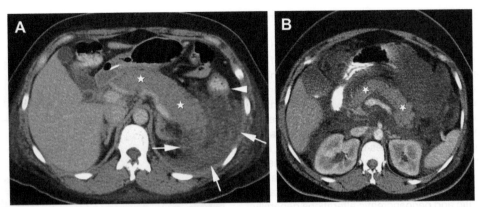

Fig. 3. Morphologically moderate severe AP (both of biliary cause) in 2 different patients. (A) Normal enhancement of the pancreas is observed (*asterisks*) with one heterogeneous peripancreatic collection in the left anterior para-renal compartment (*arrows*). There is slight wall thickening of the adjacent splenic flexure of the colon (*arrowhead*). Grade D, no parenchymal necrosis; CTSI 3. (B) Slightly swollen but normal enhancing pancreas is seen (*asterisks*), sur-rounded by multiple heterogeneous peripancreatic collections. Grade E, no parenchymal necrosis; CTSI 4.

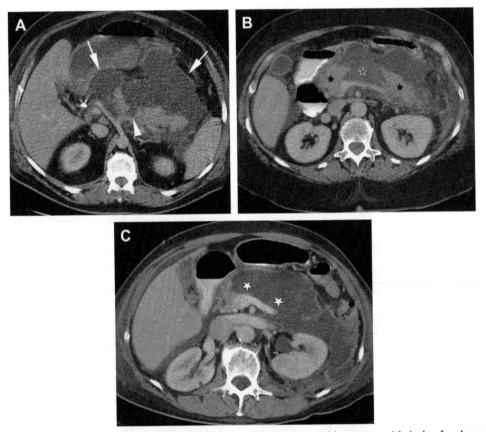

Fig. 4. Necrotizing pancreatitis in 3 different patients. (A) A 57-year-old woman with lack of enhancement (*arrowhead*) of a small part of the body of the pancreas (<30%) with surrounding acute necrotic collections (*arrows*) in lesser sac and left anterior pararenal compartment. Grade E, less than 30% parenchymal necrosis; CTSI 6. (B) A 45-year-old woman with biliary pancreatitis. CT reveals perfusion defect of approximately 30% to 50% at the body of the pancreas (*white asterisk*) with preserved enhancement of head and tail (*black asterisks*), surrounded by heterogeneous acute necrotic collections. Grade E, 30% to 50% parenchymal necrosis; CTSI 8. (C) A 44-year-old man with extensive necrosis of body and tail (*asterisks*) with surrounding partially encapsulated acute necrotic collections. Grade E, greater than 50% parenchymal necrosis; CTSI 10.

ATLANTA CLASSIFICATION: THE NEED FOR REVISION

The 1992 Atlanta symposium defined AP and classified complications of AP based on clinical criteria (**Table 2**).[9] The AC attempted to offer a universally applicable classification system for AP, and represented an important step forward in defining and classifying the severity of AP. Before this symposium, most terms used to describe the morphologic entities (seen on imaging modalities and at operation) were understood differently among different pancreatologists, especially relating to pancreatic and peripancreatic collections.

Although the AC was useful for the successive 2 decades, many of the definitions proved confusing. A primary reason for this confusion has only become apparent over time: the AC is a clinical classification system that has been used by treating pancreatologists and radiologists to define the morphologic manifestations as depicted by radiologic imaging, in particular CECT. The communication problem that results not only is an issue between clinicians and radiologists but also is evident within the radiology community. A recent interobserver study using the AC to classify local complications found that when 5 abdominal radiologists did a blinded review of CT scans from 70 patients with severe AP, agreement on the appropriate definition occurred in only 3 cases (**Fig. 5**).[21] Furthermore, several literature reviews showed that large variation existed in the interpretation of the Atlanta definitions[22,23]; many reports on AP used alternative schema for predicting severity or terms to categorize actual severity and organ failure, and different definitions were applied to the contents of peripancreatic collections. For example, because of a lack of a precise morphologic description of the Atlanta terms pancreatic pseudocyst and pancreatic abscess, interpretation between pancreatologists varied widely, depending on the presence or

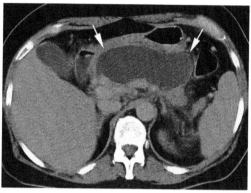

Fig. 5. CECT in a 39-year-old man with acute necrotizing pancreatitis 31 days after onset of symptoms. According to the original 1992 AC, this homogeneous and fully encapsulated collection (*arrows*) could be classified as pancreatic necrosis, pseudocyst, or even pancreatic abscess (all may have a similar appearance on CT). The patient suffered from fever despite antibiotic treatment. At surgery, infected necrosis was debrided and pus was drained.

absence of necrotic tissue as part of the collection.[23] Also, new descriptive terminology, such as extrapancreatic necrosis, necroma, organized necrosis, and other terms, have been suggested in the time after the AC in an attempt to reconcile the confusion but without success.[22]

Insights in pathophysiology and treatment of AP have improved substantially in the past decades. Several studies showed that persistent rather than transient organ failure has a significant impact on patients' morbidity and mortality.[24,25] With the introduction of new treatment modalities, such as percutaneous catheter drainage and transgastric and retroperitoneal minimally invasive necrosectomy, it has become essential in making decisions for patients with severe AP to provide accurate clinical staging, localization, and classification of morphologic changes in addition to defining the

Table 2	
The original 1992 Atlanta Classification: local complications	
Acute peripancreatic fluid collection	Occur early in the course of acute pancreatitis; are located in or near the pancreas; and always lack a wall of granulation or fibrous tissue
Pancreatic necrosis	A diffuse or focal area(s) of nonviable pancreatic parenchyma, which is typically associated with peripancreatic fat necrosis
Acute pseudocyst	A collection of pancreatic juice enclosed by a wall of fibrous or granulation tissue that arises as a consequence of acute pancreatitis or pancreatic trauma, or chronic pancreatitis
Pancreatic abscess	A circumscribed intra-abdominal collection of pus, usually in proximity to the pancreas, containing little or no pancreatic necrosis, which arises as a consequence of acute pancreatitis or pancreatic trauma

interrelationships between pancreatic collections and adjacent structures.[26]

FUNDAMENTAL CONCEPTS

AP is conceptualized as a dynamic, evolving disease process. Patients with mild AP often have only transient SIRS with no significant systemic or local sequelae.[27] Two distinct phases, however, can be distinguished in patients presenting with nonmild AP.

In the early phase of nonmild AP, the clinical severity is dominated by the extent and duration of SIRS and organ failure that may result in death.[5,6,24,27] At this stage, intervention is usually not performed unless an emergency laparotomy is indicated for complications such as abdominal compartment syndrome, bowel ischemia, or bowel perforation.[26] In the later phase of nonmild AP, morphologic changes of the pancreatic/peripancreatic region (ie, local complications) can become manifest systemically (ie, infected necrosis giving rise to bacteremia, organ failure, and sepsis), which may result in late mortality.[7,8] This is the stage at which aggressive interventional (operative or minimally invasive) management has its benefits.[26] Thus, clinical severity parameters include death and the persistence rather than transient SIRS and organ failure, whereas morphologic severity is characterized by the presence of pancreatic parenchymal necrosis and peripancreatic collections, especially when superimposed by infection. However, the working group on the revised AC is still debating the clinical aspects of defining the severity of AP, and the reader is advised to consult the final version that will probably be published later in 2012.

Interrelation Between Clinical and Morphologic Severity

It is crucial to acknowledge that clinical and morphologic severity do not necessarily overlap and do not necessarily correlate with one another. Patients with clinically mild AP may show severe morphologic manifestations on CT (Fig. 6). Conversely, patients may sustain clinically severe disease whereas CT only shows minimal inflammatory changes. In these patients, clinical severity is often mainly driven by the presence of significant comorbid disease.[27]

MORPHOLOGIC CLASSIFICATION

AP is subdivided into 2 morphologic types: acute interstitial edematous pancreatitis and acute necrotizing pancreatitis. Both types can be assessed using CECT or contrast-enhanced MR imaging.

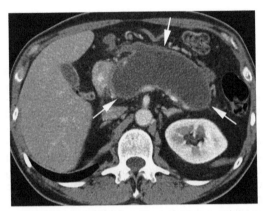

Fig. 6. Clinically mild AP in a 53-year-old man with acute necrotizing pancreatitis. CT was performed for continuing mild discomfort after a clinically mild AP. CT shows an encapsulated collection (*arrows*) located in the pancreatic bed with extensive parenchymal necrosis (>50% necrosis).

Morphologic Types of Acute Pancreatitis

Acute interstitial edematous pancreatitis

Most patients with AP will have diffuse or localized enlargement of the pancreas as a result of interstitial or inflammatory edema. On CECT, patients with interstitial edematous pancreatitis demonstrate diffuse or localized enlargement of the pancreas and normal enhancement of the pancreatic parenchyma. The pancreas often remains homogeneous, but at times can have a heterogeneous appearance depending on the amount of interstitial fluid (Fig. 7). Similarly, the retroperitoneal and peripancreatic tissues usually appear normal or show mild inflammatory changes characterized by haziness or mild stranding densities and varying but

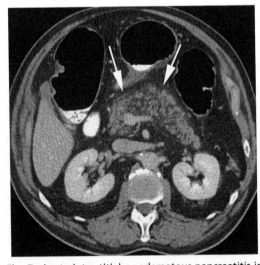

Fig. 7. Acute interstitial or edematous pancreatitis in a 65-year-old man. CT shows heterogeneous enhancement of an enlarged pancreatic gland with little surrounding fat stranding (*arrows*).

small amounts of nonenhancing areas of fluid density (acute peripancreatic fluid collections are discussed later). On occasion, an early CECT (done within the first days after onset of pancreatitis) exhibits diffuse heterogeneity in pancreatic parenchymal enhancement, which cannot be characterized definitively as interstitial edematous pancreatitis or patchy necrosis; with these findings, the presence or absence of pancreatic necrosis may have to be classified initially as indeterminate. A CECT done 3 to 7 days later should allow definitive classification.

Acute necrotizing pancreatitis

Necrosis can involve the pancreatic parenchyma and/or the peripancreatic tissues. The presence of necrosis in either the pancreatic parenchyma or the peripancreatic tissues defines the process as necrotizing pancreatitis and differentiates necrotizing pancreatitis from interstitial edematous pancreatitis. Necrotizing pancreatitis involves 1 of 3 subtypes: pancreatic parenchymal necrosis with peripancreatic necrosis (most common), pancreatic parenchymal necrosis alone (least common), or peripancreatic necrosis alone (without any discernible pancreatic parenchymal necrosis).

Pancreatic necrosis

Most patients with necrotizing pancreatitis have a variable extent of pancreatic parenchymal necrosis on CECT, evident by the lack of parenchymal enhancement after intravenous contrast administration.[15] Pancreatic necrosis usually is associated with a variable extent of peripancreatic necrosis, but on rare occasions pancreatic necrosis alone is observed. At CECT, the pancreas shows diffuse or localized enlargement with one or more areas of nonenhancing pancreatic parenchyma (Fig. 8). The extent of pancreatic parenchymal necrosis is traditionally quantified in 3 categories: less than 30%, 30% to 50%, and greater than 50% of the total pancreatic parenchyma. CECT within a few days from onset of disease may underestimate the presence and true extent of parenchymal necrosis (Fig. 9) and, therefore, CECT should be preferably performed 3 to 7 days after onset of symptoms in patients with predicted severe AP (based on established clinical and biochemical systems, such as Marshall or APACHE II score, Glasgow criteria, and C-reactive protein level, among others).[15,28]

Peripancreatic necrosis alone

The presence of (extensive) retroperitoneal peripancreatic fatty tissue necrosis secondary to AP, but with no recognizable pancreatic parenchymal necrosis on imaging and/or at operation, is recognized with increasing frequency.[29–31] Peripancreatic necrosis may result from spread of inflammation from the surface of the pancreas or disruption of small

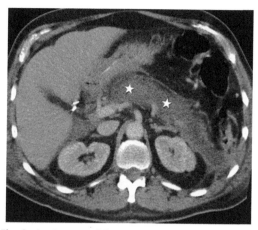

Fig. 8. Acute necrotizing pancreatitis in a 50-year-old woman with a prior history of cholecystectomy and choledocholithiasis. After endoscopic retrograde cholangiopancreatography, the patient developed extensive parenchymal necrosis of body and tail of the pancreas (*asterisks*) with accompanying acute necrotic collection in the left anterior pararenal compartment.

peripheral ductules with extravasation of activated pancreatic enzymes. This entity is recognized in up to 20% of the patients who require operative or interventional management of necrotizing pancreatitis.[31] The distinction proves important clinically, because patients without recognizable pancreatic gland necrosis have a better prognosis and outcome than patients with pancreatic parenchymal necrosis.[31]

The presence or absence of necrosis in the peripancreatic tissues is more difficult to ascertain by CECT, especially early in the course of the disease. CECT may suggest peripancreatic necrosis by the presence of heterogeneous areas of variable density containing liquid and nonliquid components in one or more areas, especially in the regions of the retroperitoneum and subperitoneal spaces of the mesenteries (Fig. 10). If concern is great enough, MR imaging or ultrasonography may aid in the recognition of nonliquid, necrotic components within the peripancreatic collection.

Characteristics of necrosis

The relative amount of liquid versus nonliquid components within areas of necrosis may vary with the time from onset of necrotizing pancreatitis. Necrosis should be thought of as a continuum; as time evolves, the necrosis that is initially nonliquid is believed to liquefy or reabsorb gradually. Thus, early in the course of the disease (in the first 1–2 weeks), the necrosis may appear as a nonenhancing area of variable density on CECT. Later in the course of the disease (≥4 weeks), it may appear as homogeneous (Fig. 11) and low in attenuation. During this stage, CECT may not be able to

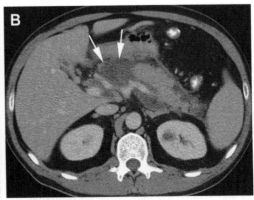
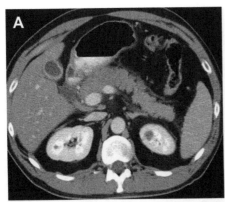

Fig. 9. False-negative parenchymal necrosis on early CT. (*A*) CECT on day of admission shows minimal hypoperfusion of the neck of the pancreas compared with the remainder of the pancreas. Parenchymal necrosis was not reported in the radiologic report. (*B*) Follow-up CT examination 7 days later reveals definitive perfusion defects of the neck and small part of the body of the pancreas (*arrows*), indicating parenchymal necrosis.

differentiate nonliquid, necrotic content from liquid content; MR imaging or ultrasonography may be necessary to do so if deemed necessary clinically. Complete resolution of necrosis (weeks or months to years later) may occur through complete liquefactive necrosis and reabsorption (**Fig. 12**). In some patients, complete liquefaction or reabsorption may never occur. This phenomenon relates to the amount of necrotic debris; up to 2 cm of necrotic tissue is reabsorbed or liquefied, but necrotic tissue that is larger than 5 cm rarely completely disappears (**Fig. 13**).[32]

Sterile and infected necrosis
According to the absence or presence of infection in the necrotic pancreatic and/or peripancreatic

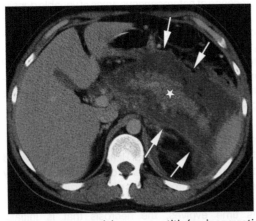

Fig. 10. Acute necrotizing pancreatitis (peripancreatic necrosis alone) in a 40-year-old man. CT shows normal enhancing pancreas (*asterisk*) surrounded by heterogeneous acute necrotic collections (*arrows*) with fluid and nonliquid (fat) densities, suggestive for peripancreatic necrosis alone. Two weeks later, operative debridement of necrotic peripancreatic tissues was performed because of infection of peripancreatic tissues.

areas, the entities of sterile and infected necrosis are distinguished. Distinction between sterile and infected necrosis is essential because they have different natural history, treatment, and prognosis.[8,26] Patients with sterile necrosis rarely need surgery or intervention except in the few patients who may remain persistently unwell after the initial SIRS phase despite optimized intensive medical management. Conversely, most patients with infected necrosis require long-term antibiotic therapy and some kind of interventional treatment.[26] Infection of necrosis can be diagnosed based on image-guided fine-needle aspiration and culture, or on the presence of extraluminal gas bubbles within pancreatic or peripancreatic collections on CECT (**Fig. 14**). This finding is virtually pathognomonic and reflects the presence of a gas-forming organism. In rare cases, perforation and spontaneous fistulization of an adjacent hollow viscus will produce gas locules in peripancreatic collections.[15]

Definition of Peripancreatic Collections

In the nonmild forms of AP, peripancreatic collections arise that may develop into local complications requiring supportive measures or interventional treatment. The morphologic characteristics are well depicted by CECT, and this modality forms the basis of the new definitions. The latest version of the revised AC discerns 4 distinct types of peripancreatic collections in the acute and subacute phase of AP and 1 type of collection that may occur during long-term follow-up after an episode of AP (**Table 3**). Differences between each of the 5 peripancreatic collections depend on:

1. The morphologic type of AP (interstitial edematous or necrotizing pancreatitis)

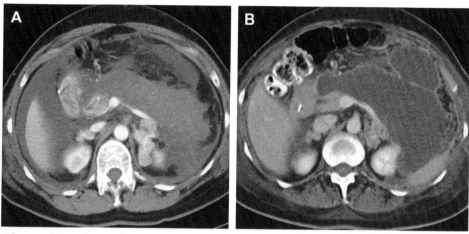

Fig. 11. Characteristics of parenchymal necrosis in a 35-year-old woman with drug-induced pancreatitis, on serial CT scans. (*A*) Initial CT study shows a heterogeneous appearance of the necrotic pancreatic neck, body, and tail caused by severe hypoperfusion (necrosis). Note the hyperenhancement of hyperplastic adrenal glands, probably stress related. (*B*) Follow-up examination performed 17 days later reveals a more homogeneous appearance, likely attributable to liquefaction necrosis.

2. The location (pancreatic, peripancreatic, or both)
3. The presence and degree of encapsulation (none, partially, or complete)
4. The contents (fluid and/or nonliquid necrotic debris)
5. The bacterial status (sterile or infected)
6. Prior interventional therapy (necrosectomy)
7. The age of the collection, a factor that relates to the degree of encapsulation.

For assessment at CECT, the most important determinants distinguishing each definition relate to the collections' contents (fluid alone vs a combination of fluid and nonliquid, necrotic debris) and the degree of encapsulation.

In interstitial edematous pancreatitis, collections composed only of fluid are termed acute peri-

pancreatic fluid collection and pseudocyst, depending on the age of the collection. In acute necrotizing pancreatitis, collections composed of necrotic material and fluid in varying degrees are termed acute necrotic collection and walled-off necrosis, depending on the age of the collection. The collection termed postnecrosectomy pseudocyst occurs in the setting of prior necrosectomy. All of these entities can be either sterile or infected, although it is highly unusual for an acute peripancreatic fluid collection to be infected.

Acute peripancreatic fluid collection

Acute peripancreatic fluid collections result from local edema related to parenchymal and/or peripancreatic inflammation (exudate); they either have no connection with the ductal system or they occur

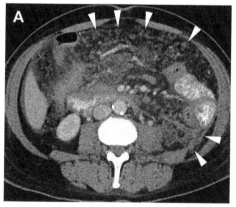
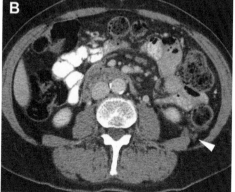

Fig. 12. Reabsorption of fat necrosis. (*A*) Multiple ill-defined nodules are seen scattered throughout the mesenteries, greater omentum (*4 arrowheads*), and retroperitoneal region, particularly on the left (*2 arrowheads*). (*B*) Follow-up CT 2 weeks later reveals resolution of the nodules, except for small residual nodules in the left anterior pararenal compartment (*arrowhead*).

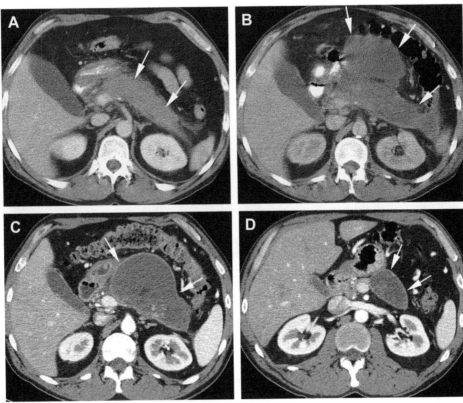

Fig. 13. Serial CT scans in a patient with persistent necrotic collections. (*A*) Initial CT shows extensive necrosis of body and tail (*arrows*). (*B*) Two weeks later, progressive peripancreatic collections are observed (*arrows*). Patient recovered without need for intervention during hospitalization. (*C*) One year after onset of acute necrotizing pancreatitis a large, slightly heterogeneous peripancreatic collection is seen with a well-defined thin wall (*arrows*). The patient was asymptomatic. (*D*) Two years after the acute attack a persistent heterogeneous collection is observed (*arrows*), although remarkably diminished in size.

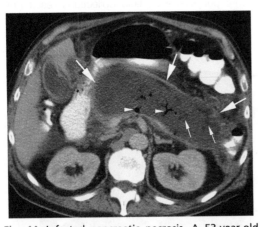

Fig. 14. Infected pancreatic necrosis. A 53-year-old woman with necrotizing pancreatitis developed spiking fever and impending organ failure 29 days after onset of symptoms. CT shows extensive necrosis (>50%) and an encapsulated heterogeneous collection (*arrows*) with liquid and nonliquid (fat) densities (*small arrows*), as well as impacted gas bubbles (*arrowheads*), indicative of infected necrosis.

from rupture of a small, peripheral, pancreatic duct side branch. These collections arise within a few days of onset of interstitial edematous pancreatitis and may persist for several weeks. Acute peripancreatic fluid collections contain fluid only and thus, per definition, have no necrotic components. Most acute peripancreatic fluid collections remain sterile and are reabsorbed spontaneously within the first several weeks after onset of AP.[33]

At CECT, acute peripancreatic fluid collections exist predominantly adjacent to the pancreas (peripancreatic), have homogeneous fluid density, have no complete definable wall (partial encapsulation is, however, allowed), and are confined by the normal peripancreatic fascial planes (Fig. 15). These acute peripancreatic fluid collections should be differentiated from areas where ascites resides (perihepatic and perisplenic spaces, paracolic gutters, and pelvic region).

Acute necrotic collection

Early pancreatic and peripancreatic collections in patients with acute necrotizing pancreatitis are

Table 3
Revised Atlanta Classification: CT criteria for local pancreatic complications

Local Complication	Morphologic CT Criteria
Acute peripancreatic fluid collection	Typically less than 4 weeks old after onset of symptoms Occurs in interstitial edematous pancreatitis Homogeneous collection with fluid density Confined by normal peripancreatic fascial planes No fully definable wall encapsulating the collection Adjacent to pancreas (no intrapancreatic extension)
Pseudocyst	Typically older than 4 weeks after onset of symptoms Occurs in interstitial edematous pancreatitis Homogeneous collection (round or oval) with fluid density Well-defined wall (ie, completely encapsulated) Absence of nonliquid component Adjacent to pancreas (no intrapancreatic extension)
Acute necrotic collection	Typically less than 4 weeks old after onset of symptoms Occurs in necrotizing pancreatitis Heterogeneous collection with liquid and nonliquid density and varying degrees of loculation No fully definable wall encapsulating the collection Located intrapancreatic and/or extrapancreatic
Walled-off necrosis	Typically older than 4 weeks after onset of symptoms Occurs in necrotizing pancreatitis Heterogeneous collection with liquid and nonliquid density and varying degrees of loculations Well-defined wall (ie, completely encapsulated) Located intrapancreatic and/or extrapancreatic
Post-necrosectomy Pseudocyst	Occurs after necrosectomy for necrotizing pancreatitis Homogeneous collection (round or oval) with fluid density Well-defined wall (ie, completely encapsulated) Absence of nonliquid component Located intrapancreatic and/or extrapancreatic

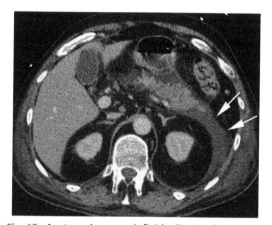

Fig. 15. Acute peripancreatic fluid collection (<4 weeks). CT shows normal enhancement of the pancreas with a fluid collection extending into the left anterior pararenal compartment (*arrows*). The fluid collection lacks a well-defined wall and conforms to the anatomic space in which it arises. The acute peripancreatic fluid collection resolved spontaneously.

termed acute necrotic collections. Acute necrotic collections represent a combination of parenchymal and/or peripancreatic fat necrosis together with pancreatic secretions. It is believed that the necrotic component of acute necrotic collections occurs following the liberation of activated pancreatic enzymes in the pancreatic and peripancreatic area, leading to (peri)pancreatic fat saponification and necrosis. Thus, the contents of acute necrotic collections are a spectrum ranging from predominantly necrotic (nonliquid) to both fluid and necrotic material (with varying degrees of each component), and generally also contain areas of loculations or septa.

On CECT, acute necrotic collections are depicted as homogeneous (fluid density) or heterogeneous (combination of fluid and nonliquid densities) in the pancreatic and/or peripancreatic area (Fig. 16). An acute necrotic collection has no capsule or is only partially encapsulated. It remains uncertain as to what proportion of peripancreatic fluid collections contains necrotic debris because CECT, the most

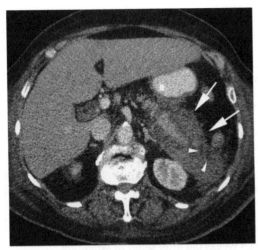

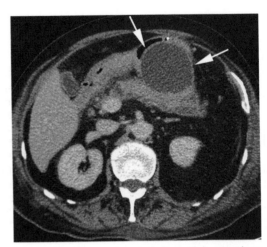

Fig. 16. Acute necrotic collection (<4 weeks). At the tail of the pancreas a heterogeneous, poorly encapsulated collection is observed (*arrows*) with fluid and nonliquid (fat) densities (*arrowheads*), indicative of peripancreatic tissue necrosis.

Fig. 17. Acute pseudocyst (>4 weeks). CT shows a normal enhancing pancreas with a homogeneous fully encapsulated collection, with fluid density in the lesser sac abutting the stomach (*arrows*).

commonly used imaging tool in AP, does not reliably depict necrotic debris inside collections, especially within the first week after onset of AP. This shortcoming implies that peripancreatic collections often cannot be categorized readily into an acute peripancreatic fluid collection or an acute necrotic collection. Both may appear as homogeneous, nonenhancing areas of low (fluid) density; these collections should then be termed indeterminate peripancreatic collections. After the first week or two, however, acute necrotic collections should become evident on CECT, MR imaging, transabdominal ultrasonography, or EUS.

Pseudocyst

The definition of a pseudocyst remains the same: a collection of pancreatic juice (analysis usually shows increased amylase and lipase level) enclosed by an encapsulated wall of granulation tissue, with little or no associated necrotic material (<5%). Pseudocysts develop from acute peripancreatic fluid collections (not from acute necrotic collections). Thus they occur in the setting of interstitial edematous pancreatitis. In general, more than 4 weeks are required for formation of a well-defined wall that differentiates a pseudocyst from an acute peripancreatic fluid collection.

At CECT, a pseudocyst is depicted as well-circumscribed, usually round or oval, homogeneous peripancreatic collection with fluid attenuation, surrounded by a well-defined wall (**Fig. 17**); an MR image or ultrasonography may be required to confirm the absence of necrosis within the fluid collection. The identification of a recognizable ductal communication can sometimes, but not reliably, be determined by

CECT. MR imaging or EUS may allow this communication to be identified; the presence or absence of ductal communication may be important in determining appropriate therapy but is not required as a criterion for a pseudocyst in this classification. It must be stressed that in AP, as opposed to chronic pancreatitis, pseudocysts are rare because most persistent peripancreatic collections contain necrotic material.

Walled-off necrosis

As the necrosis in necrotizing pancreatitis matures, the interface between the necrosis and the adjacent viable fatty tissue becomes established by an encapsulating thickened wall without an epithelial lining. The term walled-off necrosis is introduced to describe this evolution of necrosis to an encapsulated, well-defined collection of pancreatic fluid and necrotic debris. This entity, referred to previously in the literature often as organized pancreatic necrosis,[10,34] necroma,[35,36] or pseudocyst associated with necrosis,[37] represents the end stage of an acute necrotic collection. This entity was not recognized in the original AC. Just as with acute necrotic collections, walled-off necrosis more commonly involves the pancreatic parenchyma with areas of peripancreatic necrosis as well, the peripancreatic tissues alone or, on rare occasion, the pancreatic parenchyma alone.

On CECT, walled-off necrosis manifests as a full encapsulated collection with varying densities (fluid and/or nonliquid attenuation) in, around, or remote from the pancreatic area (**Fig. 18**). A complete encapsulating wall (often requiring more than 4 weeks) differentiates walled-off necrosis from an acute necrotic collection.

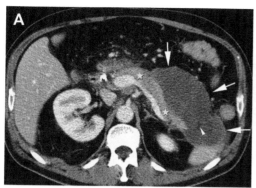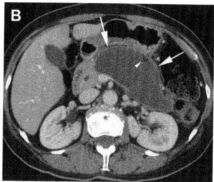

Fig. 18. Walled-off necrosis in peripancreatic necrosis alone (>4 weeks) (*A*) and pancreatic necrosis (*B*). (*A*) CT depicts adjacent to a normally perfused body and tail of the pancreas (*asterisks*), a well-defined heterogeneous collection (*arrows*) with primarily fluid density and scattered areas of fat density (*arrowhead*), indicative of necrosis of peripancreatic tissues. (*B*) A large, heterogeneous fully encapsulated collection is seen (*arrows*) with predominantly fluid density mixed with nonliquid (fat) density (*arrowhead*). The collection replaces the greater part of the pancreatic parenchyma. Because of the heterogeneity and presence of pancreatic necrosis, this is not a pseudocyst.

The CECT differentiation between a pseudocyst and walled-off necrosis is probably the most difficult, and a source of common mistakes made by radiologists because both entities may have a similar appearance.[35,36] The term pseudocyst is often applied to every collection in and around the pancreas, even to cystic pancreatic neoplasms, leading to significant problems in patient management; symptomatic pseudocysts require only simple drainage, whereas walled-off necrosis frequently but not always requires removal of necrotic material. The term pseudocyst should be applied only to patients with interstitial edematous pancreatitis (with one exception, discussed later)

who have an acute peripancreatic fluid collection evolving into a round or oval collection with a well-defined wall, whereas walled-off necrosis arises in necrotizing pancreatitis. MR imaging, transabdominal ultrasonography, or EUS may be a valuable complementary test for differentiation between pseudocysts and walled-off necrosis by documenting the presence of necrotic material within the collection (**Fig. 19**).

Postnecrosectomy pseudocyst
An exception of a pseudocyst arising in acute necrotizing pancreatitis is in the setting of a condition termed disconnected duct syndrome.[38] These

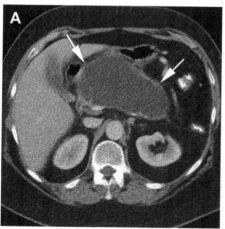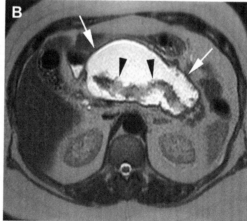

Fig. 19. CT (*A*) and corresponding MR imaging (*B*) in a 45-year-old woman who was thought to have a large symptomatic pseudocyst after acute gallstone-induced pancreatitis. (*A*) CT reveals a well-circumscribed homogeneous collection (*arrows*) in the pancreatic region exerting mass effect on the stomach. (*B*) Corresponding T2-weighted MR imaging discloses the heterogeneity of the thin-walled collection (*arrows*) with fluid intensity and dark material, most likely representing necrotic pancreatic tissue (*arrowheads*), which was not recognized by CT (note also the presence of gallstones). Consequently, endoscopic necrosectomy (rather than simple drainage) was performed, with subsidence of patient's symptoms.

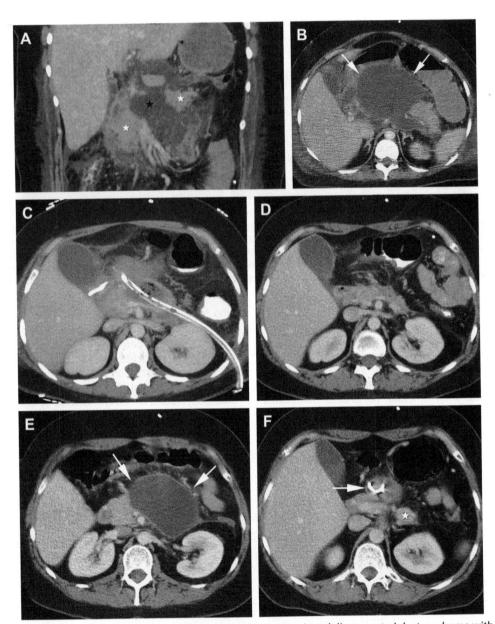

Fig. 20. Typical sequence of events in a case of central gland necrosis and disconnected duct syndrome with post-necrosectomy pseudocyst formation. (*A*) Coronal reconstructed CT depicts necrosis of the pancreatic neck and part of the body (*black asterisk*) among the viable head and tail (*white asterisks*). (*B*) Axial CT, performed 12 days later, shows an increase of the partially encapsulated acute necrotic collection (*arrows*). The patient developed fever and elevated white blood cell count, suggestive of infected necrosis. Subsequently, CT-guided percutaneous drainage was performed. (*C*) Axial thick-slab maximum-intensity projection CT shows the percutaneous drain from the left retroperitoneal compartment into the area of infected necrosis. After additional endoscopic necrosectomy, the patient recovered completely. (*D*) Axial CT obtained 6 months after removal of the drains shows pancreatic necrosis has resolved. (*E*) Follow-up CT 1 year later shows a recurrent collection, which is homogeneous and surrounded by a thin wall; a postnecrosectomy pseudocyst (*arrows*). (*F*) Endoscopic pigtail drainage (*arrow*) was performed, with complete resolution of the collection. Note the viable remnant pancreatic tail (*asterisk*).

patients have necrosis of the central portion of the pancreatic gland with a viable pancreatic tail remnant. Initially, a walled-off necrosis is formed and potentially requires necrosectomy. When the residual cavity (devoid of necrotic material) continues to have ductal communication with the remnant secreting pancreatic tail, the cavity fills with pancreatic fluid, forming a postnecrosectomy pseudocyst (Fig. 20). These recurrent collections appear months to years after the onset of AP, and thus do not occur during the acute or subacute phase of AP. A prior history of some kind of (surgical or endoscopic) necrosectomy is a prerequisite for diagnosis of this type of collection. Rarely, a pseudocyst may develop during long-term follow-up when walled-off necrosis undergoes complete liquefaction or reabsorption of necrotic material.

RADIOLOGIC EVALUATION ON CECT: PANCODE SYSTEM

Prior studies have shown that interobserver agreement for characterization of the original Atlanta definitions by CECT was poor,[21] as opposed to the excellent interobserver agreement when applying morphologic terms for describing findings in and around the pancreas using the PANCODE system (Table 4).[39] PANCODE is an acronym that stands for pancreatic nonenhancement, collections, and description, and can be used to assist in complete and systematic reporting of all pancreatic and extrapancreatic abnormalities in patients with AP.

Pancreatic Nonenhancement

The first assessment is the presence or absence of areas of pancreatic nonenhancement (indicative of parenchymal necrosis). Note the sites of perfusion defects and estimate the percentage of involved necrotic parenchyma.

Collections

The next assessment concerns the presence of pancreatic and peripancreatic collections. Peripancreatic collection refers to any (fluid) collection that exceeds peripancreatic fat stranding.

Description

Describe the sites of collections and their relation with the pancreas or other organs, the degree of encapsulation, the homogeneity and attenuation, mass effect on surrounding structures, and their shape and size, and note the presence of gas bubbles. Note and describe extrapancreatic complications, such as gastrointestinal, biliary, and vascular complications, as well as involvement of adjacent parenchymal abdominal organs

Table 4	
CT description using the PANCODE system	
1. Pancreatic nonenhancement	
Assess perfusion defects	No pancreatic perfusion defects, uniform contrast enhancement Pancreatic perfusion defect(s): Location: head, neck, body, tail Extent: <30%, 30%–50%, >50% Patchy or full width
2. Collections	
Assess presence of peripancreatic collections	No collections, only enlarged pancreas with or without peripancreatic fat stranding Presence of one or more peripancreatic collections
3. Description	
Peripancreatic collections	Assess: Location: intrapancreatic and/or extrapancreatic or separate Anatomic site(s) (eg, lesser sac, anterior pararenal space) Shape and maximum size (if possible) Homogeneity and attenuation (explicitly note hemorrhage) Degree of encapsulation (none, partial, or complete) Presence of (impacted) gas bubbles or gas-fluid levels
Extrapancreatic complications	Gastrointestinal (gastric outlet obstruction, bowel ischemia, ileus) Vascular (venous thrombosis/compression with collateralization or segmental portal hypertension, hemorrhage, and arterial pseudoaneurysm) Biliary (cholecystolithiasis, choledocholithiasis, dilation of biliary system, signs of cholecystitis) Solid organ involvement (eg, liver, spleen, kidney) Ascites Pleural effusion

(liver, spleen, and kidney) by the inflammatory process and effects of systemic complications (ascites and pleural fluid).

SUMMARY

This review presents an update rather than a final version of the revised AC that replaces the 1992 Atlanta definitions on AP; in any case, terms such as pancreatic abscess, and other antiquated terms such as phlegmon and hemorrhagic pancreatitis, are not advised for use, and therefore should no longer appear in radiologic reports. Incorporation of fundamental concepts on clinical and morphologic grounds, new insights into the pathophysiology, and the recognition of the dynamic nature of severe AP will be among the important features of this revised classification.

The clinical severity of AP is still under debate by the members of the working group, and the reader is advised to consult the final version of the revised AC, likely to be published later in 2012.

Fluid and/or necrotic collections developing in the pancreas and peripancreatic region as shown on imaging, notably CECT, are classified as early (<4 weeks) and late (>4 weeks) collections. The proposed terms of the local pancreatic complications use morphologic descriptors based on CECT criteria and age.

The early collections are classified as either an acute peripancreatic fluid collection, which develops in the course of interstitial edematous pancreatitis and represents a collection of fluid without associated necrosis, or an acute necrotic collection, which occurs in acute necrotizing pancreatitis that may involve necrosis of the pancreatic parenchyma plus the peripancreatic tissues, the peripancreatic tissue alone, or the pancreatic parenchyma alone. In the first week after onset of AP, it may be difficult to accurately classify collections located exclusively in the peripancreatic region on CECT, and these are then referred to as indeterminate peripancreatic collections. A persistent, late collection with a complete encapsulating wall on imaging should be called a pseudocyst if the collection contains only fluid; it should be called walled-off necrosis if it arose in the setting of necrotizing pancreatitis and contains variable amounts of necrosis and fluid involving the pancreatic parenchyma and the peripancreatic tissues, the peripancreatic tissues alone, or the pancreatic parenchyma alone. Postnecrosectomy pseudocyst is a recurrent fully encapsulated collection, composed only of fluid that arises after necrosectomy for necrotizing pancreatitis.

Imaging is an important feature of this revised AC, and radiologists are important members of the multidisciplinary team of specialists involved in the care and treatment of patients with this potentially devastating disease. Correct use of the revised AC definitions should allow objective communication and conveyance of CT findings to clinicians. In the end, patients with severe AP are best served by close collaboration between radiologists and clinicians for planning the appropriate treatment.

REFERENCES

1. Frossard JL, Steer ML, Pastor CM. Acute pancreatitis. Lancet 2008;371(9607):143–52.
2. Spanier BW, Dijkgraaf MG, Bruno MJ. Epidemiology, aetiology and outcome of acute and chronic pancreatitis: an update. Best Pract Res Clin Gastroenterol 2008;22(1):45–63.
3. Vollmar B, Menger M. Microcirculatory dysfunction in acute pancreatitis. Pancreatology 2003;3:181–90.
4. Cuthbertson CM, Christophi C. Disturbances of the microcirculation in acute pancreatitis. Br J Surg 2006;93(5):518–30.
5. Mofidi R, Duff MD, Wigmore SJ, et al. Association between early systemic inflammatory response, severity of multiorgan dysfunction and death in acute pancreatitis. Br J Surg 2006;93:738–44.
6. Singh VK, Wu BU, Bollen TL, et al. Early systemic inflammatory response syndrome is associated with severe acute pancreatitis. Clin Gastroenterol Hepatol 2009;7(11):1247–51.
7. Werner J, Feuerbach S, Uhl W, et al. Management of acute pancreatitis: from surgery to interventional intensive care. Gut 2005;54:426–36.
8. Petrov MS, Shanbhag S, Chakraborty M, et al. Organ failure and infection of pancreatic necrosis as determinants of mortality in patients with acute pancreatitis. Gastroenterology 2010;139(3):813–20.
9. Bradley EL III. A clinically based classification system for acute pancreatitis. Summary of the International Symposium on Acute Pancreatitis, Atlanta, GA, September 11 through 13, 1992. Arch Surg 1993;128:586–90.
10. Morgan DE, Baron TH, Smith JK, et al. Pancreatic fluid collections prior to intervention: evaluation with MR imaging compared with CT and US. Radiology 1997;203:773–8.
11. Trout AT, Elsayes KM, Ellis JH, et al. Imaging of acute pancreatitis: prognostic value of computed tomographic findings. J Comput Assist Tomogr 2010;34(4):485–95.
12. Bharwani N, Patel S, Prabhudesai S, et al. Acute pancreatitis: the role of imaging in diagnosis and management. Clin Radiol 2011;66(2):164–75.

13. Morgan DE. Imaging of acute pancreatitis and its complications. Clin Gastroenterol Hepatol 2008; 6(10):1077–85.

14. Brun A, Agarwal N, Pitchumoni CS. Fluid collections in and around the pancreas in acute pancreatitis. J Clin Gastroenterol 2011;45(7):614–25.

15. Balthazar EJ. Acute pancreatitis: assessment of severity with clinical and CT evaluation. Radiology 2002;223:603–13.

16. Balthazar EJ, Freeny PC, vanSonnenberg E. Imaging and intervention in acute pancreatitis. Radiology 1994;193:297–306.

17. Besselink MG, van Santvoort HC, Boermeester MA, et al. Timing and impact of infections in acute pancreatitis. Br J Surg 2009;96(3):267–73.

18. Balthazar EJ, Robinson DL, Megibow AJ, et al. Acute pancreatitis: value of CT in establishing prognosis. Radiology 1990;174:331–6.

19. Balthazar EJ. Staging of acute pancreatitis. Radiol Clin North Am 2002;40:1199–209.

20. Johnson CD, Stephens DH, Sarr MG. CT of acute pancreatitis: correlation between lack of contrast enhancement and pancreatic necrosis. AJR Am J Roentgenol 1991;156:93–5.

21. Besselink MG, Van Santvoort HC, Bollen TL, et al. Describing computed tomography findings in acute necrotizing pancreatitis with the Atlanta classification: an interobserver agreement study. Pancreas 2006;33:331–5.

22. Bollen TL, Besselink MG, van Santvoort HC, et al. Towards an update of the Atlanta classification on acute pancreatitis: review of new and abandoned terms. Pancreas 2007;35(2):107–13.

23. Bollen TL, van Santvoort HC, Besselink MG, et al. The Atlanta classification on acute pancreatitis revisited: review of the literature. Br J Surg 2008;95(1):6–21.

24. Johnson CD, Abu-Hilal M. Persistent organ failure during the first week as a marker of fatal outcome in acute pancreatitis. Gut 2004;53:1340–4.

25. Buter A, Imrie CW, Carter CR, et al. Dynamic nature of early organ dysfunction determines outcome in acute pancreatitis. Br J Surg 2002;89:298–302.

26. van Santvoort HC, Bakker OJ, Bollen TL, et al. A conservative and minimally invasive approach to necrotizing pancreatitis improves outcome. Gastroenterology 2011;141(4):1254–63.

27. Singh VK, Bollen TL, Wu BU, et al. An assessment of the severity of interstitial pancreatitis. Clin Gastroenterol Hepatol 2011;9(12):1098–103.

28. Bollen TL, van Santvoort HC, Besselink MG, et al. Update on acute pancreatitis: US, CT, and MRI features. Semin Ultrasound CT MR 2007;28(5):371–83.

29. Howard JM, Wagner SM. Pancreatography after recovery from massive pancreatic necrosis. Ann Surg 1989;209:31–5.

30. Madry S, Fromm D. Infected retroperitoneal fat necrosis associated with acute pancreatitis. J Am Coll Surg 1994;178:277–82.

31. Sakorafas GH, Tsiotos GG, Sarr MG. Extrapancreatic necrotizing pancreatitis with viable pancreas: a previously under-appreciated entity. J Am Coll Surg 1999;188:643–8.

32. Kloppel G. Acute pancreatitis. Semin Diagn Pathol 2004;21(4):221–6.

33. Lenhart DK, Balthazar EJ. MDCT of acute mild (non-necrotizing) pancreatitis: abdominal complications and fate of fluid collections. AJR Am J Roentgenol 2008;190(3):643–9.

34. Baron TH, Thaggard WG, Morgan DE, et al. Endoscopic therapy for organized pancreatic necrosis. Gastroenterology 1996;111(3):755–64.

35. Bradley EL III. Atlanta redux. Pancreas 2003;26:105–6.

36. Bradley EL 3rd. Confusion in the imaging ranks: time for a change? Pancreas 2006;33(4):321–2.

37. Hariri M, Slivka A, Carr-Locke DL, et al. Pseudocyst drainage predisposes to infection when pancreatic necrosis is unrecognized. Am J Gastroenterol 1994;89:1781–4.

38. Sandrasegaran K, Tann M, Jennings SG, et al. Disconnection of the pancreatic duct: an important but overlooked complication of severe acute pancreatitis. Radiographics 2007;27(5):1389–400.

39. van Santvoort HC, Bollen TL, Besselink MG, et al. Describing computed tomography findings in severe acute pancreatitis using morphologic terms: a multidisciplinary, international interobserver agreement study. Pancreatology 2008;8(6):593–9.

Imaging of Chronic Pancreatitis (Including Groove and Autoimmune Pancreatitis)

Rocio Perez-Johnston, MD[a], Nisha I. Sainani, MD[b], Dushyant V. Sahani, MD[a],*

KEYWORDS

- Chronic pancreatitis • Calcifying • Autoimmune • Groove

IMAGING OF CHRONIC PANCREATITIS

Chronic pancreatitis (CP) is an inflammatory disease process that leads to progressive and irreversible structural damage of the pancreas resulting in permanent dysfunction of both endocrine and exocrine pancreatic function. The incidence of CP ranges from 3.5 to 10.0 per 100,000 people in industrialized countries.[1] Multiple etiologic factors have been implicated in the causation of CP, such as alcohol abuse, genetic factors, hypertriglyceridemia, hypercalcemia, autoimmunity, and pancreatic ductal obstruction (Table 1).[2]

Histologic changes seen in CP include acinar cell loss, islet cell loss, inflammatory cell infiltrates, and eventually irregular fibrosis. Many theories about the pathogenesis of the disease have been proposed:

- The *ductal theory* suggests that the ducts are the primary target of the disease, with the stagnation of pancreatic juice, formation of protein plugs, and reflux of bile and duodenal juice. Protein plugs within the ducts then undergo calcium carbonate deposition resulting in intraductal calculi formation, which leads to obstruction, ectasia, and periductal fibrosis.
- The *metabolite theory* proposes that toxic metabolites induce the production of profibrotic cells and inflammation inducing periacinar fibrosis.
- According to the *necrosis-fibrosis theory*, chronic obstruction of the acini likely caused by stone obstruction leads to ulceration, scarring, and chronic inflammatory response.
- The *oxidative stress theory* suggests that excess free radicals result in the peroxidation of lipid components of the membrane of the acinar cells leading to inflammatory response.
- The *multiple-cause theory* implicates different and multiple causative factors that lead to damage through different pathways.

The diagnosis of CP is based on clinical symptoms, imaging, and the assessment of pancreatic function. The correlation between structural damage and functional impairment is poor because patients with severe exocrine insufficiency may have structurally normal pancreatic parenchyma and vice versa.[3] The main clinical manifestations of chronic pancreatitis include chronic recurrent abdominal pain, diabetes, and steatorrhea.

Disclosure: The authors have nothing to disclose.

[a] Division of Abdominal Imaging and Intervention, Harvard Medical School, Massachusetts General Hospital, 55 Fruit Street, White 270, Boston, MA 02114, USA; [b] Division of Abdominal Imaging and Intervention, Harvard Medical School, Brigham and Women's Hospital, 75 Francis Street, Boston, MA 02115, USA
* Corresponding author.
E-mail address: dsahani@partners.org

Table 1
Causes of CP

Toxic	Alcohol, cigarette smoking, drugs (valproate, thiazide, azathioprine, estrogens, phenacetin)
Metabolic	Hypercalcemia, hyperparathyroidism, hyperlipidemia, chronic renal failure
Infectious	HIV, mumps virus, Coxsackie virus, cryptosporidium
Genetic/hereditary	CFTR mutation (cystic fibrosis) PRSS1 mutation SPINK1 mutation
Obstruction of the main pancreatic duct	Gallstones Neoplasms: pancreatic/periampullary Posttraumatic scarring Sphincter of Oddi dysfunction Pancreas divisum
Autoimmune	Manifestation of immunoglobulin G4–related sclerosing disease
Recurrent acute pancreatitis	Postnecrotic Recurrent acute pancreatitis
Other	Idiopathic Tropical pancreatitis Radiation therapy Vascular disease/ischemic

Imaging studies play an important role in the diagnosis and assessment of CP, particularly in early stages of the disease, by detecting early parenchymal or ductal changes or predisposing structural abnormalities. In advanced stages of CP, imaging supports management decisions, preoperative planning, and the detection of complications.

Alcoholic Pancreatitis or Chronic Calcifying Pancreatitis

Alcohol abuse is the most common cause of CP in Western countries, accounting for 70% to 90% of cases. However, only a minority of heavy drinkers develops CP, suggesting that additional cofactors, such as smoking, genetics, and a high fat-protein diet, are necessary to develop the disease.[4]

Pathogenesis
The pathogenesis of CP secondary to alcoholism is not fully understood. Experimental studies have demonstrated that the pancreas processes ethanol efficiently; however, its metabolites injure the acinar cells.[5] In addition to the acinar cell injury, it is thought that other mechanisms, such as bile duct hypotheses (biliary-pancreatic reflux, sphincter of Oddi [SO] obstruction, duodeno-pancreatic reflux) and small duct hypotheses (increased viscosity and hypersecretion of proteins), contribute to the disease.[6]

Imaging
On abdominal radiographs, calcifications projecting over the epigastrium can be seen in 30% to 70% of patients. Pancreatic calcification is specific but poorly sensitive (30%–70%). Parenchymal or ductal calcification should be differentiated from calcified solid masses, calcified cysts, or vascular calcifications.

The evaluation of the pancreas with ultrasound is limited because of overlying bowel gas, body habitus, and operator dependence. Pancreatic calcifications can be detected in up to 40% of patients and may be focal or diffuse. These calcifications appear as punctuate, hyperechoic foci and, depending on their size, may reveal posterior acoustic shadowing or twinkling. Pancreatic enlargement or atrophy, ductal dilatation, and pseudocysts may be observed.[7]

Wide availability and high spatial resolution make computed tomography (CT) generally the first imaging study in assessing patients with CP. However, early changes may not be seen, there is no functional evaluation component, and patients are exposed to radiation. Table 2 summarizes CT protocol and usefulness.

Classical CT features of CP include scattered parenchymal or intraductal calcifications in approximately 50% of patients, parenchymal atrophy in 54% of patients, and ductal dilatation in up to 68% of patients (Fig. 1).[8] Dilatation of the main pancreatic duct or side branches is the most

Table 2
MR imaging and CT protocols

	Protocols	Indication
CT	Unenhanced MDCT arterial phase Pancreatic/venous phase Postprocessing: curved CPR, coronal and sagittal MPR, MIP, VR	Detection of calcifications Arterial mapping for surgical planning, arterial complications of CP Assessment of pancreatic parenchyma, detect hypovascular lesions as adenocarcinoma of the pancreas, venous complications of CP, pseudocysts Assessment pancreatic duct and vascular structures
MR imaging	• Thin-slice T2-weighted in axial and coronal or T2-weighted fat suppressed • T1 FSE or GRE, with fat suppression • Contrast-enhanced MR imaging: high-resolution T1-weighted 3D GRE • DWI	• Assess pancreatic and bile duct, cystic lesions • Assess pancreatic mass or focal pancreatitis • Assess inflammatory process, neoplasm and vascular involvement • Estimation of exocrine functional capacity
MRCP	2D MRCP: • Thin-slice axial, oblique, and coronal SSFSE T2 weighted 3D MRCP	Assess ductal abnormalities and filling defects
S-MRCP	• Administration of IV secretin 1 mL/10 kg of body weight • Thick-slab MRCP SSFSE axial, coronal, and oblique, every 30 sec for 10–15 min	Better delineation of the pancreatic duct Pancreatic duct anatomic variants Increases accuracy in detecting main pancreatic duct strictures Indirect assessment of pancreatic exocrine reserve

Abbreviations: CPR, curved planar reformation; DWI, diffusion-weighted imaging; FSE, fast spin echo; GRE, gradient echo; IV, intravenous; MIP, maximum intensity projection; MPR, multiplanar reformat; MR, magnetic resonance; SSFSE, single-shot fast spin echo; 3D, 3 dimensional; VR, volume rendering.

common finding in chronic pancreatitis, and the ductal contour may be smooth, beaded, or irregular. Parenchymal calcifications involve the head of the pancreas more frequently, may vary in morphology (punctuate, stippled, or coarse) and size, and may be multiple or scattered throughout the pancreas. The degree of calcification seems to be directly proportional to the course of the

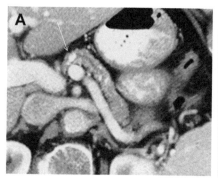 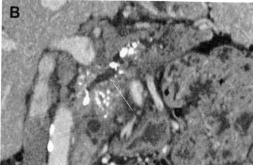

Fig. 1. Two different examples of CP. (*A*) Axial contrast-enhanced CT (CECT) of 63-year-old patient with atrophy of the pancreatic parenchyma, main pancreatic ductal prominence, and intraductal calculi (*arrow*). (*B*) Coronal reformatted image of CECT of a 56-year-old patient with dilatation (*arrow*) and irregularity of the main pancreatic duct, parenchymal calcifications, and intraductal calculi.

disease.[9] Intraductal calculi are the most reliable sign of chronic pancreatitis and can range from millimeters to more than a centimeter. Parenchymal atrophy often coexists with ductal dilatation. Most patients with exocrine insufficiency have parenchymal atrophy; nevertheless, 22% of patients with exocrine insufficiency might not show atrophy on CT.[8]

CT also allows adequate assessment of complications of chronic pancreatitis. Pseudocysts are detected in 25% of cases. They are well-defined, fluid density collections that may be localized within the pancreas, in the retroperitoneum, or in distant locations.

Some patients with CP develop pseudocysts from the evolution of peripancreatic fluid collections that complicate a severe episode of acute pancreatitis. However, in some patients, obstruction of the pancreatic duct or one of its side branches leads to a retention-type cyst upstream to the obstruction (Fig. 2). In this situation, there is no preceding history of an acute flare of complicating preexisting CP.

The development of pseudocysts, peripancreatic fluid collections, and necrosis of the gland all contribute to inflammatory phlebitis, predisposing to thrombosis and its complications. As a result, chronic inflammation in the pancreas can lead to venous thrombosis of the splenic, superior mesenteric, or portal veins. The prevalence of splenic vein thrombosis in CP is estimated to be 11%.[10] On contrast-enhanced images, filling defects within the vessel or complete obliteration of the vessel may be seen. Collateral vessels may be noted, and signs of portal hypertension, predominantly left-sided, can develop.

Chronic inflammation and spillage of pancreatic enzymes into the retroperitoneum also causes damage to the arterial structures, which may lead to the formation of pseudoaneuryms (Fig. 3). Pseudoaneurysms are more frequently noted adjacent to the pancreatic head or splenic hilum. Often, these are incidentally detected on imaging studies, but when symptomatic they manifest because of rupture and hemorrhage into the bowel, peritoneum, retroperitoneum, or biliary ducts. Patients present with intense right upper quadrant/epigastric pain or gastrointestinal (GI) bleeding (hemosuccus pancreaticus). On contrast-enhanced CT, pseudoaneurysms appear as fusiform dilatation of the vessel or as a saccular arterial enhancing structure arising from the splenic artery, pancreaticoduodenal artery, gastroduodenal artery, or less frequently from the middle colic artery.[11] Early detection and localization of a pseudoaneurysm is crucial for further treatment planning with surgery or embolization.

Another complication of CP is fistula formation, which may reach either the abdominal cavity producing pancreatic ascites or the pleural space with subsequent pancreatic pleural effusion. Fistulae can also be secondary to rupture of a pseudocyst. Ascites can be seen in 15% of patients. When sampled, both pleural and peritoneal fluids are rich in amylase.[12]

Magnetic resonance (MR) imaging is being increasingly used for the evaluation of CP. MR imaging–MR cholangiopancreatography (MRCP) provides noninvasive biliary and pancreatic duct imaging, adequate characterization of the pancreatic parenchyma, and the depiction of peripancreatic pathologic conditions (see Table 2). The

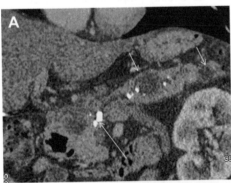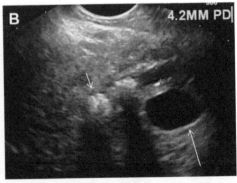

Fig. 2. A 55-year-old patient with history of alcohol consumption and CP. (A) Curved reformatted image of a contrast-enhanced CT, demonstrating atrophy of the pancreatic parenchyma, intraductal calculi (*long arrow*), and retention cysts in the body and tail of the pancreas (*short arrows*). (B) Endoscopic ultrasound demonstrated dilatation of the pancreatic duct and intraductal hyperechoic foci with shadowing, corresponding to calculi (*short arrow*). A well-defined anechoic lesion is seen adjacent to the main pancreatic duct (*long arrow*) representing a retention cyst.

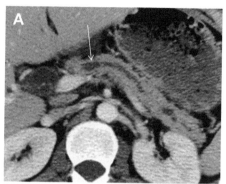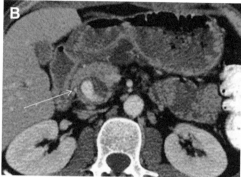

Fig. 3. (A, B) A 34-year-old man with history of prior episode of acute pancreatitis, currently present with upper gastrointestinal tract hemorrhage. Axial contrast-enhanced CT demonstrates atrophy of the pancreatic parenchyma, ductal dilatation (*arrow* in A), and a partially thrombosed pseudoaneurysm in region of head of pancreas (*arrow* in B). Pseudoaneurysm was confirmed by conventional angiography to be arising from branch of the gastroduodenal artery.

diagnosis of chronic pancreatitis on MR imaging is based on morphologic changes in the parenchyma, such as changes in signal intensity and enhancement pattern, and ductal changes on MRCP (Table 3).

Parenchymal changes In the early stages of the disease, the parenchyma reveals loss of normal hyperintense signal on T1-weighted images because of a decrease in the proteinaceous fluid content within the parenchyma caused by chronic inflammation and fibrosis.[13] The normal enhancement of the parenchyma is avid and uniform in the late arterial phase with wash out on delayed images. With CP, even in early stages, there is decreased and heterogeneous enhancement in the early phases with delayed increased enhancement (Fig. 4).[14,15] The abnormal pattern of enhancement is likely secondary to arteriolar damage and fibrosis, which reduces the blood vessels density.[16] The most sensitive parameter for early diagnosis of chronic pancreatitis is delayed parenchymal enhancement.[15] In the later stage of CP, the pancreatic parenchyma reveals atrophy in addition to altered signal and enhancement.[13]

Ductal abnormalities MRCP offers a noninvasive method to image the pancreatic ducts. Abnormalities of the ductal system are better displayed on the heavily T2-weighted images. Three-dimensional (3D) MRCP images can be acquired by using fast recovery sequences with breath hold or with the respiratory-gated technique.

In early stages of the disease, MRCP demonstrates dilatation and irregularity of the side branch ducts. In later phases, dilatation and irregularity of the main pancreatic duct, strictures, and pseudocyst may be seen (see Fig. 4). The beaded main pancreatic duct with its dilated side branches may have a chain-of-lakes appearance. Intraductal calcifications are seen as hypointense filling defects within the hyperintense fluid of the duct. MRCP has a sensitivity of 60% to 80% and a high specificity of 95% to 100% in detecting filling defects.[17] MRCP is also highly accurate in diagnosing anatomic variants, such as pancreas divisum that may be associated with CP.[18]

Table 3
MR imaging parenchymal and ductal changes in CP

Changes in CP	Early	Late
Parenchymal	Loss of normal hyperintensity Decreased and heterogeneous early enhancement Delayed enhancement	Altered signal intensity and enhancement Atrophy
Ductal	Normal main pancreatic duct Dilatation and irregularity of side branches	Main pancreatic duct dilatation Strictures of the main pancreatic duct Pseudocysts Intraductal filling defects/calculi

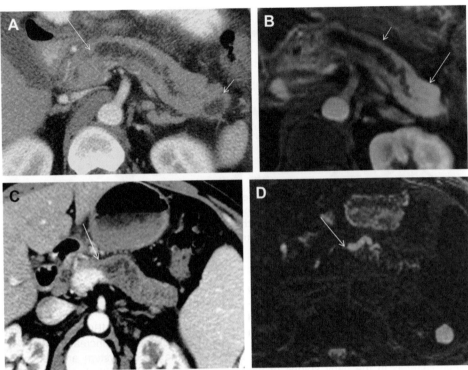

Fig. 4. Pancreatic ductal strictures caused by CP. (*A*) Axial contrast-enhanced CT (CECT) of a 52-year-old patient with history of heavy alcohol consumption and persistent abdominal pain. The main pancreatic duct is irregular and dilated up to 11 mm, with an abrupt cutoff in the neck of the pancreas (*arrow*). In addition, there is a small pseudocyst in the tail of the pancreas (*short arrow*). (*B*) T1-weighted enhanced image demonstrated main pancreatic duct (MPD) dilatation and heterogeneous enhancement of the parenchyma, with delayed enhancement of the atrophied parenchyma (*short arrow*) when compared with the rest of the parenchyma (*long arrow*). The patient had subsequent ERCP, EUS, and follow-up scans over 3 years, which demonstrated stability of the ductal stricture and no evidence of pancreatic mass. (*C*) CECT and (*D*) 2-dimensional MRCP of a 61-year-old patient with CP and stricture of the MPD in the body of the pancreas (*arrows*) with upstream dilatation of the MPD and side branches.

MRCP reveals ductal size in a more physiologic condition when compared with ERCP, but diameters may be underestimated due to signal loss, lack of resolution and blurring. MRCP can show upstream dilatation of the main pancreatic duct in the setting of obstruction, another advantage over endoscopic retrograde cholangiopancreatography (ERCP). As for pathologic findings, agreement between MRCP and ERCP has been determined to be 83% to 92% for ductal dilatation, 70% to 92% for ductal narrowing, and 92% to 100% for filling defects.[19] MRCP is 86% to 88% sensitive, 98% specific, and 91% accurate in detecting abnormalities of the main pancreatic duct.[20]

Patients with abnormal MR imaging findings but with normal MRCP may benefit from dynamic secretin-MRCP (S-MRCP), which may reveal ductal abnormalities otherwise not detected on MRCP.[21] S-MRCP can be performed dynamically after the intravenous administration of secretin. Secretin is a 27-amino-acid peptide hormone that is excreted by the duodenum in response to food, stimulating the production of bicarbonate and water by the pancreas (**Fig. 5**). Within 2 to 6 minutes of secretin injection, significant dilatation of the main pancreatic duct is observed secondary to both accumulation of pancreatic fluid secreted into the ductal system by ductal cells and increased tone of the SO. The increased tone of the sphincter prevents the release of the fluid through the papilla. Following this, the tone of the sphincter decreases resulting in flow of pancreatic secretions from the duct through the papilla into the duodenum and gradual return of the main pancreatic duct (MPD) caliber to baseline (around 10 minutes after injection).[22] By increasing the exocrine secretion, S-MRCP improves the ductal visualization and evaluation of ductal abnormalities and gives an indirect measure of

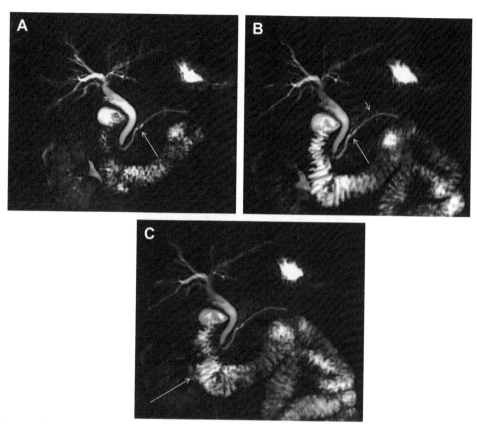

Fig. 5. S-MRCP. (*A*) Presecretin administration MRCP image, there is irregularity of the main pancreatic duct (*long arrow*). (*B*) Three minutes after secretin administration. There is slight increase in the caliber of the pancreatic duct with better visualization of the irregular segment (*long arrow*) of the pancreatic duct and the side branches (*short arrow*). (*C*) Ten minutes after secretin administration. The pancreatic duct has slightly decreased in caliber, and there is filling of pancreatic fluid in the duodenum (*long arrow*).

the pancreatic exocrine function (**Fig. 6**).[23] In patients with CP, the baseline diameters of the main pancreatic ducts are larger than the control population. On dynamic assessment, the time to reach the peak diameter is longer and the percentage of increase in the diameter is lower.[22]

In addition, diffusion-weighted (DW) images have been shown to provide information regarding the exocrine function, through stimulated with secretin.[24] Apparent diffusion coefficient values are lower in patients with CP when compared with those in normal pancreases. This finding is thought to be secondary to the replacement of normal parenchyma by fibrous tissue, which may reduce the amount of diffusible tissue water. The exocrine functional capacity can also be estimated by DW imaging after secretin stimulation. In the normal pancreas, the apparent diffusion coefficient (ADC) values after secretin administration increase from baseline; in patients with CP, no fluctuations of the ADC values are observed.[24]

Endoscopic procedures

Endoscopic retrograde cholangiopancreatography ERCP allows the detection of dilatation and stenosis of the pancreatic duct and side branches and is considered the gold standard for diagnosing CP. ERCP is specifically considered a useful tool in diagnosing early CP because the changes may not be evident on cross-sectional imaging examinations, such as CT or MR imaging. The average diameter of the duct is 3 to 4 mm in the head, 2 to 3 mm in the body, and 1 to 2 mm in the tail. The side branches range in number from 20 to 30 and join the main pancreatic duct at right angles, alternating above and below.

Early features of CP in ERCP include the dilatation and irregularity of side branches. As the disease progresses, the main pancreatic duct reveals dilation, irregularity, loss of normal tapering, focal stenosis, and filling defects (**Fig. 7, Table 4**). ERCP may also demonstrate pseudocysts communicating with the main pancreatic duct. Because

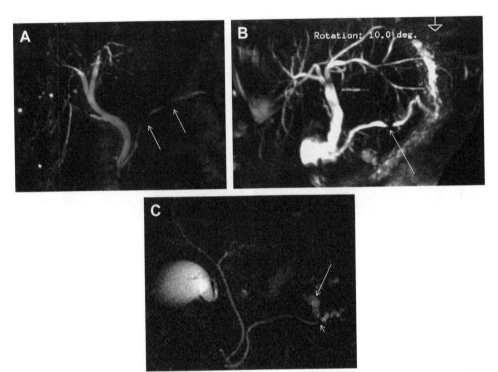

Fig. 6. (A) A 38-year-old patient with history of multiple episodes of acute pancreatitis. The S-MRCP demonstrated 2 smooth, benign strictures in the body and tail of the pancreas (*arrows*). (B) A 69-year-old patient with known history of CP. S-MRCP demonstrated dilatation of the MPD and a focal stricture in the body (*arrow*). (C) S-MRCP in a patient with CP and persistent ascites. There is segmental dilatation and irregularity of the pancreatic duct in the tail with a focal stricture (*short arrow*). Adjacent to the stricture, a pancreatic leak is noted (*long arrow*).

ERCP is an invasive procedure, one disadvantage is that it can precipitate acute pancreatitis in up to 4% of patients.[25]

Endoscopic ultrasound Endoscopic ultrasound (EUS) is commonly used to diagnose and assess

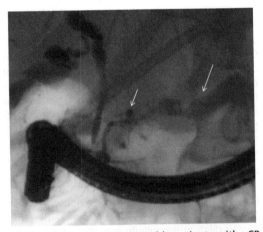

Fig. 7. ERCP of a 67-year-old patient with CP. Segmental dilatation of the MPD in the body and tail (*long arrow*) and dilatation of multiple side branches (*short arrow*) are seen in the neck of the pancreas.

the severity of CP. The proximity of the stomach and duodenum allow high-resolution imaging. The normal parenchyma is homogeneous with fine granularity and reticulation.

An international consensus resulted in the Rosemont criteria, a categorization scheme that is endorsed by the American Society for Gastrointestinal Endoscopy and that unifies the criteria to diagnose CP on EUS, thereby standardizing the nomenclature and various quantitative criteria. EUS features are categorized into major and minor criteria (**Table 5**).[26]

Differential diagnosis
In the setting of focal or segmental mass-forming pancreatitis, there can be morphologic overlap with pancreatic adenocarcinoma. Patients with malignancy have fewer ductal calculi and less side-branch dilatation but larger-caliber pancreatic ducts with abrupt cutoff in the mass without the duct penetrating sign; also, these patients may present with vascular invasion, which is not seen in CP.

In patients with CP, the cumulative incidence of pancreatic cancer is 1.1% at 5 years and 1.7% at 10 years, with a standardized incidence ratio of

Table 4
Classification of CP on ERCP (Cambridge classification)

Group	MPD	Side Branches
		Findings
Equivocal	Normal	<3 abnormal side branches
Mild	Normal	≥3 abnormal side branches
Moderate	Abnormal	≥3 abnormal side branches
Marked	Abnormal	Moderate disease with one of the following: Large cavities (>1 cm) Intraductal filling defects or calculi Ductal obstruction or strictures Gross irregularity Severe dilatation

26.7.[27] Thus, patients with CP should be closely monitored; and when in doubt, evaluation with percutaneous or EUS biopsy should be performed.

Pancreatic calcification is most commonly associated with chronic pancreatitis, presenting in up to 90% of patients with alcoholic pancreatitis. However, calcifications have also been described in certain neoplasms, such as intraductal papillary mucinous neoplasms (IPMN). Calcifications within side-branch or main-duct IPMN, although rare, have been reported.[28,29] CP and IPMN may have overlapping imaging findings: patients with main-duct IPMN present with ductal dilatation that may be associated with parenchymal atrophy; patients with side-branch IPMN present with cystic lesions often confused with pseudocysts; and patients with combined IPMN present with cystic lesion and ductal dilatation and parenchymal atrophy. IPMN should be favored as a diagnosis when a solid component is noted within the main duct or when complex features, such as pseudoseptations and nodules, are noted within

Table 5
Parenchymal and ductal features of CP on EUS

	Characteristics	Major Criteria	Minor Criteria
Parenchymal			
Hyperechoic foci with shadowing	At least 3 hyperechoic foci, >2 mm, with shadow	Yes	
Lobularity	At least 3 lobules, also defined ≥5 mm, with echogenic rim • If ≥3 contiguous lobules+ Honeycombing • If ≥3 noncontiguous lobules	Yes	Yes
Hyperechoic foci, nonshadowing	At least 3 hyperechoic foci ≥3 mm		Yes
Cysts	Anechoic, rounded/elliptical, ≥2 mm		Yes
Stranding	At least 3 hyperechoic lines ≥3 mm in length		Yes
Ductal			
MPD calculi	Echogenic structure within the MPD with shadowing	Yes	
Irregular MPD contour	Uneven or irregular outline and ecstatic course in the body and tail		Yes
Dilated side branches	At least 3 tubular anechoic structures ≥1 mm, communicating with the MPD in the body and tail		Yes
MPD dilatation	≥3.5 mm in the body or ≥1.5 mm in the tail		Yes
Hyperechoic MPD margin	Hyperechoic duct wall in >50% of MPD in the body and tail		Yes

the cysts. EUS with fine-needle aspiration (FNA) may confirm the diagnosis of IPMN by demonstrating mucin within the fluid.

Pearls: chronic calcifying pancreatitis

- Related to chronic alcohol abuse, in addition to other predisposing factors, such as smoking
- Coarse parenchymal or intraductal calcifications
- Irregular dilatation of the main pancreatic duct and side branches with chain of-lakes appearance
- Pancreatic atrophy
- Pseudocysts/retention cysts
- Differentials: pancreatic adenocarcinoma, main-duct IPMN neoplasm.

Obstructive Chronic Pancreatitis

Persistent obstruction of the pancreatic duct may lead to chronic inflammation and atrophy of the parenchyma. The obstruction can be caused either by tumors (primary or secondary) or by traumatic or inflammatory strictures.

Pathogenesis

Common neoplasms that may lead to chronic pancreatitis or recurrent acute pancreatitis are either pancreatic in origin, such as adenocarcinoma or IPMN neoplasms, or nonpancreatic, such as metastasis, duodenal adenocarcinoma, ampullary carcinoma, or adenoma. Benign conditions, such as SO dysfunction (SOD), pancreas divisum, duplication cysts, and iatrogenic or pancreatitis-related strictures, can result in chronic ductal obstruction.

Histopathology

In obstructive chronic pancreatitis (OCP), the pancreatic parenchyma reveals inflammation and fibrosis uniformly and diffusely upstream from the obstruction point, which eventually leads to diffuse atrophy. The main pancreatic duct is diffusely dilated without intraductal calculi or protein plugs.[30]

Imaging

Findings on imaging studies will vary according to the obstructive cause and the severity of the disease. On CT and MR imaging, the obstructive changes are reflected by parenchymal atrophy and upstream main ductal dilation. Dilation of the common bile duct may be seen if the obstruction is in the ampullary region or the head of the pancreas. Pseudocysts may be present in OCP; however, intraductal or parenchymal calcifications are generally not observed.[31]

ERCP and MRCP will present with irregular upstream ductal dilatation in a chain of lakes as seen in chronic calcifying pancreatitis without filling defects. However, ERCP may not opacity the upstream duct beyond an area of stenosis, in which case MRCP is more helpful.

A small or intraductal malignant neoplasm may not be visible on cross-sectional imaging, and the diagnosis is suspected based on secondary signs, such as parenchymal atrophy and loss of lobularity with significant ductal dilatation, abrupt cutoff of an upstream dilated pancreatic duct, distant metastases, and vascular involvement.[32] Acute pancreatitis may present in 3.0% to 13.8% of cases of pancreatic cancer, with inflammatory changes being the predominant finding, masking the neoplasms and delaying the diagnosis.[33]

Duodenal villous adenomas are the most common lesion of the ampulla of Vater, accounting for 1% of all duodenal tumors.[34] These adenomas may be asymptomatic or may present with obstructive jaundice, GI bleeding, or bowel obstruction.[35] Small adenomas confined to the ampulla may not be detected on cross-sectional imaging. An upper-GI barium swallow may demonstrate a filling defect in the second portion of the duodenum. In larger lesions, CT with adequate distension of duodenum with neutral oral contrast may show a soft tissue arising from the duodenal wall and OCP signs. However, endoscopy should be performed in all cases of suspected duodenal tumors with histologic sampling because endoscopic findings may be insufficient for excluding cancer.[36]

Benign strictures of the main pancreatic duct may be secondary to recurrent acute pancreatitis or trauma, leading to OCP. Benign strictures are usually smooth as opposed to malignant strictures that may have abrupt cutoff.[37] Symptomatic benign strictures may be managed with therapeutic ERCP using balloon dilatation and stent placement; however, long-term efficacy of this procedure is unclear.[38]

SOD is a benign entity secondary to abnormal contractility of the sphincter that leads to obstruction of the flow of bile and pancreatic juice through the pancreaticobiliary junction. SOD may clinically manifest as pancreatitis, abdominal pain, or abnormal liver or pancreatic function tests. SOD has 2 primary abnormalities: dyskinesia, which is mainly a motor abnormality leading to hypotonic or hypertonic sphincter, and structural abnormality caused by stenosis secondary to fibrosis and inflammation.[39] SO manometry is considered the gold standard for diagnosing SOD (diagnostic criteria: pressure of SO more than 40 mm Hg and abnormal number and duration of contractions).[40]

Nevertheless, it is a difficult test to perform and is associated with a high complication rate. S-MRCP can noninvasively, although indirectly, assess the SO function by measuring the MPD diameter. The diagnosis is suspected when the physiologic increase in caliber of the MPD from baseline persists throughout 15 minutes after secretin administration.[41]

Differential diagnosis

Because OCP can be secondary to a variety of obstructing causes, including malignancy, the imaging differentiation between pancreatic adenocarcinoma and mass-forming chronic pancreatitis can be challenging. Both entities present with parenchymal atrophy, ductal dilatation, and mass lesions that are hypodense on CT or T1 hypointense on MR imaging, with both tests showing delayed enhancement after intravenous contrast administration. Among imaging findings, morphologic changes of the MPD are the most useful to distinguish between these 2 pathologic conditions. In pancreatic adenocarcinoma, ductal dilatation is more severe, the duct is smoothly dilated without dilatation of the side branches, and when associated with the dilatation of the common bile duct with abrupt cutoff double-duct

sign, the constellation of findings is 77% sensitive and 80% specific for malignancy (**Fig. 8**).[37]

In mass-forming chronic pancreatitis, the ductal dilatation is less severe and irregular, with multiple ductal strictures and the dilatation of side branches. In addition, the visualization of the main pancreatic duct traversing the mass, the so-called duct penetrating sign, is a specific and sensitive sign (96% specificity and 85% sensitive).[42]

Nevertheless, in many cases, CT and MR imaging might not adequately differentiate malignancy from mass-forming CP, and further evaluation with EUS-FNA may be necessary.

When cross-sectional imaging and biopsy are nondiagnostic, 18F-fluorodeoxyglucose (FDG) positron emission tomography (PET) has an established role in the diagnosis of pancreatic carcinoma. The reported sensitivities range from 85% to 100% and specificities range from 67% to 99% for differentiating benign from malignant masses.[43] However, FDG PET detectability depends on the size of the lesion and the degree of uptake and surrounding background uptake. It is known that inflammatory tissue can also exhibit FDG activity. However, in the setting of chronic pancreatitis, FDG PET is able to detect pancreatic

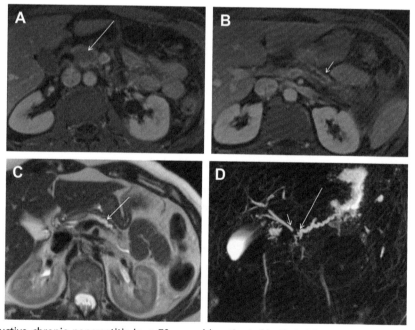

Fig. 8. Obstructive chronic pancreatitis in a 70-year-old patient. (*A, B*) Axial T1 weighted enhanced images demonstrate a hypointense mass in the head of the pancreas (*long arrow*) with upstream pancreatic duct dilatation and atrophy of the parenchyma (*short arrow*). (*C*) 2D MRCP allows better visualization of the dilatated main pancreatic duct (*arrow*). (*D*) 3D MRCP demonstrated diffuse upstream dilatation of the pancreatic duct, with no visualization of dilated side branches. There is abrupt cut-off of the common bile duct (*short arrow*) and the pancreatic duct (*long arrow*) at the level of the pancreatic head. The patient underwent EUS guided FNA biopsy after which the diagnosis of pancreatic adenocarcinoma was made.

adenocarcinoma with a sensitivity of 92% and negative predictive value of 87%.[44] If acute pancreatitis is present, specificity can be as low as 50%.[45]

Pearls: OCP

- It is related to chronic obstruction caused by a benign or malignant pathologic condition.
- There is upstream dilatation of the main pancreatic duct with diffuse atrophy of the parenchyma.
- There is no evidence of intraductal calculi or protein plugs.
- Assess the cause of the obstruction: pancreatic adenocarcinoma, duodenal adenoma, benign postinflammatory stricture, stricture secondary to trauma, or SO dysfunction.

MISCELLANEOUS PANCREATITIS
Autoimmune Pancreatitis

Autoimmune pancreatitis (AIP) is a manifestation of an immunoglobulin G4 (IgG4) systemic disease, characterized by a systemic chronic fibro-inflammatory process that affects multiple organs, including the pancreas, salivary glands, bile ducts, kidneys, lungs, retroperitoneum, and lymph nodes (Table 6).

The clinical presentation of AIP is varied, ranging from painless jaundice secondary to a pancreatic mass to a more chronic clinical condition caused by exocrine and endocrine insufficiency that leads to steatorrhea and diabetes. The presentation as acute or chronic pancreatitis is thought to be uncommon. In a recent review, 4% of patients evaluated for the cause of suspected pancreatitis had AIP, 24% of the patients with AIP had acute pancreatitis, and 11% presented as chronic pancreatitis. The age of presentation ranges from 14 to 85 years, with a mean of 60 years.[46]

Histopathology

In the pancreas, the histology is characterized by lymphoplasmacytic infiltrate around the small ducts, swirling fibrosis centered around the veins and ducts, and obliterative phlebitis sparing the arterioles.[47,48] Immunostaining of AIP is diagnostic and demonstrates abundant IgG4 positive cells, distinguishing AIP from alcoholic pancreatitis and inflammatory infiltrates surrounding pancreatic cancer.[49]

Table 6
Extrapancreatic manifestations of autoimmune pancreatitis

Organ	Frequency (%)	Findings
Biliary duct: sclerosing cholangitis	77–88	Thickening, stenosis, irregularity, abnormal enhancement Most common involvement: of the intrapancreatic portion of the common bile duct Less common multifocal intrahepatic involvement
Renal	33–35	Round or wedge-shape renal cortical nodules Peripheral cortical lesions Masslike lesion Renal pelvis involvement Frequently bilateral involvement
Salivary glands	14–24	Bilateral painless swelling of salivary and lacrimal glands
Retroperitoneum: retroperitoneal fibrosis	10–20	Thick soft tissue mass around aorta and its branches May result in hydronephrosis
Mesentery: sclerosing mesenteritis	4–33	Involvement of small bowel mesentery Soft tissue mass encasing the mesenteric vessels
Bowel: inflammatory bowel disease	10–17	12- to 5-fold increase risk factor for inflammatory bowel disease More frequently associated with AIP-PD Ulcerative colitis (more frequent), Crohn disease
Pulmonary	5–13	Solid parenchymal nodules Alveolar-interstitial pattern Bronchovascular pattern

Data from Vlachou PA, Khalili K, Jang HJ, et al. IgG4-related sclerosing disease: autoimmune pancreatitis and extrapancreatic manifestations. Radiographics 2011;31:1379–402.

Depending on the areas of involvement, histologically AIP can be classified as predominant lobular involvement (AIP-PL or type I) and predominant ductal involvement (AIP-PD or type II). The AIP-PL has predominant lobular inflammation and septal fibroblastic proliferation, presents with higher numbers of IgG4 positive cells, and is most commonly seen in Asian and male populations. The AIP-PD has predominant ductocentric inflammation, and ductocentric granulomas may be seen. This variety more commonly presents as a pseudotumor and is seen in the Western population.[50]

Imaging

Imaging plays an important role in the diagnosis of AIP; however, by itself it is not diagnostic. Commonly used diagnostic criteria for AIP include the Japan Pancreas Society criteria and the Mayo Clinic HISORt criteria (Table 7).[46,51]

There are 3 recognized patterns of autoimmune pancreatitis: diffuse, focal, and multifocal. Diffuse disease is the most common type presenting with diffuse sausagelike parenchymal enlargement seen in 40% to 60% of patients. The pancreatic contour becomes featureless and effaced (Fig. 9). Focal disease is less common and manifests as

Table 7
Diagnostic criteria for autoimmune pancreatitis

Japanese Pancreas Society Criteria:	Diagnosis is established when criteria 1 with criteria 2 or 3 are present	
	1. Typical imaging	Diffuse or segmental narrowing of the pancreatic duct with irregular wall and diffuse or localized enlargement of pancreas on US, CT, and MR imaging.
	2. Serology	Autoantibodies (antinuclear antibodies and rheumatoid factor), elevated γ-globulins, or IgG or IgG4
	3. Histopathology	Marked interlobular fibrosis and prominent infiltration of lymphocytes and plasma cells in the periductal area, occasionally with lymphoid follicles in the pancreas
HISORt Criteria: (Mayo Clinic criteria)	Diagnosis of AIP: Group A: diagnostic pancreatic histology Group B: typical imaging + serology Group C: response to steroids (pancreatic or extrapancreatic) + negative workup for cancer + elevated serum IgG4	
	Histology	Periductal lymphoplasmacytic infiltrate with obliterative phlebitis and storiform fibrosis Lymphoplasmacytic infiltrate with storiform fibrosis showing IgG4 positive cells
	Pancreatic imaging	
	Typical	Diffusely enlarged gland with delayed rim enhancement, diffusely irregular attenuated main pancreatic duct
	Other	Focal pancreatic mass/enlargement, focal pancreatic duct stricture, pancreatic atrophy, pancreatic calcifications
	Serology	Elevated IgG4 level
	Other organs involvement	Hilar/intrahepatic biliary strictures, persistent distal biliary stricture, parotid/lacrimal gland involvement, mediastinal lymphadenopathy, retroperitoneal fibrosis
	Response to therapy	Resolution/marked improvement of pancreatic or extrapancreatic manifestations with steroid therapy

Data from Okazaki K, Kawa S, Kamisawa T, et al. Research committee of intractable diseases of the Pancreas. Clinical diagnostic criteria of autoimmune pancreatitis: revised proposal. J Gastroenterol 2006;41:626–31; and Kamisawa T, Egawa N, Nakajima H, et al. Clinical difficulties in the differentiation of autoimmune pancreatitis and pancreatic carcinoma. Am J Gastroenterol 2003;98:2694–9.

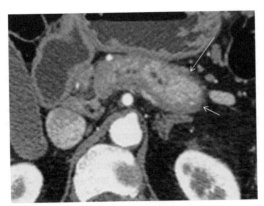

Fig. 9. AIP. CECT axial image demonstrates swelling of the pancreas with loss of lobulations, retraction of the pancreatic tail (*short arrow*) and a smooth hypodense rim around the pancreas "halo" (*long arrow*).

a well-defined hypodense mass, often involving the head and mimicking pancreatic adenocarcinoma. Upstream dilatation of the main pancreatic duct may be seen; however, it is usually less severe than with pancreatic malignancy.[52] The affected areas of the pancreas usually appear hypoechoic on ultrasound (US) and hypodense on CT. On contrast-enhanced CT there is decreased enhancement of the involved parenchyma in the arterial phase and delayed enhancement in the late phase.[53,54]

A morphologic evolution of the imaging findings in AIP has been reported. Through the analysis of the course of events, it has been suggested that AIP may start as focal swelling and progresses into a diffuse form. Without treatment, there is worsening of the parenchymal swelling with loss of parenchymal lobularity, resulting in a featureless, sausage-shaped pancreas. Subsequently, the progression of the disease leads to pancreatic tail retraction, peripancreatic findings, and ductal involvement.[55]

On MR imaging, the pancreas is diffusely hypointense on T1-weighted images and slightly hyperintense on T2-weighted images. There is diminished enhancement during early phases and delayed venous enhancement.[53,54] A low-attenuation halo around the parenchyma is present in 12% to 40% of patients and thought to represent an inflammatory cell infiltration.[56] This capsulelike rim is hypointense on both T1- and T2-weighted images and has delayed enhancement on contrast-enhanced images. On MRCP, diffuse or segmental narrowing and irregularity of the MPD are characteristic.[57] Sclerosing cholangitis is present in up to 88% of patients with AIP, stenosis, irregularity, and increased enhancement of the bile ducts. The most common segment involved is the intrapancreatic common bile duct, and less frequently multifocal intrahepatic biliary strictures are noted.[58]

Rare findings associated with autoimmune pancreatitis are pseudocysts and peripancreatic fat stranding. These features are more frequently seen in chronic alcoholic pancreatitis and acute pancreatitis respectively. Previously, the absence of pancreatic stones was thought to be characteristic of AIP. However, it has been noted that 18% of patients with AIP may have pancreatic stone formation, predominantly those with recurrent symptoms. The formation of stones might be related to incomplete obstruction and irregularity of the MPD, leading to stasis of pancreatic juices.[59]

After corticosteroid therapy, the morphology of the pancreas and the narrowing and irregularity of the pancreatic duct usually resolve. In some cases, atrophy of the affected parenchyma is noted on follow-up scans and indicates a late phase of the disease (**Fig. 10**).[60]

Differential diagnosis

The focal form of AIP can be difficult to differentiate from pancreatic adenocarcinoma, and 2% to 6% of patients who undergo pancreatic resection for suspected malignancy have AIP.[61] Focal masslike enlargement of the pancreas can be seen in up to 49% of patients with AIP (**Fig. 11**).[62] On CT, the enlarged pancreas is isoattenuating or hypoattenuating on pancreatic phase compared with the rest of the parenchyma, making it indistinguishable from pancreatic carcinoma. However, it gradually enhances on delayed phases.[54,56,63] Other findings that favor AIP over malignancy are concurrent diffuse changes or multifocality; lack of upstream pancreatic ductal dilatation; and absence of parenchymal atrophy, vascular encasement, and metastatic disease.

The diffuse form of AIP may mimic diffuse disorders like lymphoma, metastases, or other diffuse infiltrative processes. In most of these disorders, in contrast to AIP, the parenchyma is heterogeneous and has irregular contours.[55]

Pearls: AIP

- Also known as lymphoplasmacytic or sclerosing pancreatitis
- Part of IgG4-related systemic disease, which can be associated with sclerosing cholangitis, renal lesions, sialadenitis, inflammatory bowel disease, retroperitoneal fibrosis, autoimmune hepatitis, and others
- Can present as diffuse, focal, or multifocal involvement of the pancreas
- Types: lobular or ductocentric involvement
- Imaging: diffuse pancreatic swelling, sausage-shaped appearance, peripancreatic halo,

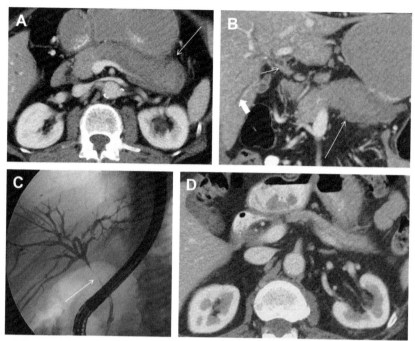

Fig. 10. AIP in a 72-year-old patient. (A) At presentation, CECT demonstrated swelling of the parenchyma, attenuation of the main pancreatic duct and peripheral hypodense "halo" (long arrow). (B) Coronal reformatted image demonstrates mild intrahepatic ductal dilatation (thick arrow) and stricture of the common bile duct, with abnormal enhancement (short arrow). The peripheral hypodense halo is again visualized (long arrow). (C) ERCP confirms the common bile duct stricture and mild intrahepatic ductal dilatation. A biliary stent was placed (not shown). (D) 3 months post corticosteroid therapy follow-up; CECT, revealing resolution of the swelling and atrophy of the pancreas.

diffuse or segmental ductal narrowing, focal masslike swelling without vascular invasion, extrapancreatic involvement
- Response to steroid treatment
- Differential diagnosis: pancreatic adenocarcinoma

Groove Pancreatitis

Groove pancreatitis is an uncommon type of focal chronic pancreatitis affecting the pancreaticoduodenal groove, located between the head of the pancreas, the duodenum, and the common bile duct.

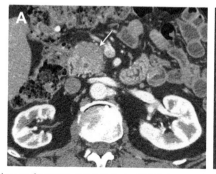

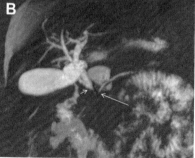

Fig. 11. Focal mass forming AIP. (A) Axial CECT shows a hypodense lesion in the head of the pancreas (arrow). (B) MRCP demonstrated mild dilatation of the main pancreatic duct and dilatation of the intra and extrahepatic biliary ducts, with abrupt-cut off of both ducts at in the head of the pancreas (short and long arrows). The patient was believed to have a pancreatic neoplasm and underwent a Whipple procedure, which revealed focal AIP.

Pathogenesis

Two patterns of groove pancreatitis have been described: the pure form, in which there is scar tissue in the groove without involvement of the pancreatic parenchyma, and the segmental form, in which the scarring involves the groove and the pancreatic head.[64] In most cases, on histopathology, hyperplasia of Brunner glands and small cysts/pseudocysts are seen within the groove. The pathogenesis remains unclear. Several factors, such as pancreatic heterotopia, true duodenal cysts, peptic ulcer disease, dorsal dominant drainage, alcohol abuse, and gastric surgery, have been related to groove pancreatitis. It is unclear if groove pancreatitis and cystic dystrophy of the duodenum are part of the same spectrum or different entities. More recently, paraduodenal pancreatitis is a term that has been proposed to include cystic dystrophy of the duodenal wall, paraduodenal wall cysts, and groove pancreatitis.[65]

Imaging

The classic MDCT features in the pure form are ill-defined soft tissue within the pancreaticoduodenal groove, with or without delayed enhancement. Small cysts may be seen along the medial wall of the duodenum or in the pancreatic groove (Fig. 12).

On MR imaging, groove pancreatitis is characterized by a sheetlike mass in the groove that is hypointense on T1-weighted images and slightly hyperintense on T2-weighted images relative to the pancreas and may show delayed enhancement.[66] In the segmental form, the pancreatic parenchyma in the head is hypointense, associated with atrophy and ductal dilatation. Duodenal thickening and cysts within the duodenal wall may also be found; these are better displayed on T2-weighted images. In addition, tapering of the common bile duct and irregularity and narrowing of the main pancreatic duct in the head is usually seen.[66] In the segmental form, involvement of the head of the pancreas produces on CT a hypodense masslike ppearance of the parenchyma, which MR imaging appears hypointense on T1 weighted images.

Differential diagnosis

With the segmental form, the most important differential diagnosis is pancreatic adenocarcinoma.[67] The presence of an abrupt cutoff of the pancreatic duct and the common bile duct and the presence of vascular invasion are considered the most useful signs in differentiating pancreatic malignancy from groove pancreatitis. In contrast, in patients with groove pancreatitis, ductal narrowing and irregularity are seen.

The disorders that may mimic the pure form of groove pancreatitis are groove carcinoma, pancreatic groove neuroendocrine tumors, duodenal or periampullary carcinoma, and acute pancreatitis with inflammatory changes in the groove. Differentiating these lesions from groove pancreatitis based only on imaging findings may be difficult; however, the presence of cysts within the lesion and thickening of the duodenal wall favors groove pancreatitis.[67]

Pearls: groove pancreatitis

- Chronic inflammatory pancreatitis affecting the pancreaticoduodenal groove
- Two forms: pure form, which only affects the groove with sparing of the pancreatic head parenchyma, and segmental form, which involves the groove and the pancreatic head
- Manifests as soft tissue in the pancreatic groove, duodenal wall thickening, smooth ductal narrowing, cystic and inflammatory

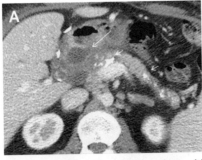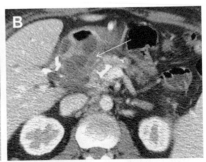

Fig. 12. Axial CECT images of a 47-year-old patient with chronic intermittent pancreatitis. (A, B) show multiple cystic changed between the duodenum and the head of the pancreas (arrows), causing compression of the duodenum and common bile duct. Atrophy of the pancreatic parenchyma with multiple parenchymal calcifications are noted (short arrow in A). The patient underwent surgical resection after which the diagnosis of groove pancreatitis was made on histopathological evaluation.

changes in the groove; no evidence of vascular invasion

- Differentials: pancreatic adenocarcinoma, duodenal carcinoma, common bile duct malignancy, peripancreatic lymphadenopathy, or extrapancreatic neuroendocrine tumors.

Tropical Pancreatitis

Tropical pancreatitis is a variant of CP presenting in young patients and is characterized by a rapidly progressive course, severe pancreatitis, and increased risk of pancreatic adenocarcinoma.

A regional predisposition has been established. Multiple cases have been reported in Asia and Africa, with a large number occurring in India. However, even in those predisposing areas of the world, idiopathic and alcoholic pancreatitis remain the primary causes of chronic pancreatitis. Recent reports from India found an incidence of tropical pancreatitis of 3.9% of the population.[68]

Pathogenesis

Multiple predisposing factors are related to the pathogenesis of tropical pancreatitis, including protein malnutrition, pancreatic ductal anomalies, cyanide toxicity, and genetic mutations (SPINK1 and CFTR).[69] To establish the diagnosis, the absence of alcohol consumption, biliary tract disease, and other biochemical or structural predisposing factors need to be corroborated. Nearly two-thirds of affected patients develop fibro-calculous pancreatic diabetes within a decade of onset.[70]

Imaging

On imaging, multiple, large pancreatic calculi (up to 5 cm) with dilatation of the pancreatic duct are noted in more than 80% of patients, and parenchymal atrophy is seen in nearly half of patients.[71]

There is a strong association with pancreatic adenocarcinoma, resulting in death in 25% of patients at an average age of 45 years. The cancer occurs most frequently in the body and tail and should be suspected clinically with symptoms of progressive weight loss or when a discrete mass is observed on imaging studies.[72]

Pearls: tropical pancreatitis

- CP in young patients in tropical countries
- Associated with malnutrition, infection, cyanide toxicity, and genetic mutations
- Multiple, large, coarse intraductal calculi (up to 5 cm), main and side-branch ductal dilatation, parenchymal atrophy
- All progress to fibro-calculous pancreatic diabetes.

Hereditary Pancreatitis

Hereditary pancreatitis is a rare cause of recurrent and CP (<1%). It is an autosomal dominant disease, with acute recurrent pancreatitis attacks usually manifesting during childhood.

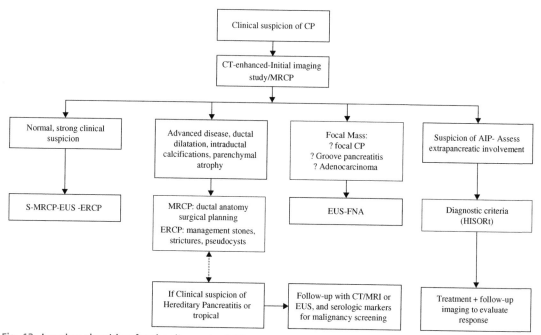

Fig. 13. Imaging algorithm for the diagnosis of CP.

Pathogenesis

The genetic disorder is secondary to various gene mutations, such as mutations of the PRSS1 gene on the long arm of the chromosome 7, which encodes for the cationic trypsinogen, or mutations in the CFTR gene.[73] In the second and third decades of life, atrophy of the parenchyma associated with exocrine and endocrine insufficiencies are encountered.

Imaging

The imaging findings are similar to those described in tropical pancreatitis, with atrophy of the parenchyma, parenchymal calcifications, and intraductal calculi. Hereditary pancreatitis should be suspected in patients who have manifested a least 2 episodes of acute pancreatitis in the absence of any predisposing factors. The diagnosis should also be considered in patients with idiopathic CP, in patients with a family history of chronic pancreatitis in first- and second-degree relatives and in children with unexplained episodes of pancreatitis.[74] Imaging plays an important role in excluding structural causes of pancreatitis and in follow-up of the disease because of the 50- to 70-fold increased risk of pancreatic malignancy. The cumulative risks of pancreatic cancer at 50 and 75 years of age are 11% and 49% for men and 8% and 55% for women and may increase in both genders if smoking coexists.[73]

Pearls: hereditary pancreatitis

- Recurrent acute pancreatitis in young patients with positive family history without anatomic explanation
- Associated with multiple genetic mutations
- Coarse intraductal and parenchymal calcifications, with parenchymal atrophy
- Increased risk of pancreatic adenocarcinoma.

SUMMARY

CP remains a complex and challenging disease. Imaging is not only used to confirm the diagnosis of CP but also looks for anatomic or pathologic causes of CP and assesses the severity of the disease and involvement of other organs. Imaging studies are important in directing patients with clinical suspicion to invasive procedures, such as ERCP or EUS, medical treatment, and follow-up (Fig. 13).

In patients with suspected CP, CT continues to be the first-line study, which is helpful in the diagnosis of moderate to severe CP and its complications.

MR imaging/MRCP plays an important role in CP because it is more sensitive in detecting mild disease. MR imaging/MRCP allows the visualization of parenchymal signal changes, abnormal enhancement pattern, and ductal changes; and S-MRCP can also indirectly estimate exocrine function of the pancreas.

REFERENCES

1. Pandol SJ, Saluja AK, Imrie CW, et al. Acute pancreatitis: bench to the bedside. Gastroenterology 2007; 132:1127–51.
2. Etemad B, Whitcomb DC. Chronic pancreatitis: diagnosis, classification, and new genetic developments. Gastroenterology 2001;120:682–707.
3. Bozkurt T, Braun U, Leferink S, et al. Comparison of pancreatic morphology and exocrine functional impairment in patients with chronic pancreatitis. Gut 1994;35:1132–6.
4. Levy P, Mathurin P, Roqueplo A, et al. A multidimensional case-control study of dietary, alcohol, and tobacco habits in alcoholic men with chronic pancreatitis. Pancreas 1995;10:231–8.
5. Pandol SJ, Rarity M. Pathobiology of alcoholic pancreatitis. Pancreatology 2007;7:105–14.
6. Pitchumoni CS. Pathogenesis of alcohol-induced chronic pancreatitis. Surg Clin North Am 2001;81: 379–90.
7. Steer ML, Waxman I, Freedman S. Chronic pancreatitis. N Engl J Med 1995;332:1482–90.
8. Luetmer PH, Stephens DH, Ward EM. Chronic pancreatitis: reassessment with current CT. Radiology 1989;171:353–7.
9. Lesniak RJ, Hohenwalter MD, Taylor A. Spectrum of causes of pancreatic calcifications. AJR Am J Roentgenol 2002;178:79–86.
10. Bernades P, Baetz A, Levy P, et al. Splenic and portal vein obstruction in chronic pancreatitis. A prospective longitudinal study of a medical-surgical service of 266 patients. Dig Dis Sci 1992;37:340–6.
11. Hsu JT, Yeh CN, Hung CF, et al. Management and outcome of bleeding pseudoaneurysm associated with chronic pancreatitis. BMC Gastroenterol 2006;6:3.
12. Bedingfield JA, Anderson MC. Pancreatopleural fistula. Pancreas 1986;1:283–90.
13. Miller FH, Keppe AL, Wadhwa A, et al. MRI of pancreatitis and its complications. AJR Am J Roentgenol 2004;183:1645–52.
14. Semelka RC, Shoenut JP, Kroeker MA, et al. Chronic pancreatitis: MR imaging features before and after administration of gadopentetate dimeglumine. J Magn Reson Imaging 1993;3:79–82.
15. Zhang XM, Mitchell DG, Dohke M, et al. Suspected early or mild chronic pancreatitis: signal intensity changes on gadolinium chelate dynamic MRI. J Magn Reson Imaging 2003;17:86–94.
16. Lewis MP, Lo SK, Reber PU, et al. Endoscopic measurement of pancreatic tissue perfusion in

patients with chronic pancreatitis and control patients. Gastrointest Endosc 2000;51:195–9.

17. Varghese JC, Masterson A, Lee MJ. Value of MR pancreatography in the evaluation of patients with chronic pancreatitis. Clin Radiol 2002;57:393–401.

18. Bret PM, Reinhold C, Taourel P, et al. Pancreas divisum: evaluation with MR cholangiopancreatography. Radiology 1996;199:99–103.

19. Takehara Y, Ichijo K, Tooyama N, et al. Breath-hold MR cholangiopancreatography with a long-echo-train fast spin-echo sequence and a surface coil in chronic pancreatitis. Radiology 1994;192:73–8.

20. Tamura R, Ishibashi T, Takahashi S. Chronic pancreatitis: MRCP versus ERCP for quantitative caliber measurement and qualitative evaluation. Radiology 2006;238:920–8.

21. Balci NC, Alkaade S, Magas L, et al. Suspected chronic pancreatitis with normal MRCP: findings on MRI in correlation with secretin MRCP. J Magn Reson Imaging 2008;27:125–31.

22. Ceppelliez O, Delhaye M, Deviere J, et al. Chronic pancreatitis: evaluation of pancreatic exocrine function with MR pancreatography after secretin stimulation. Radiology 2000;215:358–64.

23. Manfredi R, Costamagna G, Brizi MG, et al. Severe chronic pancreatitis versus suspected pancreatic disease: dynamic MR cholangiopancreatography after secretin stimulation. Radiology 2000;214: 849–55.

24. Erturk SM, Ichikawa T, Motosugi U, et al. Diffusion-weighted MR imaging in the evaluation of pancreatic exocrine function before and after secretin stimulation. Am J Gastroenterol 2006;101:133–6.

25. Mitchell RM, Byrne MF, Baillie J. Pancreatitis. Lancet 2003;361:1447–55.

26. Catalano MF, Sahai A, Levy M, et al. EUS-based criteria for the diagnosis of chronic pancreatitis: the Rosemont classification. Gastrointest Endosc 2009;69:1251–61.

27. Malka D, Hammel P, Maire F, et al. Risk of pancreatic adenocarcinoma in chronic pancreatitis. Gut 2002; 51:849–52.

28. Ogawa H, Itoh S, Ikeda M, et al. Intraductal papillary mucinous neoplasms of the pancreas: assessment of the likelihood of invasiveness with multisection CT. Radiology 2008;248:876–86.

29. Taouli B, Vilgrain V, Vullierme MP, et al. Intraductal papillary mucinous tumors of the pancreas: helical CT with histopathologic correlation. Radiology 2000; 217:757–64.

30. Suda K, Mogaki M, Oyama T, et al. Histopathologic and immunohistochemical studies on alcoholic pancreatitis and chronic obstructive pancreatitis: special emphasis on ductal obstruction and genesis of pancreatitis. Am J Gastroenterol 1990;85:271–6.

31. Kim T, Murakami T, Takamura M, et al. Pancreatic mass due to chronic pancreatitis: correlation of CT

and MR imaging features with pathologic findings. AJR Am J Roentgenol 2001;177:367–71.

32. Prokesh RW, Chow LC, Beaulieu CT, et al. Isoattenuating pancreatic adenocarcinoma at multidetector row CT: secondary signs. Radiology 2002;224: 764–8.

33. Köhler H, Lankisch PG. Acute pancreatitis and hyperamylasaemia in pancreatic carcinoma. Pancreas 1987;2:117–9.

34. Sakorafas GH, Friess H, Dervenis CG. Villous tumors of duodenum: biological characters and clinical implications. Scand J Gastroenterol 2000; 35:337–44.

35. Chappuis CW, Divincenti FC, Cohn I Jr. Villous tumors of duodenum. Ann Surg 1989;209:593–8.

36. Braga M, Stella M, Zerbi A, et al. Giant villous adenoma of duodenum. Br J Surg 1986;73:924.

37. Kalady MF, Peterson B, Baillie J, et al. Pancreatic duct strictures: identifying risk of malignancy. Ann Surg Oncol 2004;11:581–8.

38. Nguyen-Tang T, Dumonceau JM. Endoscopic treatment in chronic pancreatitis, timing, duration and type of intervention. Best Pract Res Clin Gastroenterol 2010;24:281–98.

39. Sherman S, Lehman G. Sphincter of Oddi dysfunction: diagnosis and treatment. JOP 2001;2:382–400.

40. Guelrud M, Mendoza S, Rossiter G, et al. Sphincter of Oddi manometry in healthy volunteers. Dig Dis Sci 1990;35:38–46.

41. Aisen AM, Sherman S, Jennings SG, et al. Comparison of secretin-stimulated magnetic resonance pancreatography and manometry results in patients with suspected sphincter of Oddi dysfunction. Acad Radiol 2008;15:601–9.

42. Ichikawa T, Sou H, Araki T, et al. Duct-penetrating sign at MRCP: usefulness for differentiating inflammatory pancreatic mass from pancreatic carcinomas. Radiology 2001;221:107–16.

43. Gambhir SS, Czernin J, Schwimmer J, et al. A tabulated summary of the FDG PET literature. J Nucl Med 2001;42(S1):1S–93S.

44. van Kouwen MC, Jansen JB, van Goor H, et al. FDG-PET is able to detect pancreatic carcinoma in chronic pancreatitis. Eur J Nucl Med Mol Imaging 2005;32:399–404.

45. Zimny M, Bares R, Fass J, et al. Fluorine-18 fluorodeoxyglucose positron emission tomography in the differential diagnosis of pancreatic carcinoma: a report of 106 cases. Eur J Nucl Med 1997;24: 678–82.

46. Chari ST, Smyrk TC, Levy MJ, et al. Diagnosis of autoimmune pancreatitis: the Mayo Clinic experience. Clin Gastroenterol Hepatol 2006;4:1010–6.

47. Weber SM, Cubukcu-Dimopulo O, Palesty JA, et al. Lymphoplasmacytic sclerosing pancreatitis: inflammatory mimic of pancreatic carcinoma. J Gastrointest Surg 2003;7:129–37.

48. Notohara K, Burgart LJ, Yadav D, et al. Idiopathic chronic pancreatitis with periductal lymphoplasmacytic infiltration: clinicopathologic features of 35 cases. Am J Surg Pathol 2003;27:1119–27.

49. Kamisawa T, Funata N, Hayashi Y. Lymphoplasmacytic sclerosing pancreatitis is a pancreatic lesion of IgG4-related systemic disease. Am J Surg Pathol 2004;28:1114.

50. Deshpande V, Mino-Kenudson M, Brugge W, et al. Autoimmune pancreatitis: more than just a pancreatic disease? A contemporary review of its pathology. Arch Pathol Lab Med 2005;129:1148–54.

51. Okazaki K, Kawa S, Kamisawa T, et al. Research committee of intractable diseases of the pancreas. Clinical diagnostic criteria of autoimmune pancreatitis: revised proposal. J Gastroenterol 2006;41:626–31.

52. Kamisawa T, Egawa N, Nakajima H, et al. Clinical difficulties in the differentiation of autoimmune pancreatitis and pancreatic carcinoma. Am J Gastroenterol 2003;98:2694–9.

53. Irie H, Honda H, Baba S, et al. Autoimmune pancreatitis: CT and MR characteristics. AJR Am J Roentgenol 1998;170:1323–7.

54. Sahani DV, Kalva SP, Farrell J, et al. Autoimmune pancreatitis: imaging features. Radiology 2004;233:345–52.

55. Sahani VD, Sainani N, Deshpande V, et al. Autoimmune pancreatitis: disease evolution, staging, response assessment and CT features that predict response to corticosteroid therapy. Radiology 2009;250:118–29.

56. Takahashi N, Fletcher JG, Fidler JL, et al. Dual-phase CT of autoimmune pancreatitis: a multireader study. AJR Am J Roentgenol 2008;190:280–6.

57. Kamisawa T, Chen PY, Tu Y, et al. MRCP and MRI findings in 9 patients with autoimmune pancreatitis. World J Gastroenterol 2006;12:2919–22.

58. Kamisawa T, Egawa N, Nakajima H, et al. Extrapancreatic lesions in autoimmune pancreatitis. J Clin Gastroenterol 2005;39:904–7.

59. Kawa S, Hamano H, Ozaki Y, et al. Long-term follow-up of autoimmune pancreatitis: characteristics of chronic disease and recurrence. Clin Gastroenterol Hepatol 2009;7:S18–22.

60. Kamisawa T, Okamoto A. Prognosis of autoimmune pancreatitis. J Gastroenterol 2007;42(S18):59–62.

61. Yadav D, Notahara K, Smyrk TC, et al. Idiopathic tumefactive chronic pancreatitis: clinical profile, histology, and natural history after resection. Clin Gastroenterol Hepatol 2003;1:129–35.

62. Vlachou PA, Khalili K, Jang HJ, et al. IgG4-related sclerosing disease: autoimmune pancreatitis and extrapancreatic manifestations. Radiographics 2011;31:1379–402.

63. Wakabayashi T, Kawaura Y, Satomura Y, et al. Clinical and imaging features of autoimmune pancreatitis with focal pancreatic swelling or mass formation: comparison with so-called tumor-forming pancreatitis and pancreatic carcinoma. Am J Gastroenterol 2003;98:2679–87.

64. Stolte M, Weiss W, Volkholz H, et al. A special form of segmental pancreatitis: "groove pancreatitis." Hepatogastroenterology 1982;29:198–208.

65. Adsay NV, Zamboni G. Paraduodenal pancreatitis: a clinico-pathologically distinct entity unifying "cystic dystrophy of heterotopic pancreas," "para-duodenal wall cyst," and "groove pancreatitis." Semin Diagn Pathol 2004;21:247–54.

66. Blasbalg R, Hueb Baroni R, Nobrega Costa D, et al. MRI features of groove pancreatitis. AJR Am J Roentgenol 2007;189:73–80.

67. Shanbhogue AK, Fasih N, Surabhi VR, et al. A clinical and radiological review of uncommon types and causes of pancreatitis. Radiographics 2009;29:1003–26.

68. Balakrishnan V, Unnikrishnan AG, Thomas V, et al. Chronic pancreatitis. A prospective study nationwide of 1086 subjects from India. JOP 2008;9:593–600.

69. Bhatia E, Choudhuri G, Sikora SS, et al. Tropical calcific pancreatitis: strong association with SPINK 1 trypsin inhibitor mutations. Gastroenterology 2002;123:1020–5.

70. Petersen JM. Tropical pancreatitis. J Clin Gastroenterol 2002;35:61–6.

71. Moorthy TR, Nalini N, Narendranathan M. Ultrasound imaging in tropical pancreatitis. J Clin Ultrasound 1992;20:389–93.

72. Chari ST, Mohan V, Pitchumoni CS, et al. Risk of pancreatic cancer in tropical calcifying pancreatitis: an epidemiologic study. Pancreas 1994;9:62–6.

73. Rebours V, Boutron-Ruault MC, Schnee M, et al. Risk of pancreatic adenocarcinoma in patients with hereditary pancreatitis: a national exhaustive series. Am J Gastroenterol 2008;103:111–9.

74. Ellis I, Lerch MM, Whitcomb DC, Consensus Committees of the European Registry of Hereditary Pancreatic Diseases, Midwest Multi-Center Pancreatic Study Group, International Association of Pancreatology. Genetic testing for hereditary pancreatitis: guidelines for indications, counseling, consent and privacy issues. Pancreatology 2001;1:405–15.

Cystic Tumors of the Pancreas: Imaging and Management

Catherine E. Dewhurst, MB BCh, BAO, BMedSc[a],
Koenraad J. Mortele, MD[b],*

KEYWORDS

• Pancreas • Cystic lesions • Mucinous • MR imaging

Cystic tumors of the pancreas are a diverse group of lesions that vary from benign to premalignant to frankly malignant entities. There has been a 20-fold increase in the detection of cystic pancreatic lesions in the last 15 years, most notably by cross-sectional modalities such as computed tomography (CT) and magnetic resonance (MR) imaging.[1] The true prevalence of pancreatic cystic lesions is unknown but has previously been reported to be in the range 2.4% to 16.0%, and they are detected more with increasing age.[2,3] One study reported prevalence of incidental pancreatic cystic lesions on MR imaging to be in the order of 13.5% and showed that the prevalence and cyst size also increased with age.[4] These findings have been corroborated at autopsy with the prevalence of cystic lesions approaching 25%.[5]

Given that the prevalence of pancreatic cystic lesions is increasing because of increased detection by cross-sectional imaging, and that most cystic pancreatic lesions are neoplastic, accurate diagnosis via clinical information, radiological images, and endoscopic ultrasound (EUS) with cyst fluid analysis may play an important role.[6–8] Most of these lesions, especially when large, have characteristic imaging features at radiology, and accurate differentiation between them is

Differential diagnosis of cystic pancreatic lesions
Common
Serous microcystic pancreatic adenoma
Mucinous cystic tumor
Intraductal papillary mucinous neoplasm (IPMN)
Solid pseudopapillary tumor (SPT)
Uncommon
Cystic endocrine tumor
Cystic metastases to the pancreas
Cystic teratoma of the pancreas
Pancreatic lymphangiomas/lymphoepithelial cyst of the pancreas

The authors have no conflicts of interest and nothing to disclose.
[a] Division of Abdominal Imaging and MRI, Department of Radiology, Beth Israel Deaconess Medical Center, 330 Brookline Avenue, Boston, MA 02115, USA; [b] Abdominal Imaging and MRI, Division of Clinical MRI, Harvard Medical School, Beth Israel Deaconess Medical Center, 330 Brookline Avenue, Ansin 224, Boston, MA 02115, USA
* Corresponding author.
E-mail address: kmortele@bidmc.harvard.edu

Radiol Clin N Am 50 (2012) 467–486
doi:10.1016/j.rcl.2012.03.001

Key Points: SEROUS MICROCYSTIC PANCREATIC ADENOMA

- They are benign lesions and often discovered incidentally
- 80% are found in women, average age 60 years (grandmother lesion)
- Increased incidence in von Hippel-Lindau disease
- Solitary, large (>5 cm)
- Well-circumscribed, but not encapsulated, lobulated lesion
- Cysts more than 6 in number, measure less than 2 cm
- Central stellate scar, calcifications centrally 30%

---

important to help guide future treatment and management.[9,10] Nevertheless, smaller lesions may appear indeterminate and the management pathways of these may be confusing and variable. This article reviews the histopathologic features and common imaging findings for an array of cystic pancreatic neoplasms, including the common cystic tumors of the pancreas: serous microcystic adenoma, mucinous cystic tumor (MCT), IPMN, and SPT. Uncommon cystic tumors of the pancreas include cystic endocrine tumors, cystic metastases, cystic teratomas, and lymphangiomas. This article also provides comprehensive algorithms on how to manage the individual lesions, with recommendations on when to reimage patients.

COMMON CYSTIC TUMORS OF THE PANCREAS
Serous Microcystic Adenoma

Serous microcystic adenoma is an uncommon tumor of the pancreas making up 1% to 2% of exocrine pancreatic tumors.[11] Eighty percent of these occur in women more than 60 years old, hence the term grandmother lesion.[12] Serous microcystic adenomas are benign and many are found incidentally. There is a slight predominance of occurrence in the pancreatic head, but they have been reported to occur throughout the pancreas. Atrophy of pancreatic tissue and dilatation of the pancreatic or biliary ductal systems proximal to the lesion are not commonly seen because of the tumor's tendency to displace surrounding structures rather than invade them. The tumor tends not to cause many clinical symptoms, and so can become large before being detected. Mass effect, caused by larger tumors on surrounding structures, may lead to symptoms such as nausea or nonspecific abdominal discomfort.[11–13] Larger tumors (>4 cm) may grow fast (approximately 2 cm/y) and become symptomatic. Therefore, in some institutions, these larger lesions, albeit benign, are surgically removed. Hemorrhage has occasionally been reported either from the

tumor bleeding into itself or from the gastrointestinal system secondary to ulceration from stretching of the stomach or duodenum over the tumor.[12] Whether this tumor occurs with an increased frequency in diabetics is still debated.[11,12] There is also an increased incidence of serous microcystic adenoma in patients with von Hippel-Lindau disease.[12,14,15]

Histopathologically, these lesions comprise multiple cysts (usually >6) measuring less than 2 cm and separated by thin septa lined by epithelial cells. The cysts are filled with serous fluid and the larger cysts are typically located peripherally, contributing to the lesion's lobulated contour. Grossly, the tumor has been described as having the appearance of a cluster of grapes.[16–18] In 30% of cases, the cysts are arranged around a central fibrous scar in a sunburst pattern.[19] These scars tend to have areas of coarse calcification in tumors that measure greater than 5 cm (**Fig. 1**).[16]

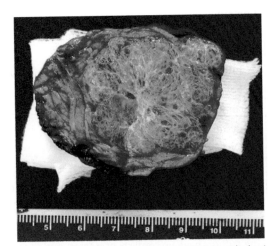

Fig. 1. Serous microcystic adenoma. Histopathologically, serous microcystic adenomas comprise multiple cysts (usually >6) measuring less than 2 cm , separated by thin septa lined by epithelial cells. The cysts are filled with serous fluid. Grossly, the tumor has been described as having the appearance of a cluster of grapes. In 30% of cases, the cysts are arranged around a central fibrous scar in a sunburst pattern.

Ultrasound of a serous microcystic adenoma typically displays a well-circumscribed, lobulated lesion with decreased through-transmission. The fibrous portion of the lesion is hyperechoic, whereas the cystic portions are hypoechoic. In lesions in which the cysts are a few millimeters in size (microcysts), the tumor can have a solid appearance caused by innumerable interfaces. Areas of calcification appear hyperechoic with decreased through-transmission and posterior acoustic shadowing.

On CT, serous microcystic adenomas most commonly have a lobular shape.[17–20] Because the tumor is primarily of water density on unenhanced CT scans, they appear hypodense. Calcifications, if present, are hyperdense and generally arranged in a stellate pattern centrally in the lesion (Fig. 2). After administration of iodinated contrast material, the fibrous portions of the lesion enhance. Serous microcystic adenomas are the only hypervascular cystic pancreatic tumors and, therefore, their enhancement pattern is an important distinguishing feature that differentiates them from other cystic neoplasms such as neuroendocrine tumors of the pancreas or hypervascular metastases. The characteristically described appearance, akin to a sponge or irregular honeycomb, is seen in only 20% of cases. Lesions with fewer fibrous septations may maintain fluid density, even after contrast administration. In lesions composed primarily of microscopic cysts, the lesions can have a solid appearance with more homogeneous enhancement after contrast administration.[21] In these cases, as with all other cystic

pancreatic neoplasms, MR imaging may be helpful to further characterize the lesion.

On T2-weighted images, the cystic fluid-filled components are hyperintense relative to adjacent pancreatic parenchyma, and the fibrous components are hypointense. The cystic portions are classically hypointense on T1-weighted imaging, but may have areas of hyperintensity if there has been previous intracystic hemorrhage.[22] The fibrous components are also hypointense on T1-weighted imaging. Any areas of calcification are hypointense on both T1-weighted and T2-weighted imaging, if visible at all. After gadolinium infusion, enhancement of the fibrous septations may be seen on early and late phases of imaging, with persistent enhancement of the central scar on more delayed phases of imaging (Fig. 3). MR imaging has increased sensitivity in detecting fluid compared with CT because the fluid components of tumors composed primarily of microcysts may not be easily detected with CT. These lesions do not show significant restricted diffusion on diffusion-weighted imaging with T2 shine-through on the corresponding apparent diffusion coefficient (ADC) map.[23]

A small number of tumors have been described with similar histologic characteristics to serous microcystic adenoma, but with different gross appearances. These tumors all contain fewer than 6 cysts and the size of the cysts has usually been described as between 1 and 2 cm, but sometimes as large as 8 cm.[18] The tumors lack a central scar, and the fibrous components may irregularly extend into the surrounding pancreatic parenchyma. Several names have been used to describe this variant: macrocystic serous cystadenoma, serous oligocystic adenoma, and ill-demarcated adenoma. Like their microcystic variant, they are benign, and do not necessitate surgical resection unless the size and/or location of the tumor causes symptoms, such as pain, pancreatitis, or jaundice (Fig. 4). Several small, retrospective reviews have attempted to define discriminating radiologic features of this lesion.[17,19] A retrospective study containing 12 cases by Cohen-Scali and colleagues[19] attained a specificity of 100% in differentiating the lesion from a mucinous cystic tumor by using a combination of any 3 of the following 4 findings on contrast-enhanced CT: location in the pancreatic head, wall thickness less than 2 mm, lobulated contour, and absence of wall enhancement. A retrospective study by Kim and colleagues[17] containing 10 cases differentiated serous oligocystic adenoma from mucinous cystadenomas and intraductal papillary mucinous tumors using contrast-enhanced CT with a specificity of 90% if the lesion was either multicystic or

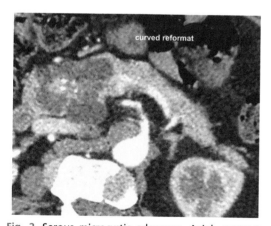
Fig. 2. Serous microcystic adenoma. Axial, contrast-enhanced, curved, reformatted CT image shows a lobulated, hypodense mass in the head of the pancreas composed of multiple small cysts with a central stellate scar containing calcifications and enhancement of the fibrous septations in a honeycomb pattern.

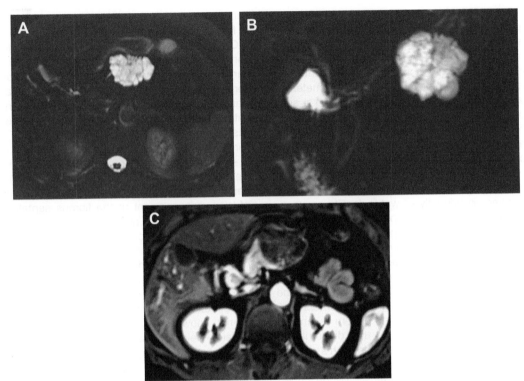

Fig. 3. Serous microcystic adenoma. (A) Heavily T2-weighted image and (B) coronal two-dimensional (2D) magnetic resonance cholangiopancreatography (MRCP) image shows a lobulated cystic lesion in the body of the pancreas that is predominantly hyperintense to pancreatic parenchyma with associated thin, fibrous septations that are hypointense. After gadolinium administration (C), during the arterial phase of imaging, there is enhancement of the fibrous septations.

lobulated cystic with or without internal septations. However, although these studies found features that may help to differentiate these lesions, definite determination based on radiologic criteria alone cannot be made in all cases. Therefore, cyst fluid analysis is important in making distinctions for this group of benign cystic lesions. For serous microcystic adenomas, cytology is positive in only 20% to 50% of cases for periodic acid-Schiff reaction, and cytokeratin AE1 and AE3. Hemosiderin-laden macrophages are seen histologically in 43% of cases and therefore still do not provide

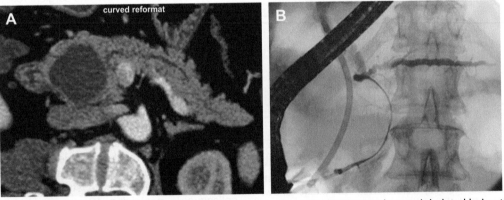

Fig. 4. Serous macrocystic (oligocystic) adenoma. (A) Curved reformatted CT image shows a lobulated lesion that is unilocular, measures greater than 2 cm, and shows no calcifications, mural nodules, or capsular enhancement. (B) Endoscopic retrograde cholangiopancreatography (ERCP) in the same patient shows external compression of the pancreatic duct by the cystic mass. The patient went to surgery and pathology revealed a serous macrocystic pancreatic adenoma.

the high diagnostic accuracy necessary for diagnosis.[24] The biochemical analysis of the fluid consists of a low amylase level (<250 IU/L), low carcinoembryonic antigen (CEA) (<5 ng/mL), and low carbohydrate antigen 19.9 (CA 19.9) (37 U/mL).[25]

Mucinous Cystic Tumor

Mucinous cystic tumors of the pancreas are rare, comprising approximately 2.5% of all exocrine pancreatic tumors.[26] Lesions within this group include the benign mucinous cystadenoma (72%), borderline mucinous cystic tumor (10.5%), mucinous cystic tumor with carcinoma in situ (5.5%), and the most aggressive form, mucinous cystadenocarcinoma (12%).[27–30]

It is not reassuring that mucinous cystadenomas occur more frequently than the other types because it has also been documented that any tumor within this group has the potential to transform into an invasive carcinoma.[26] Therefore, all are considered surgical lesions.[31]

Mucinous cystic tumors occur 99.7% of the time in women.[28,29] The mean age of occurrence is earlier than in serous adenomas, approximately age 50 years with a range from 20 to 82 years, and therefore the term mother lesion has been coined to describe them. There are only a few reported cases in men, with the mean age of presentation occurring significantly later in life, at approximately 70 years.[26] The most common locations are the pancreatic body and tail. Mucinous cystic tumors are composed of a dominant cyst that is round or oval and is encapsulated. Series have differed in the average size of mucinous cystic tumors of the pancreas at diagnosis, with average sizes being quoted from 6 cm to 11 cm.[31]

Histologically, the stromal elements of the tumor are similar to ovarian stroma. This element is important and differentiates this tumor from an IPMN, whose stromal elements are ductal in origin. The epithelial elements consist of tall columnar cells with abundant intracellular mucin. The cells can be arranged either in a single row or vertically, forming papillary or polypoid projections. Areas may have no columnar cells and only consist of atrophic epithelial cells. Importantly, the epithelium can have different configurations in different portions of the lesion, with portions of benign-appearing epithelium being adjacent to areas of invasive carcinoma.[32] This makes biopsy to determine benign versus invasive disease unreliable in virtually all cases. Coupled with the future potential for malignant conversion, all lesions are considered surgical.

Ultrasound of a mucinous cystic tumor displays a well-circumscribed cystic mass in the pancreas. Depending on the size and composition, a lesion can have an irregular contour to the wall, septations, mural nodularity, and calcifications.[33] However, because findings on ultrasound tend to overlap with those seen in other cystic tumors, further evaluation with either CT or MR imaging is necessary.

On unenhanced CT studies, the cyst contents are of fluid density, and the lesions are usually well circumscribed with a smooth morphology. Curvilinear calcifications occur along the periphery of the lesion and are seen in 15% of cases.[27,34] After administration of iodinated contrast material, enhancement of the fibrous cyst wall (capsule) along with enhancement of any septations or mural nodules can be depicted (**Fig. 5**).[33] A retrospective study by Procacci and colleagues[27] using both conventional and 2-phase helical CT scans in 52 patients with histologically proven mucinous cystic tumor found that, if a lesion contained wall or septal calcifications, septations, and a thick surrounding wall, the probability of malignancy was 94.5%. The probability of malignancy in lesions that

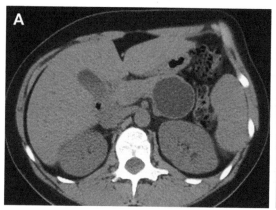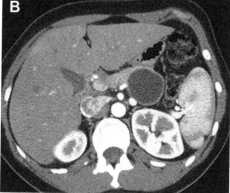

Fig. 5. Mucinous cystic tumor. Axial unenhanced (*A*) and contrast-enhanced (*B*) CT images show a unilocular, well-circumscribed, encapsulated cystic lesion in the tail of the pancreas. It has a smooth morphology.

contained any 2 of the 3 features ranged from 56% to 73.8% depending on which 2 features were present. Overall, using these features to predict malignancy, readers' ability to correctly characterize the lesions produced 81.3% sensitivity and 83.3% specificity, respectively.

MR imaging shows a cystic lesion that is hyperintense to pancreatic parenchyma on T2-weighted imaging. The capsule is T2 hypointense. It may be hypointense, isointense, or slightly hyperintense to pancreas on fat-saturated T1-weighted imaging based on the proteinaceous content of the cyst. After gadolinium infusion, enhancement of the thick cyst wall is seen on more delayed phases of imaging because it is fibrous, with associated enhancing internal septations and areas of mural nodularity (**Fig. 6**).[33] Atrophic changes in the gland with compensatory ductal dilatation, areas of decreased signal intensity on T1-weighted fat-saturated images, and heterogeneous and delayed enhancement after gadolinium administration may be seen in patients with concomitant obstructive pancreatitis. Calcifications, if visible, are hypointense on both T1-weighted and T2-weighted imaging. The use of diffusion-weighted imaging and corresponding ADC maps has been evaluated for assessment of the presence of mucin within these lesions. Mucin-producing tumors have a mean ADC value (b = 1000) of 2.7×10^{-3} mm^2/s versus pseudocyst of the pancreas and serous tumors having a mean ADC value of 3.2×10^{-3} mm^2/s and 5.8×10^{-3} mm^2/s, respectively. However, more recent studies have not been able to confirm these findings and the role of diffusion MR imaging in differentiating cystic pancreatic tumors based on ADC values remains controversial.[35–39]

The prediction of malignancy with imaging and cyst fluid analysis now approaches a sensitivity of 57% to 94% and a specificity of 85% to 97%.[40,41] Cytology is positive in 40% to 68% cases and mucinous cystic tumors stain positive for alcian blue and mucicarmine. Their fluid has a low amylase level (<250 I/L), high CEA (>800 ng/mL) and, when malignant, also a high CA 19.9 level.[42,43]

IPMN

IPMN are mucin-producing tumors arising from the epithelium of the pancreatic duct (main-duct type), its side branches (side-branch type), or both (combined type). They were first described as a distinct pancreatic neoplasm in 1982.[36] Since that time, IPMN has been diagnosed with increasing frequency with the advent of high-resolution cross-sectional imaging techniques and thus has become a more recognized pathologic entity.

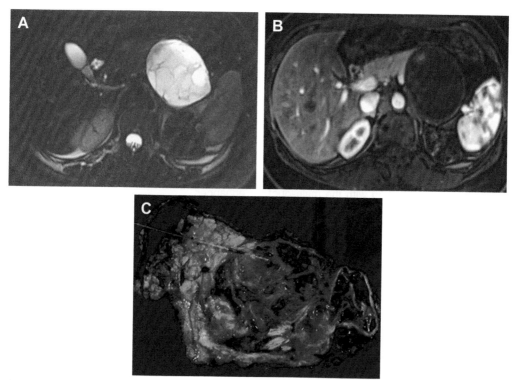

Fig. 6. Mucinous cystic tumor. Heavily T2-weighted image (*A*) shows a hyperintense cyst in the tail of the pancreas with a few internal septations. After gadolinium administration (*B*), there is enhancement of the fibrous wall with regions of internal septal enhancement and mural nodularity. Gross pathology specimen (*C*) assessment following distal pancreatectomy shows a mucinous cystadenocarcinoma.

In 1996, the lesion received formal recognition by the World Health Organization (WHO) as an "intra-ductal papillary mucin-producing neoplasm, arising in the main pancreatic duct or its major branches."[44] IPMNs have been noted to be variable in aggressiveness, from slow-growing, local lesions to invasive and metastatic tumors. This finding led to further categorization by the WHO in 2000; from least to most aggressive, the lesions are referred to as IPMN adenoma (mild dysplasia), IPMN borderline lesion (when moderate dysplasia is present), and intraductal papillary mucinous carcinoma.[45] Carcinomas are further categorized into carcinoma in situ (high-grade dysplasia) and invasive carcinoma.[46,47] IPMN typically presents in men (70%) and in the older age group, with a mean age of 65 years.[45,47] Therefore, it has been called the grandfather lesion.

Histologically, the tumor is characterized as intra-ductal with growth of mucin-producing columnar cells with differing degrees of atypia, supported by pancreatic parenchyma with fibroatrophic changes, and lack of the ovarianlike stroma typical of mucinous cystic tumors. Lesions are graded by the greatest degree of atypia present in the sample (Fig. 7).[48]

Imaging diagnosis of an IPMN is most dependent on identifying the relationship of the lesion to the pancreatic duct, especially in the case of side-branch lesions. These lesions distend the affected side branch with mucin, giving the

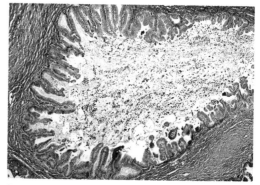

Fig. 7. IPMN. Histologically, the tumor is characterized as intraductal with growth of mucin-producing columnar cells with differing degrees of atypia (moderate dysplasia in this case), supported by pancreatic parenchyma with fibroatrophic changes, and lack of the ovarianlike stroma typical of mucinous cystic tumors. Lesions are graded by the greatest degree of atypia present in the sample.

appearance of a pleomorphic cystic mass in the pancreas that communicates with the main pancreatic duct. Identifying this communication is important, because other neoplastic cystic lesions such as mucinous cystic tumors, serous microcystic adenomas, and SPT generally do not communicate with the pancreatic duct.[15,49–52]

Ultrasound of IPMNs generally displays pancreatic duct dilatation in the case of a main-duct IPMN, or a well-circumscribed pleomorphic cystic mass in the pancreas in the case of a side-branch IPMN. Ultrasound does not generally show the communication with the main-duct of side-branch lesions. Depending on the size and composition of the lesion, other findings such as mural nodules, mucin globules, or septations may be visualized. However, ultrasound findings tend to be nonspecific and these lesions typically require imaging with other modalities for further evaluation.

On CT, a side-branch IPMN appears most commonly as a hypodense, pleomorphic lesion in close proximity to the pancreatic duct.[53] The classic location is in the uncinate process. The main pancreatic duct is usually not dilated. The communication between the lesion and the duct is best shown using curved planar reformatted images, and usually is not seen on axial imaging alone. The main pancreatic duct lesions are typified by diffuse or segmental dilatation of the duct (Figs. 8 and 9). A discrete lesion may or may not be visualized. Enhancement is generally only appreciated in lesions containing nodular foci. Assessing for enhancement is best performed by comparing the Hounsfield unit (HU) densities of the lesion before and after iodinated contrast administration to differentiate mucin globules, which are nonenhancing, from solid tumor, which enhances.

Magnetic resonance cholangiopancreatography (MRCP) has the ability to provide noninvasive, multiplanar imaging of the pancreatic ductal system, and has similar accuracy to endoscopic retrograde cholangiopancreatography (ERCP) in identifying cystic lesions.[54] Arakawa and colleagues[53] also showed that findings made on MRCP correlate with findings at histopathology. The main pancreatic duct lesions are typified by dilatation of the entire duct (see Fig. 8). A discrete lesion may or may not be visualized in these patients. Therefore, main-duct IPMN should be entertained in the differential of patients with

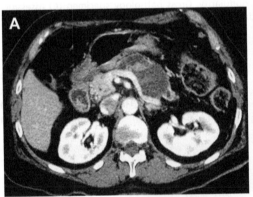
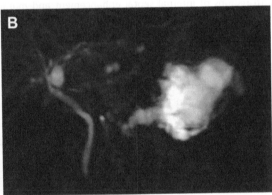
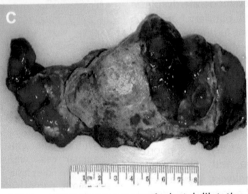

Fig. 8. IPMN. Contrast-enhanced CT image (A) shows pancreatic ductal dilatation in the region of the body and tail of the pancreas with intraductal soft tissue nodules. MRCP image (B) confirms segmental dilatation of pancreatic duct. Distal pancreatectomy (C) shows invasive carcinoma arising in combined-duct IPMN.

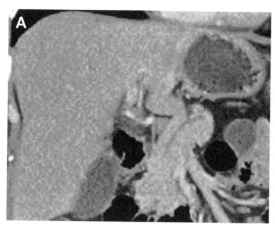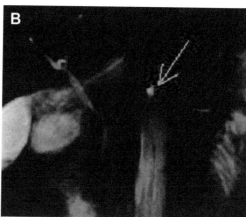

Fig. 9. IPMN. (*A*) Coronal reformatted CT image shows a small pleomorphic cystic lesion in the body of the pancreas, clearly communicating with the main pancreatic duct. MRCP image (*B*) confirms the communication (*arrow*), confirming the diagnosis of side-branch IPMN.

a dilated pancreatic duct without a visible obstructing lesion or stenosis, along with ampullary dysfunction. In these cases, an MRCP with secretin injection or ERCP may be helpful for further assessment.

Side-branch lesions are pleomorphic and are hyperintense to pancreatic parenchyma on T2-weighted imaging and hypointense on T1-weighted imaging. The lesion is either in close proximity to, or in direct communication with, the main duct (see **Fig. 9**; **Fig. 10**). The relationship of the lesion and the main pancreatic duct is generally best shown on MRCP imaging. Combined-type lesions show dilatation of both the main duct and side branches. Enhancement of nodular components or areas of wall thickening (if present) are appreciated after gadolinium infusion (**Fig. 11**).

As discussed earlier, the histologic appearances of IPMNs range from adenomas (benign) to carcinomas (malignant), with carcinomas being further subdivided into in situ and invasive lesions. The ability to reliably diagnose malignant lesions is beneficial for presurgical planning and for predicting the prognosis of patients. Several studies in the radiologic literature have thus attempted to clarify specific CT and MR imaging features that would help differentiate invasive lesions from noninvasive ones. The risk of malignancy in main-duct IPMN is 63% at 5 years and, with isolated side-branch lesions, is 15% at 5 years. Risk factors for malignancy depicted on imaging include main duct width greater than 10 mm, increasing size of side-branch lesions, side-branch lesions larger than 3 cm, presence of calcifications, common

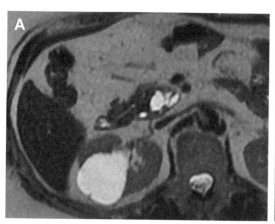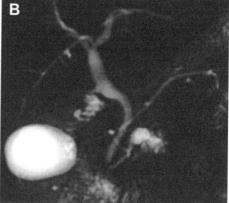

Fig. 10. Side-branch IPMN. MRCP image shows a pleomorphic lesion in the uncinate process of the pancreas, which is a classic location for a side-branch lesion. It is hyperintense relative to pancreatic parenchyma on T2-weighted imaging (*A*) and, on the coronal 2D slab MRCP sequence (*B*), communication is seen between the side-branch lesion and the duct of Wirsung. Note presence of pancreas divisum.

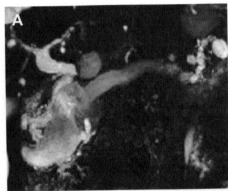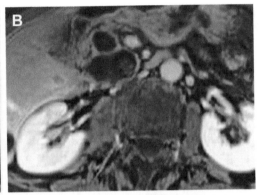

Fig. 11. IPMN. MRCP image (*A*) shows diffuse dilatation of the main pancreatic duct throughout the pancreas, greater in the head and neck compared with the body and tail of the pancreas, with associated side-branch dilatation. Fat-suppressed T1-weighted image following gadolinium administration (*B*) shows enhancement of a mural nodule in the duct in the pancreatic head. Postsurgical diagnosis was invasive carcinoma in combined-duct IPMN.

bile duct dilatation, thick septations, and/or mural nodules.[48,53,55–57] At this time, radiologic studies have not led to clearly defined criteria that reliably establish the presence of malignancy, and, even in areas of agreement between studies, differences in threshold values or the power of a finding to predict malignant disease is not well established. It is probably most helpful to have an awareness of findings that have been described in malignant disease, but not to rely too heavily on any single, specific factor in predicting the malignancy of a lesion. In general, main-duct lesions with a diameter greater than 1 cm are likely to be malignant, whereas most side-branch lesions less than 3 cm are likely benign.

IPMN cyst fluid analysis is positive for acid-Schiff reaction in 60% cases and for alcian blue and mucicarmine, just like mucinous cystic tumors. However, IPMNs have a high amylase level (>20,000 U/mL) because they communicate with the pancreatic duct, a high CEA level (>200 ng/mL), and a high CA 72.4 (>40 U/mL) when malignant.[57]

Treatment of IPMN, especially lesions involving the main pancreatic duct, is surgical resection. Preoperative imaging can both overestimate and underestimate the degree of involvement of the ductal system, and surgeons should be aware of this pitfall and be ready to modify the resection plan during surgery to ensure negative margins. In cases of invasive disease, regional lymph node dissection is also performed. The treatment of side-branch lesions without malignant features is controversial, especially asymptomatic lesions in the elderly or infirm, with increasing numbers of patients undergoing serial imaging without surgical intervention in the event of stable imaging

findings, especially if the lesion is less than 3 cm in size.

SPT

SPT, formerly known as solid and papillary epithelial neoplasm (SPEN), is a rare pancreatic tumor with less than 1000 cases described in the literature.[58] SPT occurs almost exclusively in women (85%), with most being found in younger women (mean age 25 years; age range 8–67 years).[59] Thus, the term daughter lesion has been coined to describe it among the cystic pancreatic tumors. Although some case series have reported that SPT is most commonly located in the tail of the pancreas and in patients of African and Asian descent,[60–62] other series have not confirmed these findings.[63] The pathogenesis of SPT is uncertain, but abnormalities in primordial pancreatic stem cells have been implicated as the most likely source because of the lack of endocrine or exocrine differentiation of the tumor.

SPT is usually a benign or a low-grade malignant tumor. The tumor is generally asymptomatic and, therefore, incidentally discovered in most cases. However, when it grows to a sufficient size, it may cause symptoms related to extrinsic compression on surrounding structures. It is usually solitary and large at presentation with an average size of 9.3 cm.[64] SPT tends to displace surrounding vessels and organs rather than invade them, and only rarely has encasement of vessels and involvement of the mesentery been described.[63] Rarely, dissemination has been described and, if present, is most commonly to the liver. Fifteen percent of cases are diagnosed as solid pseudopapillary carcinoma. These tumors are usually larger than

> **Key Points: SPT**
>
> - 85% are seen in women; age at diagnosis approximately 25 years; termed the daughter lesion
> - Solitary large lesion, approx 9.3 cm at diagnosis
> - No race or location predilection
> - Well demarcated on imaging and has a capsule
> - Predominantly solid and cystic components but this is variable depending on the lesion
> - May have internal hemorrhage
> - Calcification seen in 30% of lesions

5 cm , are more commonly seen in men, and are associated with vascular invasion and metastatic disease.

However if diagnosed and resected they have a 5-year survival of 96%.[64]

Ultrasound is generally not helpful in differentiating an SPT from other types of cystic pancreatic lesions. In cases in which patients underwent sonography, the presence of a large, diffusely echogenic, or complex mass that is well circumscribed in the upper abdomen was described, with or without through-transmission depending on the composition of the tumor, but findings suggesting a definitive diagnosis were not generally made, and further imaging was usually required.[61]

Tumors imaged with CT are generally described as well-demarcated, encapsulated, large, cystic, and solid masses. In cystic and solid tumors, the solid tissue components are generally noted at the periphery, with central areas of hemorrhage and cystic degeneration noted more centrally.[64–66] After contrast administration, the capsule and solid components enhance (**Fig. 12**).[66] Casadei

and colleagues[58] reported 2 tumors with calcifications, 1 with central calcifications, and 1 with both central and marginal calcifications.

MR imaging also typically shows a well-defined mass that commonly has a heterogeneous appearance on both T1-weighted and T2-weighted imaging.[66] Areas of hemorrhage appear hyperintense relative to pancreatic parenchyma on T1-weighted imaging, and hypointense on T2-weighted imaging (**Fig. 13**). After gadolinium infusion, peripheral mild enhancement is typically noted during the arterial phase with progressive enhancement of the solid portions during the portal venous and delayed phases. A key diagnostic finding of SPT is the presence of a fibrous capsule that encompasses and surrounds the tumor. In a review of 19 cases, Cantisani and colleagues[62] found that 18 contained a capsule that was hypointense on T1-weighted and T2-weighted imaging, with earlier and more intense enhancement than the rest of the tumor during the arterial phase, and progressive blending in with the rest of the enhancing components during later phases.

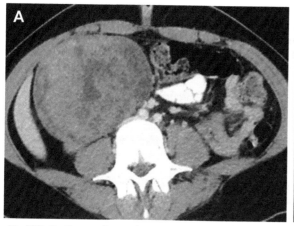 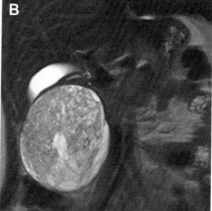

Fig. 12. SPT. Contrast-enhanced CT image (*A*) shows a well-demarcated, encapsulated, hypodense lesion in the head of the pancreas; the solid components peripherally enhance and the more central cystic components do not. T2-weighted MR imaging (*B*) confirms the cystic nature of the mass and better illustrates the T2-hypointense capsule. (*Courtesy of* Dr Jeff Mottola and Dr Dejana Radulovic, Winnipeg, MB, Canada.)

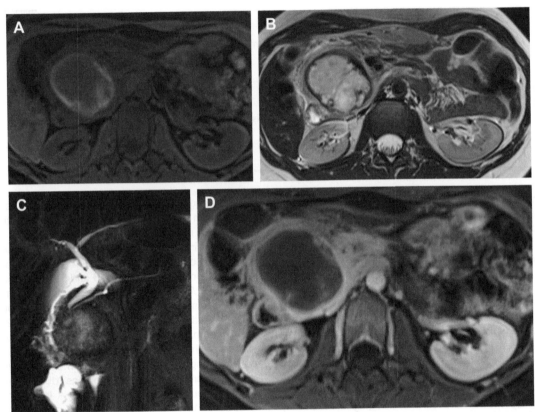

Fig. 13. SPT. (*A*) Fat-saturated, unenhanced, T1-weighted image of the pancreas shows increased signal intensity in an encapsulated, well-demarcated lesion in the head of the pancreas. The increased signal intensity is consistent with hemorrhage. (*B*) The lesion is predominantly cystic and of increased signal intensity relative to pancreatic parenchyma on T2-weighted imaging. More solid components are noted peripherally in the lesion. Note is also made of a hypointense rim corresponding with the capsule. (*C*) MRCP coronal 2D lesion showing that this lesion does not communicate with the main pancreatic duct and there is no evidence for ductal obstruction. (*D*) After gadolinium administration, there is intense progressive enhancement of the fibrous capsule and peripheral solid components of the lesion.

Treatment of SPT has generally been surgical resection but enucleation procedures have been described, made possible by the fibrous capsule encompassing the tumor. Overall, patients with this tumor have excellent survival rates, including the rarer solid pseudopapillary carcinoma (15%), which has a 5-year survival of 96%.

UNCOMMON CYSTIC PANCREATIC TUMORS
Cystic Endocrine Tumors

Endocrine tumors of the pancreas originate from the islet cells of the pancreas. As a group, they are rare, occurring at a rate of 1 case per million people per year.[67,68] They are divided into 2 main groups: syndromic (also termed hyperfunctioning) and nonsyndromic (also termed nonhyperfunctioning).[69] The cystic endocrine lesions tend to be larger than the solid lesions (8.4 cm vs 2.9 cm, respectively).[70] They tend to be nonsyndromic (64%) and, of those that were syndromic, most tended

to be of the non–insulin-producing varieties.[70] Seventy-five percent of these occur sporadically in the population but the remainder (25%) are associated with multiple endocrine neoplasia (MEN) type 1.

On ultrasound, the cystic or necrotic portion appears anechoic with posterior through-transmission.[71] In cases of cystic degeneration, there is a well-circumscribed, uniform wall, whereas, in cases of necrosis, the wall tends to be less uniform and more irregular. There are no reported ultrasound features that help to discriminate a cystic or necrotic endocrine tumor from other cystic or necrotic tumors of the pancreas.

On CT, the cystic or necrotic portion is hypodense and of fluid density. The peripheral rim of tissue typically enhances more than the pancreatic parenchyma during the arterial and venous phases, although smaller lesions may blend with the surrounding parenchyma on the venous phase.[71] Again, in lesions with necrosis, the

> **Key Points: CYSTIC ENDOCRINE TUMORS**
>
> - Rare, seen in middle-aged adults, no gender predilection
> - Usually found in body and tail of pancreas
> - 75% sporadic, 25% associated with MEN type 1
> - Most cystic endocrine tumors are nonhyperfunctioning
> - May be encapsulated
> - Solid components are hypervascular
> - Irregular solid wall, thick nodular septations
> - Round to oval shape, not lobulated

peripheral rim of tissue tends to appear less uniform and more irregular than in lesions in which there is cystic degeneration.

On MR imaging, the peripheral rim of tissue has a similar signal intensity pattern to a solid endocrine tumor, classically described as moderately hyperintense to pancreatic parenchyma on fat-saturated T2-weighted images, and hypointense on fat-saturated T1-weighted imaging.[72–74] When a capsule is present, it may appear as a T2-hypointense rim. Hypervascular enhancement is expected after gadolinium infusion, although this is not present in all cases (**Fig. 14**).[69,72,73] Dynamic acquisition of multiple contrast-enhanced images at different time points is recommended, especially for cystic or necrotic endocrine tumors, because the classic enhancement pattern helps to differentiate these lesions from other cystic tumors of the pancreas.[74]

Cystic Metastatic Disease

Some metastases present as cystic pancreatic masses. Although metastases to the pancreas are most commonly seen with renal cell carcinoma and lung carcinoma, necrotic metastases occur most often in cases of aggressive tumors such as sarcomas, melanomas, or ovarian carcinomas.[75] Metastatic disease to the pancreas occurs most often through a hematogenous route, and is generally found late in the disease process. Because of this, foci of disease in multiple organs are to be expected in patients with metastatic pancreatic lesions (**Fig. 15**).

The exception to this is renal cell carcinoma, in which cases of solitary metastatic disease to the pancreas have been described.[76] However, even in these cases, there should be a lesion in the kidney or evidence of a previous partial or total nephrectomy

Cystic Teratoma

Cystic teratoma of the pancreas is an extremely rare tumor with fewer than 20 cases being reported in the literature. Patients can be asymptomatic, with incidental discovery, to symptomatic, with detection during work-ups for vague abdominal pain. As with teratomas from other locations in the body, they can form many different tissue types including bone, cartilage, hair follicles, teeth, and sebaceous glands. They are thought to develop from epithelial inclusions, secondary to arrest in migration of pleuripotential stem cells in the process of migrating to the gonads during development, and subsequent incorporation into the tissues making up the pancreas.[77] Because the tissues comprising teratomas can be of any of the 3 germinal layers, there are different subtypes. Teratomas can be divided into mature and immature, with the mature subtype being further subdivided into solid and cystic (dermoid cyst).[78] Because there are so few cases described in the literature, the imaging findings of these tumors are discussed in this article as a group.

Pancreatic cystic teratomas appear well defined on ultrasound,[79,80] but have been described as

> **Key Points: CYSTIC METASTATIC DISEASE**
>
> - Generally seen in the setting of diffuse metastatic disease: renal, lung, bowel, breast, prostate cancer
> - Purely cystic lesions seen in cases of melanoma and sarcoma
> - Multifocal or solitary

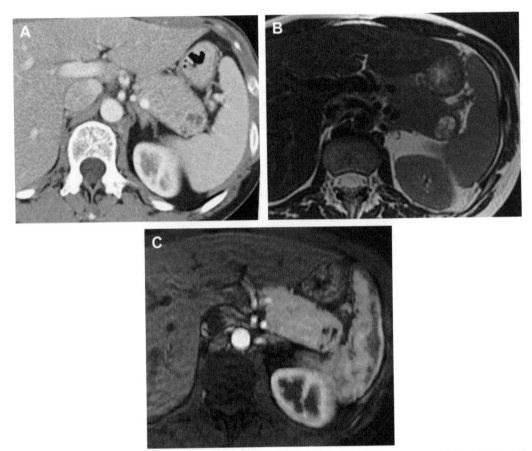

Fig. 14. Cystic pancreatic endocrine tumor. Contrast-enhanced CT image (*A*) shows a round lesion in the tail of the pancreas that shows necrosis centrally. The peripheral solid components are hypervascular. Axial T-weighted imaging of the upper abdomen (*B*) shows a lesion that is hyperintense to pancreatic parenchyma on T2-weighted imaging and (*C*) shows peripheral irregular enhancement after gadolinium on the arterial phase of imaging.

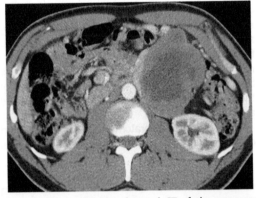

Fig. 15. Axial contrast-enhanced CT of the pancreas shows a cystic mass lesion in the tail of the pancreas. The central necrotic component of the tumor does not enhance. It is a solitary lesion. Findings at pathology were consistent with metastasis from the patient's soft tissue sarcoma.

both predominantly echogenic[79] and hypoechogenic.[80] This is likely because of the variable amount of fat and sebum that may be found in different types of lesions. Lesions containing bone or tooth elements also have areas of acoustic shadowing.[79]

On CT, teratomas have also been described as well defined.[80] The lesions are variable in appearance: low attenuation, multilocular, and cystic,[80] soft tissue with fat elements and peripheral calcification,[79] or purely soft tissue.[80] Heterogeneous enhancement after contrast has been reported.[79] Several case reports noted that, although the mass abutted vascular structures or the biliary or pancreatic ducts, there was no evidence of invasion or obstruction of these structures.[79,80]

Strasser and colleagues[77] described the appearance of teratomas on MR imaging as hyperintense to pancreatic parenchyma and well defined on T2-weighted imaging, with areas of loss of signal intensity on fat-saturated sequences consistent with bulk fat. They can have heterogeneous signal intensity on T1-weighted precontrast imaging, and there is variable heterogeneous enhancement after administration of gadolinium. Seki and colleagues[80] described the findings of 2 cases at MRCP. One appeared predominately as a soft tissue mass with a small cystic area within it, and the other was predominately cystic, with a nodular filling defect. No communication, involvement, or dilatation of the biliary or pancreatic ducts was appreciated.

Lymphangioma

Lymphangiomas are benign tumors usually found in the soft tissues of the neck and axilla in the pediatric population. Less than 1% occurs in the abdomen.[81,82] Lymphangiomas are congenital malformations of the lymphatic system, and are classified as capillary, cavernous, or cystic.[83] A review of the literature by Igarashi and colleagues[82] found that the cystic type is the most common (17 cases), followed by the cavernous type (15 cases), and the capillary type (13 cases). They also found that the lesions occur more often in women by almost a 2:1 ratio (29:16). Although they are found in all parts of the pancreas, they arise most commonly in the body and tail (30/45). There is no age predilection.[83] Lymphangiomas can grow to be large, becoming 20 cm or larger.[83] Patients may be asymptomatic, have nonspecific general symptoms, have a palpable mass, or present with acute symptoms secondary to hemorrhage, infection, torsion, or rupture.[83]

Definitive diagnosis requires surgical excision and pathologic examination.[83] Although benign, lymphangiomas can be locally invasive, but complete surgical excision is usually curative.[82,83]

Ultrasound typically shows a hypoechoic or anechoic cystic or multicystic lesion in the region of the pancreas.[82,83] Hyperechoic masses have also been reported.[83]

On CT, multiple well-circumscribed cystic masses are noted in, abutting, or attached via a pedicle to the pancreas; thin septations with a variable enhancement pattern are seen after iodinated contrast injection.[83] The cystic components are most often of fluid density, but, in cases of previous hemorrhage, the density may be higher. Phlebolithlike calcifications can occur in the dilated lymphatic spaces (Fig. 16).[83]

MR imaging also displays a well-circumscribed lesion. Because the lesion is predominantly cystic, the cystic portion of the lesion is hyperintense on T2-weighted images and hypointense on T1-weighted images. In cases of previous hemorrhage or infection, this is reflected in decreased T2

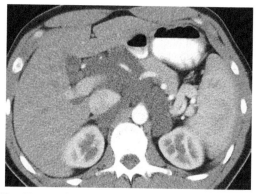

Fig. 16. Lymphangioma. There is a large cystic lesion attached to the pancreas. The most common subtype of lymphangioma is cystic malformation. They show variable enhancement after contrast administration and there may be thin septations within it.

signal, and, in the case of hemorrhage, increased T1 signal. The capsule is hypointense on T1-weighted and T2-weighted imaging, and is thin. Enhancement may or may not be found after gadolinium infusion.

(Lympho)Epithelial Cyst

Nonneoplastic epithelial cysts are seen in the following syndromes: von Hippel-Lindau disease, cystic fibrosis, hepatorenal polycystic disease, Meckel-Gruber syndrome, Saldino-Noonan syndrome, Jeune and Ivermark syndrome.[84]

On imaging, they can be indistinguishable from other cystic lesions of the pancreas. On CT imaging, the lesion is hypodense and has no capsule. Because it is entirely cystic, it does not have central enhancement (Fig. 17).

On MR imaging, the lesion can be isointense or hypointense relative to pancreatic parenchyma

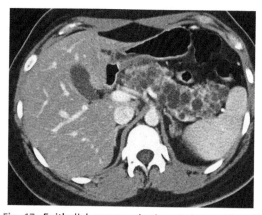

Fig. 17. Epithelial, nonneoplastic cysts in von Hippel-Lindau disease. Axial contrast-enhanced CT image shows multiple cystic lesions throughout the pancreas.

on T1-weighted imaging and hyperintense on T2-wighted imaging. There may be a thin rim of enhancement after gadolinium.

Lymphoepithelial cysts (LECs) are rare cystic lesions of the pancreas. They usually measure less than 5 cm and are usually seen in men.[85–88]

MANAGEMENT OF CYSTIC PANCREATIC LESIONS
Facts

Of all focal cystic pancreatic lesions detected incidentally on imaging, almost 75% to 90% of these lesions are stable at long-term follow-up. Of those that do progress, the mean time interval for significant growth (>20%) is longer than 2 years. The size of the lesion at first diagnosis is an important factor in determining the probability of malignancy. If a lesion measures less than 3 cm, then the likelihood of malignancy is less than 3%. It has also been shown that symptomatic focal cystic pancreatic lesions are also more likely to be malignant than nonsymptomatic lesions.[89] Therefore, we designed an in-house algorithm for the management of cystic pancreatic lesions based on size of the lesion and presence of patient symptoms (Fig. 18). Although we recognize that this algorithm requires prospective validation in patients with long-term follow-up, it has the significant advantage that patients at our institution are now undergoing an agreed-on and systematic management approach, independent of the radiologist who reads the study.[90]

In general, symptomatic lesions larger than 3 cm usually go straight for resection. An asymptomatic lesion larger than 3 cm could be further evaluated first with fine-needle aspiration (FNA) and cyst fluid evaluation (cytology, CEA, CA 19.9, presence of mucin, molecular analysis). Based on the presence of mucin, dysplasia, or cancer, the patient undergoes resection. Nonmucinous, nondysplastic lesions may be followed with short-term repeat imaging. For an asymptomatic lesion that measures less than 3 cm, observation is the recommended management. For a symptomatic lesion less than 3 cm, we recommend further evaluation with EUS and FNA to evaluate the presence of mucin, CEA, and Ca 19.9 levels, cytology, and molecular analysis. The patient can then be managed with resection or observation depending on the FNA results.

Follow-up Guidelines

Focal cystic pancreatic lesions can be followed up on imaging to ensure stability by identifying the size and other features that may be associated with malignancy (Table 1). The detection of increasing cyst size, size larger than 3 cm, suspicious features, or development of symptoms related to the lesion should prompt the reader to recognize these as risk factors for malignant change in the lesion. As to which imaging modality is the most beneficial in follow-up of lesions less than 3 cm, MR imaging and EUS seem to be the most sensitive and specific in characterizing these lesions.[91] EUS is an invasive technique and is usually reserved for when FNA is being considered. MR imaging has an accuracy of 60% to 98% in classifying lesions and a sensitivity for detection of 94.4%. Macari and colleagues[92] showed that use of gadolinium chelates has minimal impact in follow-up of focal cystic pancreatic lesions; therefore, an express cystic pancreatic

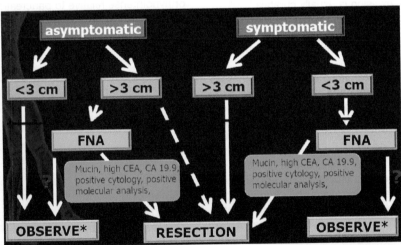

Fig. 18. Algorithm displays our standardized in-house approach to cystic pancreatic lesions. Follow-up guidelines are described in **Table 1**.

Table 1
Follow-up guidelines for focal pancreatic cystic lesions measuring less than 3 cm

Lesion Size	Recommended Follow-up
<1 cm	Every 2 y (2×) for a total of 4 y; if still stable then stop
1–2 cm	Every year for 2 y (2×), then once after 2 y; if still stable then stop
>2 cm but <3 cm	Every 6 mo for 1 y (2×), then every year for 3 y (3×); if still stable then stop

follow-up protocol without gadolinium may be used. CT is not generally used for follow-up because of radiation consideration. Ultrasound (US), although inexpensive, risk free, and widely available, is typically not used routinely for smaller lesions or lesions located more distally in the body or the tail of the pancreas because these regions become obscured by overlying bowel gas. Moreover, they may be difficult to visualize because of patient body habitus, and US is operator dependent. MR imaging has been shown to be the most consistent imaging modality for follow-up of these lesions.[92] **Table 1** lists guidelines that can be used for the follow-up of focal cystic pancreatic lesions, taking into account lesion size. When the lesion's size or appearance changes, the lesion has to be recategorized within the provided algorithm. If patients are not surgical candidates (eg, because of advanced age or comorbidities), following their cystic pancreatic lesions has minimal benefits.

SUMMARY

Cystic tumors of the pancreas represent a diverse group of pancreatic lesions, many of which have specific imaging findings that allow them to be differentiated. Accurate assessment of these lesions with US, CT, or MR imaging is important both to help guide treatment and prevent unnecessary surgical interventions. An accurate preoperative diagnosis can routinely be achieved with a combination of imaging and EUS with or without FNA. Although exact guidelines for management and follow-up of incidental and symptomatic cystic lesions in the pancreas vary widely from institution to institution, by understanding the pathology and clinical course of these lesions, only lesions with true malignant potential should be resected owing to the considerable morbidity and mortality associated with pancreatic surgery.

REFERENCES

1. Khalid A, Brugge W. ACG practice guidelines for the diagnosis and management of neoplastic pancreatic cyst. Am J Gastroenterol 2007;102: 2339–49.

2. De Jong K, Bruno MJ, Fockens P. Epidemiology, diagnosis, and management of cystic lesions of the pancreas. Gastroenterol Res Prac 2012;2012: 147465.

3. De Jong K, Nio CY, Hermans JJ, et al. High prevalence of pancreatic cysts detected by screening magnetic resonance imaging examinations. Clin Gastroenterol Hepatol 2010;8(9):806–11.

4. Lee KS, Sekhar A, Rofsky NM, et al. Prevalence of incidental population on MR imaging. Am J Gastroenterol 2010;105(9):2079–84.

5. Kimura W, Nagai H, Kuroda A, et al. Analysis of small cystic lesions of the pancreas. Int J Pancreatol 1995;18(3):197–206.

6. Jani N, Bani Hani M, Schulick RD, et al. Diagnosis and management of cystic lesions of the pancreas. Diagn Ther Endosc 2011;2011:487913. [Epub ahead of print].

7. Procacci C, Biasiutti C, Carbognin G, et al. Characterization of cystic tumors of the pancreas: CT accuracy. J Comput Assist Tomogr 1999;23: 906–12.

8. Visser BC, Yeh B, Qayyum A, et al. Characterization of cystic pancreatic masses: relative accuracy of CT and MRI. AJR Am J Roentgenol 2007;189:648–56.

9. Sahani DV, Kadavigere R, Saokar A, et al. Cystic pancreatic lesions: a simple imaging-based classification system for guiding management. Radiographics 2005;25(6):1471–84.

10. Garcea G, Ong SL, Ragesh A, et al. Cystic lesions of the pancreas: a diagnostic and management dilemma. Pancreatology 2008;8:236–51.

11. Solicia E, Capella C, Kloppel G. Tumors of the exocrine pancreas. 3rd series, fasc. 20. In: Rosai J, Sorbin L, editors. Atlas of tumor pathology. Washington, DC: Armed Forces Institute of Pathology; 1997. p. 31–144.

12. Buck JL, Hayes WS. From the Archives of the AFIP. Microcystic adenoma of the pancreas. Radiographics 1990;10(2):313–22.

13. Colonna J, Plaza JA, Frankel WL, et al. Serous cystadenoma of the pancreas: clinical and pathological features in 33 patients. Pancreatology 2008;8:135–41.

14. Kanno A, Satoh K, Hamada S, et al. Serous cystic neoplasms of the whole pancreas in a patient with von Hippel-Lindau disease. Intern Med 2011; 50(12):1293–8.

15. Sakorafas GH, Smyrniotis V, Reid-Lombardo KM, et al. Primary pancreatic cystic neoplasms revisited. Part 1: serous cystic neoplasms. Surg Oncol 2011; 20(2):e84–92.

16. Siegalman ES. Body MRI. Philadelphia: Elsevier Saunders; 2005. p. 100–1.

17. Kim SY, Lee JM, Kim SH, et al. Macrocystic neoplasms of the pancreas: CT differentiation of serous oligocystic adenoma from mucinous cystadenoma and intraductal papillary mucinous tumor. AJR Am J Roentgenol 2006;187(5): 1192–8.

18. Khurana B, Mortele KJ, Glickman J, et al. Macrocystic serous adenoma of the pancreas: radiologic-pathologic correlation. AJR Am J Roentgenol 2003; 181(1):119–23.

19. Cohen-Scali F, Vilgrain V, Brancatelli G, et al. Discrimination of unilocular macrocystic serous cystadenoma from pancreatic pseudocyst and mucinous cystadenoma with CT: initial observations. Radiology 2003;228(3):727–33.

20. Procacci C, Graziani R, Bicego E, et al. Serous cystadenoma of the pancreas: report of 30 cases with emphasis on imaging findings. J Comput Assist Tomogr 1997;21:373–82.

21. Takeshta K, Kutomi K, Takhada H, et al. Unusual imaging appearances of pancreatic serous cystadenoma: correlation with surgery and pathological analysis. Abdom Imaging 2005;30(5):610–5.

22. Sahni VA, Mortele KJ. The bloody pancreas: MDCT and MRI features of hypervascular and hemorrhagic pancreatic conditions. AJR Am J Roentgenol 2009; 192:923–35.

23. Mottola JC, Sahni VA, Erturk SM, et al. Diffusion-weighted MRI of focal cystic pancreatic lesions at 3.0-Tesla: preliminary results. Abdom Imaging 2012;37(1):110–7.

24. Belsley N, Pitman M, Lauwers G, et al. Serous cystadenoma of the pancreas: limitations and pitfalls of endoscopic ultra-sound guided fine needle aspiration biopsy. Cancer 2008;114(2):102–10.

25. Bhosale P, Balachandran A, Tamm E. Imaging of benign and malignant cystic lesions pancreatic and a strategy for follow-up. World J Radiol 2010; 28:345–53.

26. Scott J, Martin I, Redhead D, et al. Mucinous cystic neoplasms of the pancreas: imaging features and diagnostic difficulties. Clin Radiol 2000;55(3): 187–92.

27. Procacci C, Carbognin G, Accordini S, et al. CT features of malignant mucinous cystic tumors of the pancreas. Eur Radiol 2001;11(9):1626–30.

28. Crippa S, Roberta S, Warshaw A, et al. Mucinous cystic neoplasms of the pancreas is not an aggressive entity: lessons from 163 resected patients. Ann Surg 2008;247:571–9.

29. Goh BK, Tan YM, Chung YF, et al. A review of mucinous cystic tumors of the pancreas defined by ovarian type stroma: clinicopathological features in 344 patients. World J Surg 2006;30: 2236–45.

30. Nadig SN, Pedrosa I, Goldsmith JD, et al. Clinical implications of mucinous non-neoplastic cysts of the pancreas. Pancreas 2012;41(3):441–6.

31. Buetow PC, Rao P, Thompson LD. Mucinous cystic neoplasms of the pancreas: radiologic-pathologic correlation. Radiographics 1998;18:433–49.

32. Kloppel G, Solcia E, Longnecker DS, et al. Histological typing of tumors of the exocrine pancreas. World Health Organization international classification of tumors. 2nd edition. Berlin: Springer; 1996. p. 11–20.

33. Zhong N, Zhnag L, Takahashi N, et al. Histological and imaging features of mural nodules in mucinous pancreatic cysts. Clin Gastroenterol Hepatol 2011; 10(2):192–8, 198.e1-2. Epub 2011 Oct 5.

34. Chalian H, Tore HG, Miller FH, et al. CT attenuation of unilocular pancreatic cystic lesions to differentiate pseudocysts from mucin-containing cysts. JOP 2011;12(8):384–8.

35. Fatima Z, Ichikawa T, Motosugi U, et al. Magnetic resonance diffusion-weighted imaging in the characterization of pancreatic mucinous cystic lesions. Clin Radiol 2011;66(2):108–11.

36. Wang Y, Miller FH, Chen ZE, et al. Diffusion-weighted MR imaging of solid and cystic lesions of the pancreas. Radiographics 2011;31(5):1496.

37. Sandrasegaran K, Akisik FM, Patel AA. Diffusion-weighted imaging in characterization of cystic pancreatic lesions. Clin Radiol 2011;66(9): 808–81.

38. Boraschi P, Donati F, Gigoni R, et al. Diffusion-weighted MRI in the characterization of cystic pancreatic lesions: usefulness of ADC values. Magn Reson Imaging 2010;28(10):1447–55.

39. Mansour JC, Schwartz L, Pandit-Taskar N. The utility of F-18 fluorodeoxyglucose whole body PET imaging for determining malignancy in cystic lesions of the pancreas. J Gastrointest Surg 2006;10:1354–60.

40. Sperti C, Pasquali C, Chierrichetti F, et al. Value of 18-flurodeoxyglucose positron emission tomography in the management of patients with cystic tumors of the pancreas. Ann Surg 2001;234:675–80.

41. Yamashita Y, Namimoto T, Mitsuzaki K, et al. Mucin-producing tumor of the pancreas: diagnostic value of diffusion-weighted echo-planar MR imaging. Radiographics 1998;208:605–60.

42. Bhutani MS, Gupta V, Gupta S, et al. Pancreatic cyst fluid analysis–a review. J Gastrointestinal Liver Dis 2011;20(2):175–80.

43. Carrara S, Cangi MG, Arcidiacono PG, et al. Mucin-expression pattern in pancreatic diseases: findings from EUS-guided fine need aspirations. AJR Am J Gastroenterol 2011;106(7):1359–63.

44. Longnecker DS, Adler G, Hruban RH, et al. Intraductal papillary mucinous neoplasms of the pancreas. In: Hamilton SR, Aaltonen LA, editors. WHO classification of tumors of the digestive system. Lyon (France): IARC Press; 2000. p. 237–40.

45. Ohashi K, Murakami Y, Maruyama M. Four cases of mucin producing cancer of the pancreas on specific findings of the ampulla of Vater. Prog Dig Endosc 1982;20:348.

46. Nagai E, Ueki T, Chijiiwa K, et al. Intraductal papillary mucinous neoplasms of the pancreas associated with so-called "mucinous ductal ectasia". Histochemical and immunohistochemical analysis of 29 cases. Am J Surg Pathol 1995;19(5):576–89.

47. Kawamoto S, Horton KM, Lawler LP, et al. Intraductal papillary mucinous neoplasm of the pancreas: can benign lesions be differentiated from malignant lesions with multidetector CT? Radiographics 2005; 25(6):1451–68.

48. Pedrosa I, Boparai D. Imaging considerations in intraductal papillary mucinous neoplasms of the pancreas. World J Gastrointest Surg 2010;2(10): 324–30.

49. Zhang HM, Yao F, Liu GF, et al. The differences in imaging features of malignant and benign branch duct type of intraductal papillary mucinous tumor. Eur J Radiol 2011;80(3):744–8.

50. Sakorafas GH, Smyrniotis V, Reid-Lombardo KM, et al. Primary pancreatic cystic neoplasms revisited. Part III. Intraductal papillary mucinous neoplasms. Surg Oncol 2011;20(2):e109–18.

51. Taouli B, Vilgrain V, Vullierme MP, et al. Intraductal papillary mucinous tumors of the pancreas: helical CT with histopathologic correlation. Radiology 2000;217(3):757–64.

52. Hintze RE, Adler A, Veltzke W, et al. Clinical significance of magnetic resonance cholangio-pancreatography (MRCP) compared to endoscopic retrograde cholangio-pancreatography (ERCP). Endoscopy 1997;29(3):182–7.

53. Arakawa A, Yamashita Y, Namimoto T, et al. Intraductal papillary tumors of the pancreas. Histopathologic correlation of MR cholangio-pancreatography findings. Acta Radiol 2000;41(4):343–7.

54. Kawamoto S, Lawler LP, Horton KM, et al. MDCT of intraductal papillary mucinous neoplasm of the pancreas: evaluation of features predictive of invasive carcinoma. AJR Am J Roentgenol 2006; 186(3):687–95.

55. Irie H, Honda H, Aibe H, et al. MR cholangio-pancreatography differentiation of benign and malignant intraductal mucin-producing tumors of the pancreas. AJR Am J Roentgenol 2000;174(5): 1403–8.

56. Choi BS, Kim TK, Kim AY, et al. Differential diagnosis of benign and malignant intraductal papillary mucinous tumors of the pancreas: MR cholangio-pancreatography and MR angiography. Korean J Radiol 2003;4(3):157–62.

57. Maire F, Voitot H, Aubert A, et al. Intra-ductal papillary mucinous neoplasms of the pancreas: performance of pancreatic fluid analysis for positive

diagnosis and the prediction of malignancy. AJR Am J Roentgenol 2008;103(11):2871–7.

58. Casadei R, Santini D, Calculli L, et al. Pancreatic solid-cystic papillary tumor: clinical features, imaging findings and operative management. JOP 2006;7(1):137–44.

59. Choi JY, Kim MJ, Kim JH, et al. Solid pseudopapillary tumor of the pancreas: typical and atypical manifestations. AJR Am J Roentgenol 2006;187: 178–86.

60. Dong DJ, Zhang SZ. Solid-pseudopapillary tumor of the pancreas: CT and MRI features of 3 cases. Hepatobiliary Pancreat Dis Int 2006;5(2):300–4.

61. Buetow PC, Buck JL, Pantongrag-Brown L, et al. Solid and papillary epithelial neoplasm of the pancreas: imaging-pathologic correlation on 56 cases. Radiology 1996;199(3):707–11.

62. Cantisani V, Mortele KJ, Levy A, et al. MR imaging features of solid pseudopapillary tumor of the pancreas in adult and pediatric patients. AJR Am J Roentgenol 2003;181(2):395–401.

63. Lee JH, Yu JS, Kim H, et al. Solid pseudo-papillary carcinoma of the pancreas: differentiation from benign solid pseudopapillary tumor using CT and MRI. Clin Radiol 2008;63:1006–14.

64. Balthazar EJ, Subramanyam BR, Lefleur RS, et al. Solid and papillary epithelial neoplasm of the pancreas. Radiographic, CT, sonographic, and angiographic features. Radiology 1984;150(1):39–40.

65. Choi BI, Kim KW, Han MC, et al. Solid and papillary epithelial neoplasms of the pancreas: CT findings. Radiology 1988;166(2):413–6.

66. Ohtomo K, Furui S, Onoue M, et al. Solid and papillary epithelial neoplasm of the pancreas: MR imaging and pathologic correlation. Radiology 1992;184(2):567–70.

67. Ichikawa T, Peterson MS, Federle MP, et al. Islet cell tumor of the pancreas: biphasic CT versus MR imaging in tumor detection. Radiology 2000;216(1): 163–71.

68. Boninsegna L, Partelli S, D'Innocenzio MM, et al. Pancreatic cystic endocrine tumors: a different morphological entity associated with a less aggressive behavior. Neuroendocrinology 2010;92(4): 246–51.

69. Beutow PC, Miller DL, Parrino TV, et al. Islet cell tumors of the pancreas; clinical, radiological and pathologic correlation in diagnosis and localization. Radiographics 1997;17:453–72.

70. Horton KM, Hruban RH, Yeo C, et al. Multi-detector row CT of pancreatic islet cell tumors. Radiographics 2006;26(2):453–64.

71. Buetow PC, Parrino TV, Buck JL, et al. Islet cell tumors of the pancreas: pathologic-imaging correlation among size, necrosis and cysts, calcification, malignant behavior, and functional status. Am J Roentgenol 1995;165(5):1175–9.

72. Herwick S, Miller FH, Keppke AL. MRI of islet cell tumors of the pancreas. AJR Am J Roentgenol 2006;187(5):W472–80.

73. Semelka RC, Custodio CM, Cem Balci N, et al. Neuroendocrine tumors of the pancreas: spectrum of appearances on MRI. J Magn Reson Imaging 2000;11(2):141–8.

74. Thoeni RF, Mueller-Lisse UG, Chan R, et al. Detection of small, functional islet cell tumors in the pancreas: selection of MR imaging sequences for optimal sensitivity. Radiology 2000;214(2): 483–90.

75. Ferrozzi F, Bova D, Campodonico F, et al. Pancreatic metastases: CT assessment. Eur Radiol 1997;7(2): 241–5.

76. Eidt S, Jergas M, Schmidt R, et al. Metastasis to the pancreas-an indication for pancreatic resection? Langenbecks Arch Surg 2007;392(5):539–42.

77. Strasser G, Kutilek M, Mazal P, et al. Mature teratoma of the pancreas: CT and MR findings. Eur Radiol 2002;12(Suppl 3):S56–8.

78. Koomalsingh KJ, Fazylov R, Chorost MI, et al. Cystic teratoma of the pancreas: presentation, evaluation and management. JOP 2006;7(6):643–6.

79. Jacobs JE, Dinsmore BJ. Mature cystic teratoma of the pancreas: sonographic and CT findings. AJR Am J Roentgenol 1993;160(3):523–4.

80. Seki M, Ninomiya E, Aruga A, et al. Image-diagnostic features of mature cystic teratomas of the pancreas: report on two cases difficult to diagnose preoperatively. J Hepatobiliary Pancreat Surg 2005;12(4):336–40.

81. Koenig TR, Loyer EM, Whitman GJ, et al. Cystic lymphangioma of the pancreas. AJR Am J Roentgenol 2001;177(5):1090.

82. Igarashi A, Maruo Y, Ito T, et al. Huge cystic lymphangioma of the pancreas: report of a case. Surg Today 2001;31(8):743–6.

83. Bhatia V, Rastogi A, Saluja SS, et al. Cystic pancreatic lymphangioma. The first report of a preoperative pathological diagnosis by endoscopic ultrasound-guided cyst aspiration. JOP 2011;12(5):473–6.

84. Nam SJ, Hwang HK, Kim H, et al. Lymphoepithelial cysts in the pancreas: MRI of two cases with emphasis of diffusion-weighted imaging characteristics. J Magn Reson Imaging 2010;32(3): 692–6.

85. Maass J, Fronticelli CM, Macri L, et al. Lymphoepithelial cyst of the pancreas: radiological and pathological findings. Eur Radiol 1995;5:448–50.

86. Adsay NV, Hasteh F, Cheng JD, et al. Lymphoepithelial cysts of the pancreas: a report of 12 cases and a review of the literature. Mod Pathol 2002;15(5): 492–501.

87. Liu J, Shin HJ, Rubenchik I, et al. Cytological features of lymphoepithelial cyst of the pancreas: two preoperatively diagnosed cases based on fine-needle aspiration. Diagn Cytopathol 1999; 21(5):346–50.

88. Karim Z, Walker B, Lam E. Lymphoepithelial cysts of the pancreas: the use of endoscopic ultrasound-guided fine needle aspiration in diagnosis. Can J Gastroenterol 2010;24(6):348–50.

89. Lee CJ, Scheiman J, Anderson MA, et al. Risk of malignancy in resected cystic tumors of the pancreas < or = 3 cm in size: is it safe to observe asymptomatic patients? A multi-institutional report. J Gastrointest Surg 2008;12(2):234–42.

90. Ip IK, Mortele KJ, Prevedello LM, et al. Focal cystic pancreatic lesions: assessing variation in radiologists' management recommendations. Radiology 2011;259:136–41.

91. Kim YC, Choi JY, Chung Y, et al. Comparison of MRI and endoscopic ultrasound in the characterization of pancreatic cystic lesions. AJR Am J Roentgenol 2010;195:947–52.

92. Macari M, Lee T, Kim S, et al. Is gadolinium necessary for MRI follow-up evaluation of cystic lesions in the pancreas? preliminary result. AJR Am J Roentgenol 2009;912(1):159–64.

Congenital Pancreatic Anomalies, Variants, and Conditions

Lauren F. Alexander, MD

KEYWORDS

- Pancreas • Development • Pancreas divisum
- Annular pancreas • Ectopic pancreas

Understanding pancreatic development and the congenital anomalies and variants that result from alterations in normal development allows for better recognition of these anomalies at diagnostic imaging. This article reviews normal pancreatic embryology and anatomy, and the appearance of the more common developmental anomalies and ductal variants, with emphasis on CT and MRI. Common mimics of masses are also covered.

NORMAL DEVELOPMENT

The pancreas develops from dorsal and ventral buds that arise from the foregut during the fifth week of embryonic development (Fig. 1). The ventral bud forms as an outpouching of the liver diverticulum, which develops during the fourth week. The dorsal bud arises opposite and slightly cranial to the liver diverticulum. The two pancreatic buds develop independently, each with a dominant duct draining into the duodenal lumen. The main pancreatic duct forms as the dorsal pancreas grows, beginning in the tail region at the convergence of small tributaries. During the sixth week, the dorsal bud elongates and grows into the dorsal mesentery. The ventral bud is carried away from the duodenum by growth of the liver bud and development of the common bile duct. The common bile duct and the ventral bud rotate counterclockwise around the duodenum because of its eccentric growth, eventually being located just caudal and posterior to the dorsal bud.[1]

During the seventh week, the ventral and dorsal pancreas parenchymal buds fuse, with the dorsal pancreas accounting for most pancreatic tissue, including the anterior head, body, and tail. The ventral pancreas forms the posterior head and uncinate process. Shortly thereafter, the pancreatic ducts also fuse in the region of the head. The ventral duct downstream from the fusion point is called the *duct of Wirsung*. The downstream dorsal duct is known as the *duct of Santorini* or *accessory duct* (Fig. 2).[1]

NORMAL ANATOMY

The pancreas is located within the anterior pararenal space in the retroperitoneum and is divided into the head, neck, body, and tail, with the head adjacent to the left wall of the second portion of the duodenum and the tail directed toward the splenic hilum. A groove on the posterior surface accommodates the superior mesenteric artery and vein, and the latter delineates the neck, or division between the head and body. The body is arbitrarily divided from the tail using half of the distance from the left side of the superior mesenteric vein to the tip of the tail in the splenic hilum. The uncinate process is a continuation of the head caudally and is located cephalad and anterior to the third portion of the duodenum.

The main pancreatic duct runs from the tail to the pancreatic head, supplied by numerous small tributaries that enter at right angles from the pancreatic parenchyma. Most commonly, the ducts are fused at the neck, with predominant drainage through the duct of Wirsung, emptying at the major papilla. The accessory duct may contribute some drainage through the minor papilla. If the minor papilla is not patent, the duct

Department of Radiology, University of Alabama - Birmingham, 619 19th Street South, JTN355B, Birmingham, AL 35249-6830, USA
E-mail address: lfalexander@uabmc.edu

Radiol Clin N Am 50 (2012) 487–498
doi:10.1016/j.rcl.2012.03.006
0033-8389/12/$ – see front matter © 2012 Elsevier Inc. All rights reserved.

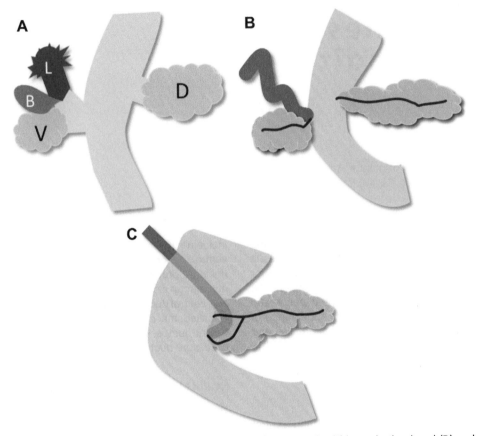

Fig. 1. Normal embryologic development of the pancreas. (*A*) During the fifth week, the dorsal (D) and ventral (V) buds arise from the foregut. The ventral bud and biliary system (B) arise from the developing liver diverticulum (L). (*B*) During the sixth week the pancreatic buds develop acini and ducts. (*C*) After rotation around the duodenum during the sixth week, the buds and ducts fuse during the seventh week.

of Santorini acts as a tributary, draining the anterior pancreatic head into the main duct.[1,2]

The duct of Wirsung and the common bile duct are linked by their common origin from the hepatic diverticulum and empty at the major papilla on the posteromedial wall of the second portion of the duodenum. These ducts pass obliquely through the wall of the duodenum with associated decrease in diameter. The ducts usually remain separated by a common adventitia for several millimeters. The ampulla of Vater is the common pancreaticobiliary channel within the papilla below the junction of the common bile duct and the duct of Wirsung, with three common arrangements (**Table 1**).[3] The sphincter of Oddi complex in the duodenal wall consists of three separate circular muscle bundles surrounding the intramural common bile duct, the main pancreatic duct, and the ampulla, respectively.[1]

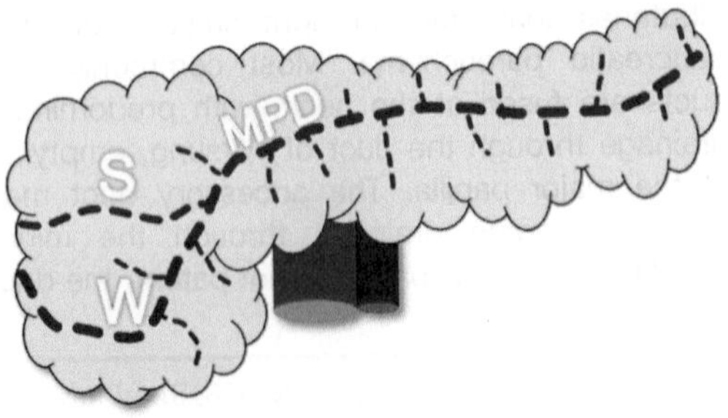

CONGENITAL ANOMALIES
Agenesis and Hypoplasia

Complete agenesis of the pancreas results in severe intrauterine growth retardation and early death. Partial agenesis more often involves the dorsal pancreas. Dorsal agenesis may be an isolated finding but has also been reported as part of heterotaxia syndromes.[4] Complete dorsal agenesis may be present, with absence of the anterior head, body, and tail, and of the duct of Santorini

Fig. 2. The normal pancreas with typical duct arrangement of the main pancreatic duct (MPD), the duct of Santorini (S), and the duct of Wirsung (W).

Table 1
Types of pancreaticobiliary union at the ampulla of Vater

Classification	Description	Incidence
Type 1	MPD duct opens into the CBD at a variable distance from the major papilla orifice	85%
Type 2	MDP and CBD open separately near one another at the major duodenal orifice	5%
Type 3	MDP and CBD open into the duodenum at separate points	9%

Abbreviations: CBD, common bile duct; MPD, main pancreatic duct.

Data From Skandalakis JE, Gray SW, Ricketts R, et al. The pancreas. In: Skandalakis JE, Gray SW, editors. Embryology for surgeons: the embryological basis for the treatment of congenital anomalies. 2nd edition. Baltimore (MD): Williams & Wilkins; 1994. p. 366–404; and Androulakis J, Colborn GL, Skandalakis PN, et al. Embryologic and anatomic basis of duodenal surgery. Surg Clin North Am 2000;80(1):171–99.

and the minor papilla. Partial dorsal agenesis involves a variable amount of absent tissue; the duct of Santorini and minor papilla are present.[5]

Partial agenesis of the pancreas may be asymptomatic depending on the volume of remaining tissues; however, some patients present with nonspecific abdominal pain.[5] Most islet cells are found in the pancreatic tail, and therefore most cases of partial dorsal agenesis are associated with diabetes mellitus. The diagnosis is suggested when pancreatic tissue cannot be seen ventral to the splenic vein at ultrasound, CT, or MRI. The potential space usually occupied by the pancreas is filled with stomach and/or bowel (**Fig. 3**). This appearance can help differentiate from pancreatic lipomatosis after pancreatic atrophy, in which fatty tissue occupies the expected location of the pancreas.[6] Visualization of the pancreatic duct system with endoscopic retrograde cholangiopancreatography (ERCP) or magnetic resonance cholangiopancreatography (MRCP) is helpful to avoid misdiagnosing fatty replacement or parenchymal atrophy of the pancreas as partial agenesis. No identifiable dorsal duct should be present within fatty tissue in the anterior pararenal space in cases of dorsal agenesis.[4,5,7]

Annular Pancreas

Annular pancreas occurs when a ring of pancreatic tissue surrounds the second portion of the duodenum. Although the embryonic development is not fully understood, annular pancreas may result from adhesion of the ventral bud to the duodenum during duodenal rotation, resulting in persistent tissue around the duodenum. Annular pancreas may be complete or incomplete, with variable incidence of 1 in 1000 to 1 in 20,000.[8–10]

Approximately 50% of all patients with annular pancreas present as neonates (mean age, 1 day) with symptoms of duodenal obstruction. Ultrasound and radiographs show a "double bubble" appearance of the obstructed stomach and duodenal bulb. Differential considerations for this appearance should also include duodenal atresia and midgut volvulus. Approximately 70% of infants with annular pancreas have associated congenital anomalies, such as duodenal stenosis/atresia, Down syndrome, tracheoesophageal fistula, and various congenital heart defects.[1,9]

The second peak presentation of annular pancreas occurs in adults in the third to sixth

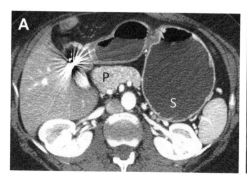
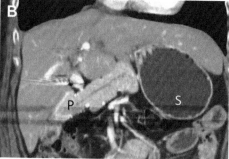

Fig. 3. Partial agenesis of the pancreas in a patient with polysplenia syndrome. Axial (*A*) and coronal (*B*) images from contrast-enhanced CT show truncated dorsal pancreas (P), with the stomach (S) extending posteriorly into the potential space usually occupied by pancreatic tissue.

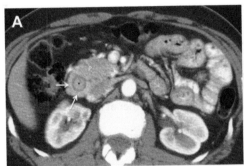
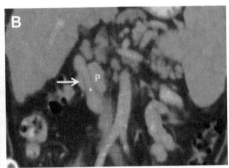

Fig. 4. Annular pancreas. Axial (*A*) and coronal (*B*) contrast-enhanced CT images show pancreatic tissue (*arrows*) surrounding the entire duodenum (*asterisk*), in continuity with the anatomic pancreas (P).

decade (median age, 47 years). Adults often present with pain or pancreatitis symptoms rather than obstructive symptoms. Only 16% of adults have associated congenital anomalies; however, approximately one-third have associated pancreas divisum.[10,11] At CT or MRI, a ring of pancreatic tissue surrounds the second portion of the duodenum, in continuity with the anatomic pancreas (**Figs. 4** and **5**). On ERCP, the duct within the encircling tissue crosses the endoscope to the patient's right. This duct usually communicates with the main pancreatic duct but may empty directly into the duodenum. Similar findings of a pancreatic duct crossing the duodenum are seen at MRCP.[12]

Congenital Cysts

Isolated congenital cysts of the pancreas are extremely rare. They are distinguished from postinflammatory pseudocysts through the presence of a cuboidal or stratified squamous epithelial lining.[1] von Hippel-Lindau disease (VHL) is associated with nonneoplastic epithelial-lined pancreatic cysts in addition to central nervous system hemangioblastomas; pheochromocytoma; renal cysts and renal

cell carcinoma; pancreatic endocrine tumors; pancreatic serous microcystic adenomas; and epididymal or broad-ligament cystadenomas. Pancreatic cysts and serous cystadenomas have been reported in 17% to 56% of patients with VHL, and 35% to 70% of patients with VHL have some sort of pancreatic involvement.[13] Most pancreatic lesions are single or multiple cysts, and multiple pancreatic cysts may be the only abdominal manifestation (**Figs. 6** and **7**).[14,15]

Ectopic Tissue

Ectopic pancreas (heterotopic pancreas) is defined as pancreatic tissue with no anatomic or vascular connection to the normal pancreas. The incidence on autopsy is variable, with reports ranging from 1% to 15%.[1,16,17] The most common locations include the gastric antrum, proximal duodenum, and jejunum, with approximately 50% of reported

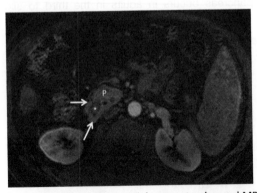

Fig. 5. Annular pancreas. Axial contrast enhanced MR images show pancreatic tissue (*arrows*) surrounding the entire duodenum (*asterisk*), in continuity with the anatomic pancreas (P).

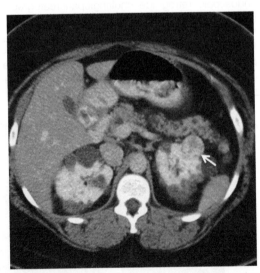

Fig. 6. von Hippel-Lindau. Axial contrast-enhanced CT shows multiple small cysts throughout the pancreas, with an enhancing mass (*arrow*) in the left kidney, and bilateral renal cysts.

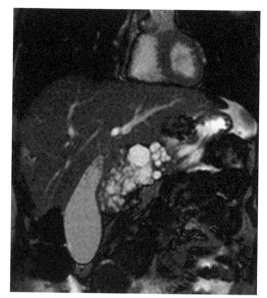

Fig. 7. von Hippel-Lindau. Coronal balance fast-field echo MR image through the pancreas shows numerous cysts with high signal intensity throughout the pancreas.

cases occurring in the stomach or duodenum. Ectopic pancreatic tissue can also be found in 6% of patients with Meckel diverticulum, and more rarely in the colon, appendix, gallbladder, and mesentery.[1,2] Microscopically, the ectopic tissue resembles normal pancreatic tissue, with small ducts draining independently or into a central rudimentary duct.[2]

Most areas of ectopic pancreatic tissue are detected incidentally and are asymptomatic; however, patients may present with epigastric pain, symptoms of peptic ulcer disease, hemorrhage, intussusception, or obstruction.[2] The ectopic pancreas is subject to the same inflammatory and neoplastic processes as the anatomic pancreas. Adenocarcinoma occurring in ectopic pancreas is

a rare occurrence, with approximately 30 cases reported in the literature.[17]

At barium upper gastrointestinal series, this lesion is usually seen as a smooth, broad-based submucosal mass, commonly in the gastric antrum or proximal duodenum. A diagnostic feature is a central umbilication containing barium, seen in up to 45% of cases (Fig. 8). This central niche is thought to represent the orifice of the rudimentary pancreatic duct. When this umbilication is not seen, the differential diagnosis includes peptic ulcer, gastric polyp, gastrointestinal stromal tumors, gastric lymphoma, or metastases to the stomach.[18] No specific diagnostic features have been shown at multiphasic CT to differentiate ectopic pancreas from other submucosal masses (Fig. 9), and endoscopic ultrasound also has low specificity.[19]

DUCTAL VARIANTS
Pancreas Divisum

Pancreas divisum is the most common ductal variant, occurring in 4% to 15% of autopsy specimens,[1,20] and seen in 2% to 8% of ERCP cases.[1,21,22] Pancreas divisum results from failed fusion of the dorsal and ventral ducts during embryonic development. Pancreatic secretions drain through the duct of Santorini at the minor papilla, whereas the common bile duct and duct of Wirsung empty normally at the major papilla (Fig. 10).[20]

On axial CT or MR images, pancreas divisum can be identified when a prominent duct of Santorini passes anterior and cranial to the common bile duct (Fig. 11). The duct of Wirsung may not be visible. At cannulation of the major papilla during ERCP, the duct of Wirsung fills but does not communicate with any duct draining the body and tail and may be short or tapered. Cannulation of the minor papilla is often performed to confirm

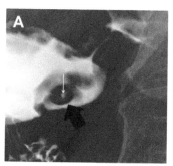
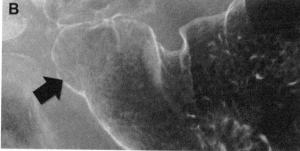

Fig. 8. (A, B) Ectopic pancreas. Two images from a double-contrast upper gastrointestinal study show a smooth, broad-based, submucosal mass (black arrow) with a central umbilication containing barium (white arrow). (Courtesy of Cheri Canon, MD, Birmingham, AL.)

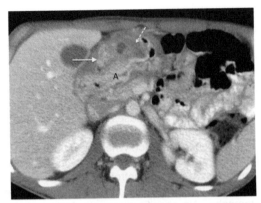

Fig. 9. Ectopic pancreas. Axial contrast-enhanced CT shows a heterogeneous mass (*arrow*) with surrounding edema (*dashed arrow*) on the anterior wall of the collapsed gastric antrum (A). At surgical resection, this mass was composed of pancreatic tissue with acute and chronic pancreatitis, abscess formation, and associated fibrosis.

the location of the main draining duct (**Fig. 12**).[21] MRCP can noninvasively confirm that the main dorsal duct is in continuity with the duct of Santorini, with the dominant dorsal pancreatic duct crossing the lower common bile duct and emptying separately into the duodenum (**Fig. 13**). No connection is seen with ventral duct of Wirsung; however, this duct is not always identified

at MRCP.[23] A santorinicele, or focal dilation of the terminal dorsal duct, may be present and is thought to develop from obstruction at the minor papilla and relative weakness at the duodenal wall.[24,25]

The clinical significance of pancreas divisum is debated in the literature, because it is often detected incidentally. Incidence is increased in patients with acute recurrent pancreatitis and chronic pancreatitis.[22] Acute recurrent pancreatitis is thought to occur because of poor drainage through the small, often stenotic minor papilla, with increasing age. Studies have shown decreased episodes of pancreatitis after endoscopic or surgical therapy. Primary therapy is usually endoscopic minor papillotomy, with or without duct stenting. Stent placement alone has not proven beneficial, and can induce duct changes similar to chronic pancreatitis. Short-term stent placement is helpful to guide sphincterotomy.[11]

Other variants of pancreatic duct configuration can occur (**Fig. 14**). Although the bifid configuration with dominant duct of Wirsung drainage is most common (60%), a rudimentary, nondraining duct of Santorini (30%), or dominant duct of Santorini without divisum (1%), may be present. A rare variant known as *ansa pancreatica* is seen at ERCP when the duct of Santorini takes a curved or looped course before its fusion with the duct of Wirsung (**Fig. 15**). This looped duct usually

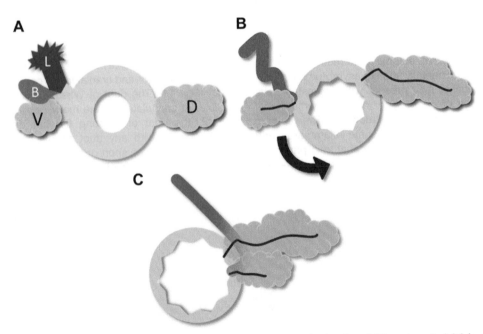

Fig. 10. Development of pancreas divisum. (*A*) During the fifth week, the dorsal (D) and ventral (V) buds arise from the foregut. The ventral bud and biliary system (B) arise from the developing liver diverticulum (L). (*B*) During the sixth week, the pancreatic buds develop acini and ducts and rotate around the duodenum. (*C*) After rotation, the pancreatic buds and ducts fail to fuse, with the dorsal duct emptying at the minor papilla and the ventral duct at the major papilla.

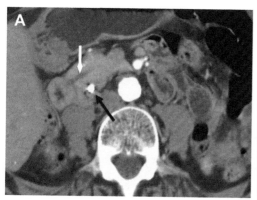
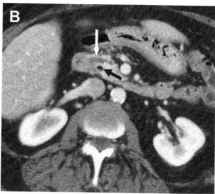

Fig. 11. Pancreas divisum. (*A*) Axial contrast-enhanced CT shows the main pancreatic duct (*white arrow*) crossing anterior to the common bile duct, which contains a stent (*black arrow*). (*B*) Similar arrangement in a different patient with chronic pancreatitis, with the dilated main pancreatic duct (*white arrow*) crossing anterior to the common bile duct (*black arrow*). Pneumobilia is present from prior sphincterotomy.

does not have an orifice into the duodenum and does not cross the duodenum, differentiating it from annular pancreas.[26,27]

Anomalous Pancreaticobiliary Junction

The anomalous pancreaticobiliary junction (pancreaticobiliary maljunction) occurs when the union of the main pancreatic duct and common bile duct occurs before the ducts enter the duodenal wall.[28] This abnormal junction is often associated with cystic dilation of the common bile duct or chole-dochochal cyst formation. Junction of the common bile duct with the dorsal pancreatic duct has never been reported, consistent with the embryologic development of the common bile duct and ventral pancreatic duct from a common hepatic bud.[29]

Because the junction of the common bile duct and main pancreatic duct occurs outside of the duodenal wall in patients with maljunction, the normal muscle complex of the sphincter of Oddi does not prevent pancreaticobiliary or biliopancreatic reflux. Additionally, when associated with congenital cyst of the common bile duct, cholestasis can occur, inducing metaplasia of the biliary tract.[30,31] Clinical features include intermittent abdominal pain, jaundice, acute cholangitis, and acute pancreatitis, although some patients are asymptomatic.[29]

The appearance of anomalous pancreaticobiliary junction is confirmed at ERCP through identifying a long common channel (>15 mm) between the duct of Wirsung and common bile duct (Fig. 16).[28] Evaluation for an anomalous pancreaticobiliary junction is more difficult at CT and requires thin-section, angled, reformatted images

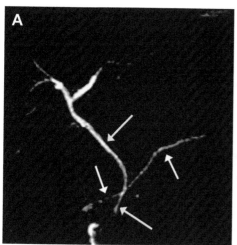
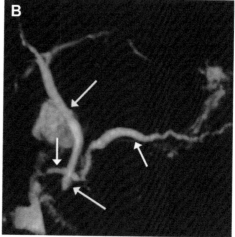

Fig. 12. Pancreas divisum at MRCP. Radial (*A*) and maximum-intensity projection (*B*) images show the dorsal duct (*white arrows*) crossing anterior to the common bile duct (*yellow arrows*) and emptying separately into the duodenum.

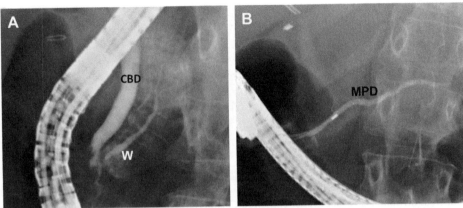

Fig. 13. Pancreas divisum at ERCP. (A) Injection of the major papilla, with filling of the duct of Wirsung (W) and the common bile duct (CBD), but no filling of the main pancreatic duct. (B) Injection of contrast at the minor papilla fills the main pancreatic duct (MPD) without any communication with the duct of Wirsung.

through the pancreatic head with optimized pancreatic enhancement. This meticulous technique can result in high sensitivity and specificity.[32] MRCP is limited by spatial resolution and has lower reported accuracy.[23] The combination of MRCP and multidetector-row CT has been shown to improve diagnostic performance compared with either option alone.[33]

MIMICS OF PANCREATIC PATHOLOGY
Fatty Change of the Pancreas

Fatty change of the pancreas (also known *adipose atrophy*, *fatty replacement*, or *lipomatosis of the pancreas*) has been associated with a variety of diseases (**Box 1**), and with obesity and aging. Fatty replacement of pancreatic tissue can develop

upstream of an obstructed pancreatic duct. When associated with obesity, fatty change can be reversed with weight loss.[34–36]

The distribution of pancreatic fatty change at imaging is often variable. In the diffuse form, pancreatic lipomatosis involves intermixed fat attenuation separating the normal parenchymal tissue. Severe, diffuse pancreatic lipomatosis is seen with cystic fibrosis (**Fig. 17**) and Shwachman-Diamond syndrome, usually with complete replacement of the normal pancreatic parenchyma with adipose tissue. Focal fatty change is most prominent in the anterior pancreatic head. Uneven fatty replacement occurs in approximately 3% of the population, usually in the sixth to seventh decades, with four usual patterns of fatty replacement (**Table 2**).[37] Focal fatty sparing often has

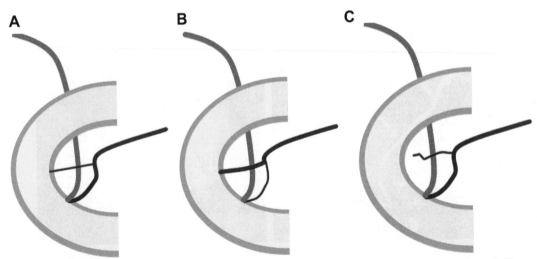

Fig. 14. Common arrangements of the pancreatic ducts. (A) Bifid arrangement with dominant duct of Wirsung drainage. (B) Dominant duct of Santorini without divisum. (C) Rudimentary, nondraining duct of Santorini.

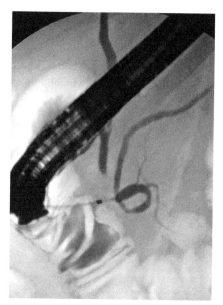

Fig. 15. Ansa pancreatica at ERCP. Injection of the major papilla shows a looped configuration of the main pancreatic duct.

a plate-like or triangular shape with higher attenuation than adjacent fatty change at CT.

Uneven fatty replacement and focal sparing can mimic a pancreatic mass. When the area is large enough, measurement of negative Hounsfield units at CT can help confirm fat density. Chemical

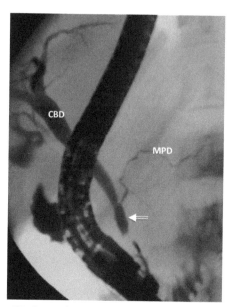

Fig. 16. Anomalous pancreaticobiliary junction at ERCP. Cannulation and contrast injection through the major ampulla shows a long common channel (*arrow*) downstream from the junction of the common bile duct (CBD) and the main pancreatic duct (MPD). (*Courtesy of* Desiree Morgan, MD, Birmingham, AL.)

> **Box 1**
> **Diseases associated with fatty change of the pancreas**
>
> Diabetes mellitus
>
> Cystic fibrosis
>
> Shwachman-Diamond syndrome
>
> Hepatic disease
>
> Viral infection
>
> Steroid therapy
>
> Chronic pancreatitis
>
> Dietary deficiency
>
> *Data from* Refs.[34–36]

shift MRI is more sensitive for detecting intravoxel lipid, with moderate to marked decrease in signal intensity in areas of fatty change on opposed-phase T1-weighted sequence compared with in-phase T1-weighted sequence (**Fig. 18**).[35] Additional confirmatory findings include the preservation of the normal pancreatic contour, lack of dilation of the common bile and/or pancreatic ducts, and no displacement, distortion, or invasion of the adjacent vessels.[35,36]

Intrapancreatic Accessory Spleen

Accessory spleens result from failed fusion of splenic buds in the dorsal mesogastrum during the fifth week of embryonic development. They are found in approximately 10% to 30% of autopsy

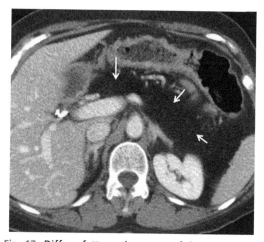

Fig. 17. Diffuse fatty replacement of the pancreas in a patient with cystic fibrosis (*arrows*). Hypoattenuating fat has replaced the normal pancreatic parenchyma, but the expected mass effect of this tissue still occurs, as would be seen with normal pancreatic tissue.

Table 2
Uneven fatty replacement of the pancreas

Classification	Description
Type Ia	Fatty change of pancreatic head with sparing of the posterior head and uncinate process No involvement of the pancreatic body or tail
Type Ib	Fatty change of pancreatic head with sparing of the posterior head and uncinate process Involvement of the pancreatic body and tail
Type IIa	Fatty change of pancreatic head with sparing around the common bile duct No involvement of the body or tail
Type IIb	Fatty change of pancreatic head with sparing around the common bile duct Involvement of the body or tail

Data From Matsumoto S, Mori H, Miyake H, et al. Uneven fatty replacement of the pancreas: evaluation with CT. Radiology 1995;194(2):453–8.

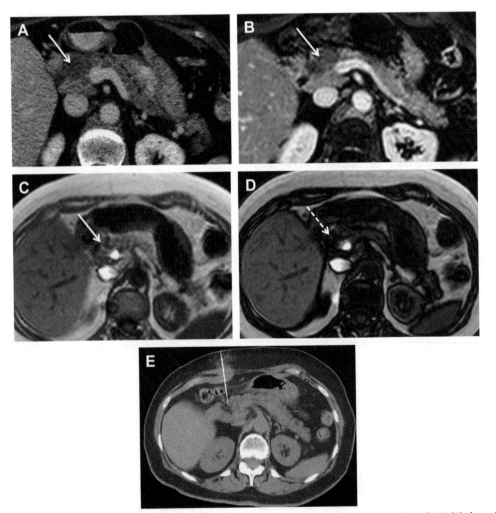

Fig. 18. Focal fatty change of the pancreatic head. Images from contrast-enhanced CT (*A*) and MR (*B*) show focal hypoenhancing area (*white arrow*) in the pancreatic head. In-phase (*C*) and opposed-phase (*D*) T1 weighted sequences show mildly heterogenous signal in the head (*white arrow*), with signal drop out on the opposed phase (*dashed arrow*) in this area. CT-guided biopsy of this area (*E*) confirmed focal fat. (*Courtesy of* Rupan Sanyal, MD, Birmingham, AL.)

cases. Approximately 17% of these accessory spleens occur in or around the tail of the pancreas. Although accessory spleens are often asymptomatic, they can be a cause of pain from torsion, rupture, or hemorrhage.[4,38,39]

At CT, the intrapancreatic accessory spleen is usually seen as a well-marginated rounded lesion, ranging from 4 to 32 mm.[38] At dynamic contrast-enhanced CT, the accessory spleen shows a variegated enhancement pattern during the arterial phase from the altered perfusion of the right and white pulp. The accessory spleen has similar enhancement to the anatomic spleen on all CT phases, although an accessory spleen smaller than 1 cm may be hypoattenuating on portal venous phase. Similarly on MRI, the accessory spleen follows the anatomic spleen signal intensity on all phases, with decreased signal intensity relative to the pancreas on T1-weighted sequences, and increased signal intensity relative to the pancreas on T2-weighted sequences. As at CT, the dynamic enhancement pattern follows the native spleen.[39]

Intrapancreatic accessory spleen must be differentiated from hypervascular endocrine tumors and metastases. Generally, endocrine tumors have more homogeneous arterial enhancement, with relative washout compared with normal pancreatic tissue on portal venous phase. A technetium 99m heat-damaged red blood cell study can be helpful to identify splenic tissue at equivocal CT and MRI cases. Approximately 90% of the heat-damaged red blood cells are trapped by splenic tissue, seen as an area of increased uptake greater than cardiac blood pool at the site of suspected accessory spleen. This study is not as useful in lesions less than a centimeter or in the presence of minimal functioning splenic tissue.[39] Some cases do require endoscopic-guided biopsy or even surgery to achieve a definitive diagnosis.

REFERENCES

1. Skandalakis JE, Gray SW, Ricketts R, et al. The pancreas. In: Skandalakis JE, Gray SW, editors. Embryology for surgeons: the embryological basis for the treatment of congenital anomalies. 2nd edition. Baltimore (MD): Williams & Wilkins; 1994. p. 366–404.
2. Cruickshank AH. Pathology of the pancreas. Berlin (Germany); New York: Springer-Verlag; 1986.
3. Androulakis J, Colborn GL, Skandalakis PN, et al. Embryologic and anatomic basis of duodenal surgery. Surg Clin North Am 2000;80(1):171–99.
4. Low JP, Williams D, Chaganti JR. Polysplenia syndrome with agenesis of the dorsal pancreas and preduodenal portal vein presenting with obstructive jaundice–a case report and literature review. Br J Radiol 2011;84(1007):e217–20.
5. Macari M, Giovanniello G, Blair L, et al. Diagnosis of agenesis of the dorsal pancreas with MR pancreatography. AJR Am J Roentgenol 1998;170(1):144–6.
6. Karcaaltincaba M. CT differentiation of distal pancreas fat replacement and distal pancreas agenesis. Surg Radiol Anat 2006;28(6):637–41.
7. Schnedl WJ, Piswanger-Soelkner C, Wallner SJ, et al. Agenesis of the dorsal pancreas and associated diseases. Dig Dis Sci 2009;54(3):481–7.
8. Sandrasegaran K, Patel A, Fogel EL, et al. Annular pancreas in adults. AJR Am J Roentgenol 2009;193:455–60.
9. Nijs E, Callahan MJ, Taylor GA. Disorders of the pediatric pancreas: imaging features. Pediatr Radiol 2005;35(4):358–73.
10. Zyromski NJ, Sandoval JA, Pitt HA, et al. Annular pancreas: dramatic differences between children and adults. J Am Coll Surg 2008;206:1019–25 [discussion: 1025–7].
11. Levy MJ, Geenen JE. Idiopathic acute recurrent pancreatitis. Am J Gastroenterol 2001;96(9):2540–55.
12. Choi JY, Kim MJ, Kim JH, et al. Annular pancreas: emphasis on magnetic resonance cholangiopancreatography findings. J Comput Assist Tomogr 2004;28(4):528–32.
13. Lonser RR, Glenn GM, Walther M, et al. von Hippel-Lindau disease. Lancet 2003;361(9374):2059–67.
14. Hough DM, Stephens DH, Johnson CD, et al. Pancreatic lesions in von Hippel-Lindau disease: prevalence, clinical significance, and CT findings. AJR Am J Roentgenol 1994;162(5):1091–4.
15. Elli L, Buscarini E, Portugalli V, et al. Pancreatic involvement in von Hippel-Lindau disease: report of two cases and review of the literature. Am J Gastroenterol 2006;101(11):2655–8.
16. Harold KL, Sturdevant M, Matthews BD, et al. Ectopic pancreatic tissue presenting as submucosal gastric mass. J Laparoendosc Adv Surg Tech A 2002;12(5):333–8.
17. Emerson L, Layfield LJ, Rohr LR, et al. Adenocarcinoma arising in association with gastric heterotopic pancreas: a case report and review of the literature. J Surg Oncol 2004;87(1):53–7.
18. Shirkhoda A, Borghei P. Anomalies and anatomic variants of the pancreas. In: Gore RM, Levine MS, editors. Textbook of gastrointestinal radiology. 3rd edition. Philadelphia: W.B. Saunders; 2008. p. 1869–84.
19. Cho JS, Shin KS, Kwon ST, et al. Heterotopic pancreas in the stomach: CT findings. Radiology 2000;217(1):139–44.
20. Yu J, Turner MA, Fulcher AS, et al. Congenital anomalies and normal variants of the pancreaticobiliary tract and the pancreas in adults: part 2, Pancreatic duct and pancreas. AJR Am J Roentgenol 2006;187(6):1544–53.

21. Agha FP, Williams KD. Pancreas divisum: incidence, detection, and clinical significance. Am J Gastroenterol 1987;82(4):315–20.

22. Morgan DE, Logan K, Baron TH, et al. Pancreas divisum: implications for diagnostic and therapeutic pancreatography. AJR Am J Roentgenol 1999; 173(1):193–8.

23. Kamisawa T, Tu Y, Egawa N, et al. MRCP of congenital pancreaticobiliary malformation. Abdom Imaging 2007;32(1):129–33.

24. Klein SD, Affronti JP. Pancreas divisum, an evidence-based review: part I, pathophysiology. Gastrointest Endosc 2004;60:419–25.

25. Hernandez-Jover D, Pernas JC, Gonzalez-Ceballos S, et al. Pancreatoduodenal junction: review of anatomy and pathologic conditions. J Gastrointest Surg 2011;15(7):1269–81.

26. Tanaka T, Ichiba Y, Miura Y, et al. Variations of the pancreatic ducts as a cause of chronic alcoholic pancreatitis; ansa pancreatica. Am J Gastroenterol 1992;87(6):806.

27. Bhasin DK, Rana SS, Nanda M, et al. Ansa pancreatica type of ductal anatomy in a patient with idiopathic acute pancreatitis. JOP 2006;7(3):315–20.

28. The Japanese study group on pancreaticobiliary maljunction. Diagnostic criteria of pancreaticobiliary maljunction. J Hepatobiliary Pancreat Surg 1994;1: 219–21.

29. Matsumoto Y, Fujii H, Itakura J, et al. Recent advances in pancreaticobiliary maljunction. J Hepatobiliary Pancreat Surg 2002;9(1):45–54.

30. Kamisawa T, Kurata M, Honda G, et al. Biliopancreatic reflux-pathophysiology and clinical implications. J Hepatobiliary Pancreat Surg 2009;16(1):19–24.

31. Kimura W. Congenital dilatation of the common bile duct and pancreaticobiliary maljunction: clinical implications. Langenbecks Arch Surg 2009;394(2): 209–13.

32. Itoh S, Takada A, Satake H, et al. Diagnostic value of multislice computed tomography for pancreas divisum: assessment with oblique coronal reconstruction images. J Comput Assist Tomogr 2005;29:452–60.

33. Nakamoto A, Kim T, Hori M, et al. Comparative study of the diagnostic ability of magnetic resonance imaging and multidetector row computed tomography for anomalous pancreaticobiliary ductal junction. J Comput Assist Tomogr 2010;34(5):725–31.

34. Patel S, Bellon EM, Haaga J, et al. Fat replacement of the exocrine pancreas. AJR Am J Roentgenol 1980;135(4):843–5.

35. Isserow JA, Siegelman ES, Mammone J. Focal fatty infiltration of the pancreas: MR characterization with chemical shift imaging. AJR Am J Roentgenol 1999; 173(5):1263–5.

36. Kawamoto S, Siegelman SS, Bluemke DA, et al. Focal fatty infiltration in the head of the pancreas: evaluation with multidetector computed tomography with multiplanar reformation imaging. J Comput Assist Tomogr 2009;33(1):90–5.

37. Matsumoto S, Mori H, Miyake H, et al. Uneven fatty replacement of the pancreas: evaluation with CT. Radiology 1995;194(2):453–8.

38. Mortelé KJ, Mortelé B, Silverman SG. CT features of the accessory spleen. AJR Am J Roentgenol 2004; 183(6):1653–7.

39. Kim HJ, Byun JH, Park SH, et al. Focal fatty replacement of the pancreas: usefulness of chemical shift MRI. AJR Am J Roentgenol 2007;188(2):429–32.

Unusual Solid Pancreatic Tumors

Alec J. Megibow, MD, MPH

KEYWORDS

- Endocrine tumor • Solid pseudopapillary tumor
- Hematogenous metastasis • Pancreas

The World Health Organization (WHO) recognizes 28 histologic classes of solid and cystic epithelial exocrine tumors and a wide variety of other tumor types, including nonepithelial tumors arising from mesenchymal elements, secondary tumors, tumorlike conditions (eg, chronic pancreatitis, pseudocysts, other cysts), ductal abnormalities, acinar changes, heterotopic pancreas, heterotopic spleen, hamartomas, inflammatory pseudotumor, lipomatous hypertrophy, and focal lymphoid hyperplasia.[1] Add to this list pancreatic tumors of endocrine origin and there becomes a huge variety of types of pancreatic neoplasms that could account for the etiology of any given pancreatic mass. Therefore, it is not surprising that a specific diagnosis of a solid pancreatic mass in an individual patient can be challenging.[2] Ductal adenocarcinoma and pancreatic cysts have been covered elsewhere in this issue. Any attempt to comprehensively review the imaging findings of the remaining subtypes would be impossible. Therefore, the following discussion is restricted to those entities that are likely to be encountered in clinical practice, specifically pancreatic endocrine tumors (PETs), solid pseudopapillary tumor (SPT), secondary pancreatic masses, and heterotopic spleen.

PANCREATIC ENDOCRINE TUMORS

Primitive neuroectodermal tumors (PNETs) are a heterogeneous group of tumors, some of which are associated with hypersecretion of hormones that produce clinically recognizable syndromes. There is controversy among pathologists as to the exact cell of origin of these tumors being either ductular cells or islet cells. Some investigators suggest that these tumors arise from a part of the endocrine cell system, being closely related to cells that give rise to carcinoid tumors, medullary thyroid cancers, melanoma, and pheochromocytoma. PETs produce gastrointestinal hormones, insulin being most common, followed, in decreasing order of frequency, by tumors secreting gastrin, vasoactive intestinal peptide (VIP), glucagon, somatostatin, and adrenocorticotrophic hormone. Case reports of renin-secreting, erythropoietin-secreting, and luteinizing hormone–secreting tumors arising in the pancreas appear in the literature.[3] The so-called nonhyperfunctioning, nonfunctional, or nonsyndromic PETs (NF-PETs) also secrete substances that display immunoreactive staining to peptides; however, these peptides are not biologically active, are secreted in amounts that are insufficient to produce clinical symptoms, or are rapidly degraded.[4]

The current WHO classification divides PETs and endocrine tumors of gastrointestinal tract origin into 3 subcategories: well-differentiated endocrine tumor, well-differentiated endocrine carcinoma, and poorly differentiated endocrine carcinoma. The well-differentiated PET is further divided into those with benign behavior (confined to pancreas, nonaggressive, <2 cm in size, functional or nonfunctional) and uncertain behavior (confined to pancreas, >2 cm in size, with angioinvasion, functional or nonfunctional). All well-differentiated endocrine carcinomas are thought to be low-grade malignancies and are categorized based on size, mitotic rate, cell proliferation

Department of Radiology, New York University Langone Medical Center, 550 First Avenue, Room HCC232, New York, NY 10016, USA
E-mail address: alec.megibow@nyumc.org

Radiol Clin N Am 50 (2012) 499–513
doi:10.1016/j.rcl.2012.03.009

(as measured by Ki-67 labeling index), and evidence of invasion.[5] Poorly differentiated PETs predominantly display small cell type histology with vascular and/or perineural invasion, regardless of the presence of distant metastases.[3] Although smaller lesions tend to be less aggressive, lesions smaller than 2 cm may present with metastases.

PETs account for only 1% to 10% of all pancreatic neoplasms. Their overall prevalence is reported to be 1 in 100,000, with an annual incidence of 1 to 4 cases per million persons per year. NF-PETs account for 14% to 30% of PET, although they have been reported in as high as 80%.[6] PETs occur with an equal frequency in men and women, with peak age being the 50s and 60s. PETs are found with equal frequency throughout the pancreas.[7] Increased frequency in patients with 4 inherited disorders is well documented: autosomal dominant multiple endocrine neoplasia (MEN-1) syndrome, von Hippel-Lindau disease, tuberous sclerosis (Fig. 1), and neurofibromatosis 1.[8] About 82% of patients with MEN-1 develop concurrent PET.[3]

There is a wide spectrum of imaging appearances of PETs, without specific features that allow for definitive diagnosis. The most widely expected imaging appearance of PET is a hypervascular focus best seen during the pancreatic phase of enhancement on multidetector computed tomography (MDCT) or as a briskly enhancing focus on fat-suppressed, gadolinium-enhanced, T1-weighted magnetic resonance imaging (MRI)

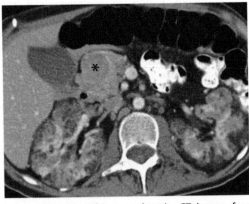

Fig. 1. PET with tuberous sclerosis. CT image from a 32-year-old man with a long history of tuberous sclerosis complex (TSC); pancreatic mass (*asterisk*) detected on surveillance. Biopsy revealed well-differentiated PET. Multiple renal hamartomas are evident. Genetic mutations in TSC activate the same molecular pathways that have been shown in pancreatic endocrine carcinogenesis.

(Fig. 2).[9–11] On cross-sectional imaging, larger lesions may be isodense/intense or hypodense/intense compared with background pancreatic parenchyma (Fig. 3). About 5% to 10% of PETs are cystic; a thick enhancing peripheral rim may allow differentiation from other pancreatic cysts. The fluid content is clear or hemorrhagic (Fig. 4).[5] Recent reports of isolated pancreatic duct strictures without apparent mass secondary to a serotonin-secreting PET have appeared (Fig. 5).[12,13]

NF-PET is more easily diagnosed, with characteristic imaging appearances in 80% of cases. These features include large masses (usually >10 cm), location in the pancreatic head, sharp definition, and lobulated borders (Fig. 6).[5,14] Differentiation of benign from malignant masses may be difficult unless distant metastases can be detected. Because the extrapancreatic metastases are frequently hypervascular (becoming isodense with brightly enhancing liver on portal venous acquisitions), dual-phase studies are particularly important (Fig. 7). Central calcifications are extremely helpful in suggesting the correct diagnosis when present in a solid-appearing pancreatic mass (Fig. 8).[15]

Other pancreatic masses that can present as solid hypervascular masses include solid serous microcystic pancreatic adenoma, SPT, peripancreatic endocrine tumors, Castleman disease, gastrointestinal stromal tumor, splenic artery aneurysm, and intrapancreatic accessory spleen (IPAS).[16]

Insulinoma is the most common hyperfunctioning PET. Patients may present with Whipple triad (hypoglycemic symptoms such as syncopy, sweatiness, and shakiness; hypoglycemia; and symptom reversal with administration of glucose). Fifty percent of the lesions are found in the head of the pancreas, the remainder elsewhere within the gland. Eighty-five percent are solitary; 0.5% of the lesions are extrapancreatic. Most lesions are 1 to 2 cm, and metastases occur in less than 15% of cases; however, 10% of the lesions are malignant. Malignant insulinomas are larger (measuring up to 8 cm) and produce extremely high levels of insulin or proinsulin, and metastases are typically present at the time of diagnosis.[17] When the lesion is solitary and localized, simple excision or enucleation is sufficient for treatment.

Gastrinoma is the second most common hyperfunctioning PNET. Most are located in the anatomic region between the pancreatic head and common bile duct and within the first or second portion of the duodenum, the so-called gastrinoma triangle.[18] The excessive gastrin production leads to the Zollinger-Ellison (Z-E)

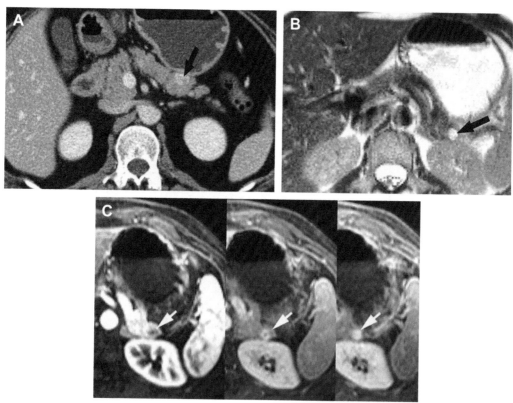

Fig. 2. (*A*) Small well-differentiated PET (*arrow*), incidental finding in a 38-year-old woman. At resection, the lesion was characterized as a well-differentiated endocrine tumor. This is the most widely recognized imaging appearance of PET. (*B*) PET MRI appearance: single-shot turbo T2 (HASTE) image reveals high–signal intensity lesion in pancreatic tail (*arrow*). (*C*) PET MRI appearance. Pancreatic, early and late portal phase images following intravenous gadolinium chelate administration shows the thick wall enhancement and progressive filling in on later images (*arrows*). The lesion was an incidental PET in a 78-year-old man.

syndrome either as a sporadic entity or as a manifestation of MEN-1. About 50% to 70% of sporadic cases of Z-E syndrome are usually the result of tumors within the pancreas, whereas the remaining cases are secondary to tumors located within the duodenum. Most gastrinomas found in patients with MEN-1 are located within the duodenum. At diagnosis, 60% of gastrinomas would already have metastasized to peripancreatic lymph nodes or, less frequently, the liver.[17]

Glucagonoma is a malignant tumor in more than 60% of patients at the time of diagnosis. These tumors are usually found in the tail of the pancreas and give rise to a clinical syndrome characterized by migratory necrolytic erythema, angular stomatitis, cheilitis, and atrophic glossitis. The patients are diabetic and have elevated serum glucagon levels. Treatment is surgical, if possible, because the tumor presents late.[3]

VIPomas produce watery diarrhea, hypokalemia, hypochlorhydria, and metabolic acidosis,

also known as the Verner-Morrison syndrome. The masses are large, solitary, and located in the pancreatic tail; 80% of these tumors will be malignant at the time of diagnosis.

Only 35% of somatostatinomas present in the pancreas, 52% in the duodenum, and the remaining 13% anywhere else. Seventy percent of tumors arising in the pancreas are malignant, whereas 50% of duodenal lesions are malignant. These tumors are extremely rare.[3]

NF-PET has a peak incidence in the sixth and seventh decades, with an equal distribution between men and women. The masses are usually larger than hyperfunctioning PNET; 60% to 83% of lesions are malignant at the time of diagnosis. Most patients present with liver metastases (see **Fig. 7**) at the time of diagnosis, but only 18% will have localized disease in the liver. Still, most experienced surgeons attempt to resect as many lesions as possible. In general, survival is excellent when compared with ductal adenocarcinoma, with

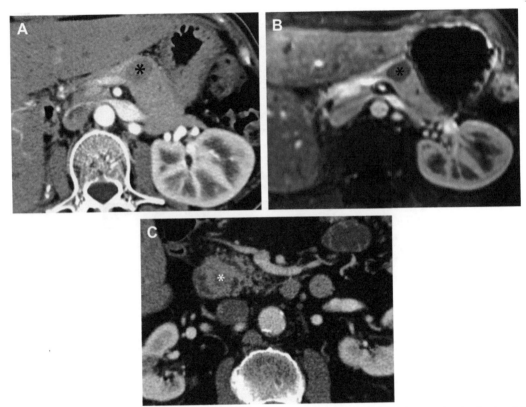

Fig. 3. (A) Hypodense PET. A homogeneous-appearing hypodense mass (asterisk) is seen in the body of the pancreas. (B) Same patient as in A. The mass (asterisk) is hypointense compared with contrast-enhanced pancreatic parenchyma on the gadolinium-enhanced gradient-recall echo image. A 2.3-cm well-differentiated PET was resected. (C) Isodense PET. Periampullary mass (asterisk) with slight decrease in central attenuation is indistinguishable from pancreatic adenocarcinoma. Biopsy of a hepatic lesion revealed metastatic endocrine tumor with positive staining for gastrin.

5-year survival rates approaching 70% and 10-year survival rates approaching 50% of patients.[19] Because these tumors are more likely to be malignant and lesions smaller than 2 cm may present with metastases, the need for imaging acquisitions in both pancreatic and portal venous phases (Fig. 9) is underscored.

Multiphase MDCT remains the first imaging choice for patients suspected of harboring hyperfunctioning PET tumors.[20] MDCT has been shown to increase the detection of insulinomas to 94% compared with single-slice CT success rate of 29%.[21] The median sensitivity of tumor detection for all subtypes is of the order of 84%. Multiple studies confirm the increased sensitivity of arterial phase images compared with portal venous phase images.[21,22] In our practice, we obtain images approximately 40 seconds (pancreatic phase) and 70 seconds (portal phase) following intravenous (IV) contrast administration. We use the narrowest detector configuration to optimize

3-dimensional (3D) visualization. IV contrast is delivered at a minimum of 3 mL/s (preferably 4–5 mL/s), and we use 1.5 mL/kg of 300-mgI/mL contrast. The overall detection rate is similar for MRI: 85%. MRI has a sensitivity of 100% for lesions larger than 3 cm but has extremely poor performance for smaller lesions.[23] During MRI, PET displays significantly higher signal intensity than normal pancreas on T2-weighted images and demonstrate a ringlike enhancement following IV contrast.[24] In our practice, we use a multisequence approach consisting of unenhanced in-phase and opposed-phase T1 images, fat-suppressed T2-weighted images, single-shot fast T2-weighted images, and magnetic resonance pancreatogram and cholangiogram images. We then administer IV gadolinium chelates and sequentially image the pancreas during early arterial, late arterial, or pancreatic, portal, and equilibrium phases using 3D volume interpolated breath-hold examination. This sequence provides

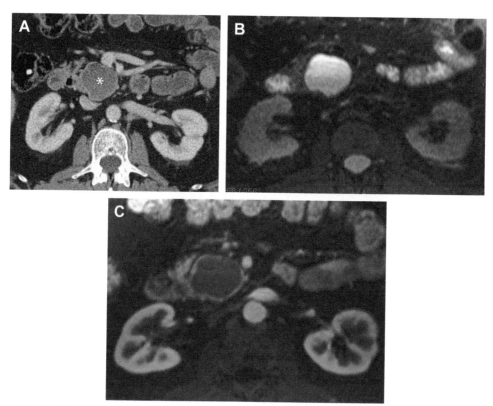

Fig. 4. (A) Cystic PET. CT in a 53-year-old man with a prior history of carcinoma of the lung reveals a low-density, but not water density, mass in the pancreatic head (*asterisk*). (B) Cystic PET: same patient as in A. T2-weighted fat-suppressed MRI reveals high signal cyst with layering debris. (C) Cystic PET: same patient as in A. No enhancing elements were detected following intravenous contrast. Surgery revealed well-differentiated PET.

isotropic data sets that facilitate 3D imaging. A dose of 0.1 mmol/kg IV gadolinium, given at 2 mL/s, produces uniformly excellent image quality. We are currently investigating the possible increased benefit of diffusion-weighted imaging with apparent diffusion coefficient (ADC) mapping.

Endoscopic ultrasonography (EUS) and molecular methods are widely used and provide a statistically incremental improvement in the imaging assessment of patients with suspected PET, particularly those who ultimately are proved to have smaller lesions.[25,26] In a series of 217 patients with 231 PETs, CT detected 84%. In this cohort, 56 patients underwent both CT and EUS. EUS detected 91.7% of PETs as opposed to 63.3% detected by CT. EUS detected 20 of 22 CT-negative tumors. The investigators conclude that MDCT can be a first-line study, but, if the results are negative, EUS can be performed. EUS may be the better first-line test for the evaluation of suspected insulinoma.[20] Use of molecular agents that target specific metabolic pathways and/or receptors is directly related to the specific tumor subtype. Somatostatin receptor scintigraphy is widely performed, indium In 111 pentetreotide (Octreoscan) being currently available for clinical use.[27] This agent is only useful in tumors with somatostatin receptor sites. Therefore, although detection rates are in the range of 80% in patients with gastrinoma, this agent is successful in the range of 60% to 70% for localizing insulinoma.[25] Newer agents, particularly those that can be used with CT/PET scanning such as 68-DOTA-NOC, display more true positive tumor foci than indium In 111 DTPA octreotide.[28] The major use of these and other newly developed molecular agents is increased detection of sites of unsuspected metastases.

Continuous improvements in MDCT and MRI technology also have resulted in improved detection and analysis of PET. Lin and colleagues[29] reported a sensitivity of 95.7% using dual energy spectral CT compared with a sensitivity of 68.8% using MDCT, the improvement being directly related to the ability to combine a monochromatic and iodine density image. Using

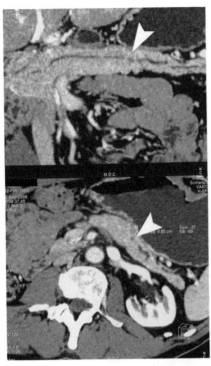

Fig. 5. PET with pancreatic duct stricture: segmental pancreatic duct dilatation in the tail of the gland is present (*arrowhead*). There is barely visible 8-mm lucency in the pancreatic body on lower image (*arrowhead*). Pathologic examination of the resected specimen revealed periductal fibrosis secondary to a small serotonin-secreting PET. (*Courtesy of M. D'Onofrio MD, Verona, Italy.*)

diffusion-weighted MRI, Wang and colleagues[30] showed higher ADC values with well-differentiated PETs as opposed to endocrine carcinoma. Most investigators of clinical reviews agree that

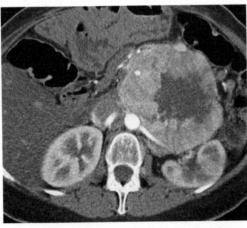

Fig. 6. NF-PET: a large, sharply circumscribed, heterogeneously enhancing mass is characteristic of NF-PET.

multimodality imaging, usually beginning with MDCT and or MRI, supplemented with EUS and nuclear studies when necessary, is the most cost-effective and accurate method to detect PET.[19,23,31]

SOLID PSEUDOPAPILLARY TUMOR

This neoplasm is considered as either a benign tumor or a tumor with low malignant potential, occurring predominantly, but not exclusively, in young women.[32] This lesion has been referred to by a variety of names; however, the term SPT has been proposed as the single best term for this lesion in both the Armed Forces Institute of Pathology (AFIP) classification of 1997 and the WHO classification of 1996.[33]

The female predominance of this lesion is well documented. Buetow and colleagues[34] reviewed the AFIP experience, which found 53 of 56 (94.6%) cases occurring in women. Martin and colleagues[35] reviewed the experience at Memorial Sloan-Kettering Cancer Center in New York, documenting 20 of 24 lesions (83.3%) occurring in females; this percentage remained constant when the analysis was updated from data in 45 patients.[32] The reason for the female predominance is unclear; despite sophisticated pathologic, genetic, and immunohistochemical analysis, no consistent evidence of hormone receptors has been found.

The age of these patients is considerably less than that typically seen in patients with pancreatic adenocarcinoma. Reported mean ages vary from 25 years (range 10–74 years),[34] 27 years,[36] 32 years (range 16–66 years)[37] to 38 years (range 12–63 years).[32] In all series, a few elderly patients are encountered. Individual case reports in patients as young as 10 years appear in the literature.[38] Metastatic disease has been reported in an 11-year-old patient,[39] although there is evidence that the tumor is more aggressive in elderly patients based on the higher prevalence of metastases and microscopic evidence of angioinvasion and perineural invasion[40,41]; however, even in the presence of these markers of advanced disease, the prognosis is extremely favorable.

Typical lesions are greater than 3 cm in diameter. On imaging studies, this lesion appears as a round encapsulated mass with variably attenuating components including hemorrhagic areas, cystic spaces, and soft tissue. The lesions demonstrate more heterogeneous enhancement on earlier acquisition phases that then progressively normalizes. Peripheral calcifications can be seen in 28% of cases[34,42]; the presence of calcifications

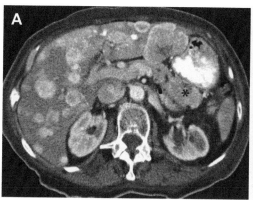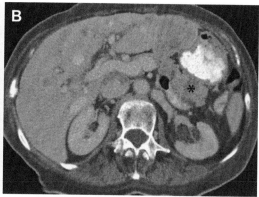

Fig. 7. (A) NF-PET, value of dual phase acquisition. The primary tumor is isodense with the pancreatic tail, recognizable as a contour defect (*asterisk*). Extensive hepatic metastases are evident. (B) NF-PET value of dual-phase acquisition, same patient as in A. During the portal phase acquisition, hepatic metastases can be identified, but the majority are now isodense during the portal phase of hepatic enhancement. The primary tumor remains isodense with the pancreas (*asterisk*).

has been associated with more aggressive tumors.[43] The presence of cystic regions within the mass is the result of hemorrhagic necrosis.[44,45] These lesions may appear anywhere within the pancreas, although there appears to be a slight predilection for the pancreatic tail (**Fig. 10**).

With improved imaging capabilities, small (<3 cm) SPTs are now becoming recognized. In a series of 45 solid pancreatic tumors, 11 (24%) were small.[46] When small, the lesions do not display the typical features of classic SPT but instead appear as sharply marginated solid tumors with no dilatation of the pancreatic duct. The lesions were shown to progressively enhance, comparing pancreatic phase with portal venous phase CT or MRI.[46,47] On MRI, the lesions display low signal on noncontrast T1-weighted images

and strikingly high signal intensity on T2-weighted images (**Fig. 11**).[46] Larger lesions (>3 cm) display bright T1 signal in regions of hemorrhage and variable enhancement during contrast phases; the presence of intratumoral hemorrhage is characteristic of SPT (**Fig. 12**).

The biological behavior of SPT is variable. Most investigators consider these lesions to be low-grade malignancies and suggest aggressive, curative resection when discovered.[37,48] In a review of 292 cases reported in the world literature, 43 (14.7%) were recognized as malignant.[49] The likelihood of malignancy increases with patient age[41] and with tumor size.[32] In the 2011 series from Memorial Sloan-Kettering of 45 patients with SPT, 9 had malignant disease defined by a locally unresectable tumor in 3, liver metastases in 3,

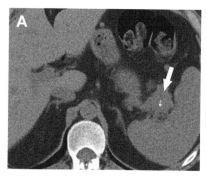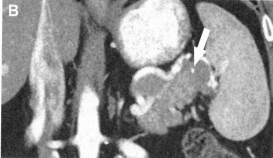

Fig. 8. PET with calcification. (A) Incidental finding in a 67-year-old patient undergoing unenhanced chest CT. Central calcification present in mass in pancreatic tail (*arrow*). (B) The calcification is difficult to detect on the arterial phase of a follow-up pancreas protocol MDCT scan (*arrow*). The diagnosis of endocrine tumor was established by cytology from endoscopic ultrasonography. PET should be the primary diagnosis in any solid pancreatic mass containing central calcification.

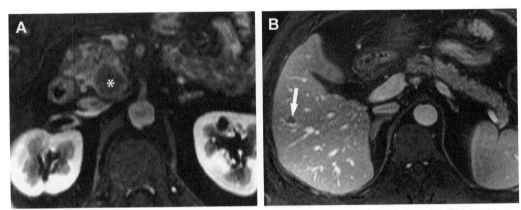

Fig. 9. Metastases from small PET. (*A*) Lesion is seen in uncinate process of pancreas on contrast-enhanced MRI (*asterisk*). (*B*) Low-signal lesion in segment 5 of liver on portal phase contrast-enhanced MRI (*arrow*) proved to be a mixed endocrine-acinar pancreatic neoplasm.

locally unresectable tumor and liver metastases in 1, local recurrence and liver metastases in 1, and local recurrence in 1. After a median follow-up of 44 months, 34 patients were without evidence of disease, 4 patients were alive with disease, 3 patients died of disease, and 4 patients died of other causes.[32]

HEMATOGENOUS METASTASES TO THE PANCREAS

The pancreas may be secondarily affected by neoplasm from direct extension from an adjacent organ or direct extension from adjacent lymph nodes or by hematogenous seeding. Autopsy studies reveal that metastases to the pancreas may be found in between 3% of 5000 patients[50] and

10.6% of 2587 patients.[51] Their presence may be underestimated by imaging studies. CT abnormalities were seen in 18(53.8%) of 34 cases of autopsy-confirmed metastatic tumors to the pancreas (8, diffuse enlargement; 9, localized mass; 1, multiple low-attenuated nodules). In the remaining 16 patients, histologic investigation revealed that metastatic carcinoma resulted in diffuse infiltration of the pancreatic lobules, not macroscopically visualized by CT.[52] Although this study from 1989 used less-sophisticated technology than presently available, it is evident that still a significant number of cases may go unrecognized.

Klein and colleagues[53] reviewed 66 patients seen at the Mayo Clinic between 1984 and 1994. Of these, 13 patients already had pancreatic

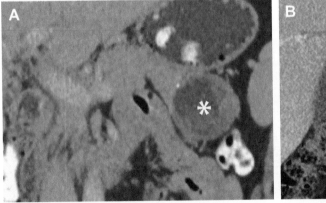
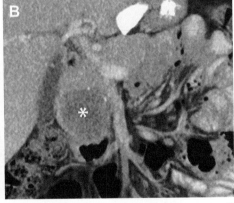

Fig. 10. SPT CT appearance. (*A*) Low-dose MDCT in a 15-year-old male patient reveals sharply circumscribed heterogeneous mass (*asterisk*) in pancreatic tail. A peripheral fleck calcification is present. (*B*) MDCT in a 19-year-old female patient who presented to emergency room with abdominal pain displays a pancreatic mass (*asterisk*) with imaging features similar to that in the patient in *A*. Note the peripheral calcifications and heterogeneous appearance.

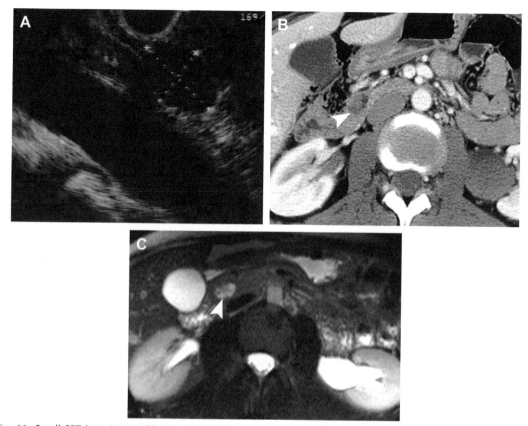

Fig. 11. Small SPT in a 4-year-old girl. (*A*) EUS image reveals a cystic mass in the head of the pancreas. (*B*) CT appearance. The lesion has a heterogeneous appearance with both lower-attenuation and higher-attenuation components (*arrowhead*). (*C*) MRI appearance. The lesion is T2 hyperintense, with some low-signal central elements (*arrowhead*).

metastases at the time of initial CT, whereas the remainder developed in the follow-up period (2–295 months; mean, 57.2 months). In more than one-third of the patients, the metastases appeared later than 60 months. Patients with pancreatic metastases from renal cell carcinoma (RCC) demonstrated the longest interval between detection of tumor and appearance of a pancreatic abnormality, 85% appearing at an interval of greater than 60 months following diagnosis. In another series, the mean time from nephrectomy to pancreatic recurrence in 10 patients with RCC was 9.8 years.[54] The pancreas is rarely the only site of metastatic dissemination; between 45% and 95% of patients are reported to have metastases to other sites.[53,55] When the pancreas is the sole site of metastasis, differentiation from primary pancreatic tumor is difficult without tissue confirmation by biopsy.

On imaging studies, pancreatic metastases can appear as localized (50%–73%) or multifocal (15%–44%) masses or can result in diffuse enlargement of the gland (5%–10%)[56,57] mimicking primary pancreatic neoplasms of a variety of morphologic appearances (**Figs. 12–14**). Although there is wide variability in the contrast enhancement characteristics between metastases of different primary tumors, the enhancement characteristics of the metastases from the same primary tumor are consistent.[58] The most frequent primary tumor to metastasize to the pancreas is RCC as evidenced in multiple series.[53,55,56,58–60] Renal cell metastases are frequently unifocal as opposed to lesions from other primary sites.[61] RCC appears as an intensely hypervascular mass when small and with bright rim enhancement when large.[58] Lung cancer and melanoma are also seen with some frequency. Virtually, any primary tumor can metastasize to the pancreas; in our practice, we have seen cases of metastatic hepatocellular carcinoma, ovarian cancer, carcinoid, breast cancer, and liposarcoma. The long-term survival of patients with metastasis to the pancreas is considerably improved over those

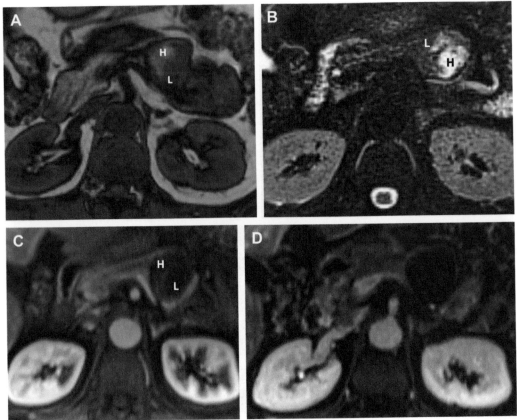

Fig. 12. SPT in a 66-year-old man. (*A*) Opposed-phase T1-weighted image reveals a mixed signal mass with both high signal (H), representing blood, and low signal (L), representing necrotic elements. (*B*) Fat-suppressed T2-weighted image reveals reversal of the T1 signal. (*C*) Gadolinium-enhanced fat-suppressed T1-weighted gradient-recalled echo image reveals the high-signal (H) and low-signal (L) components in similar relation to the noncontrast image shown in (*A*). (*D*) Subtraction image. There is no significant enhancement in the mass. The MRI appearance can be explained by the presence of intratumoral hemorrhage. Recognition of bleeding into a pancreatic tumor allowed the correct preoperative diagnosis to be made despite the "unusual" demographic.

who might have primary pancreatic cancer, and, therefore, in appropriate situations (when imaging fails to define other foci of disease), aggressive surgical therapy in patients with a low surgical risk has been shown to provide survival benefit as well as palliation.[60,62–64]

OTHER UNUSUAL SOLID PANCREATIC MASSES

As stated initially, there is a vast array of possible histologies for a given pancreatic mass. At our own institution, we have seen sporadic cases of acinar cell carcinoma, benign fibrous tumor, giant cell osteoclastoma, adenosquamous carcinoma, mature teratoma, and even an intrapancreatic amyloidoma. These masses are infrequently encountered clinically. A specific diagnosis is rarely made, although radiologists comment that the

imaging appearance is not typical for adenocarcinoma. They will not be considered further in this review.

Two other types of solid pancreatic masses need consideration in appropriate cases; mass-forming chronic pancreatitis and/or autoimmune pancreatitis is discussed in the article by Sahani and colleagues within this issue and will not be further discussed here. The other lesion is the IPAS.

IPAS is a benign lesion, but its appearance can be confused with true pancreatic neoplasms, particularly PET or small SPT.[16] The pancreatic tail is the second most common location of an accessory spleen. Of 364 accessory spleens found in an autopsy of 3000 patients, 61 (17%) were in the pancreatic tail.[65] In 1000 consecutive patients undergoing CT scanning, 156 (15.6%) had at least 1 accessory spleen, but only 2 of these

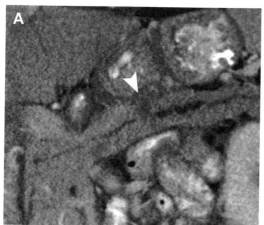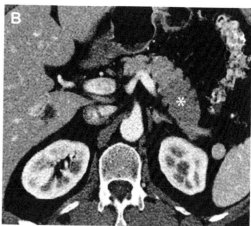

Fig. 13. (*A*) Metastatic lung carcinoma to the pancreas presenting as a low attenuation lesion (*arrowhead*) obstructing the main pancreatic duct. The appearance cannot be distinguished from a primary adenocarcinoma. A second lesion is seen in the pancreatic neck. (*B*) Metastatic lung carcinoma to the pancreas presenting as a mass diffusely infiltrating the pancreatic tail (*asterisk*). As in (*A*), the appearance cannot be distinguished from primary pancreatic adenocarcinoma. The lesion in the liver is a hemangioma.

were IPAS[66]; this discrepancy between autopsy frequency and imaging detection has been noted elsewhere.[67]

IPAS is most frequently detected by CT scanning. It belongs to the differential diagnosis of a 1- to 3-cm hypervascular mass in the pancreatic tail. If arterial phase imaging is performed, the so-called moiré-enhancement of the spleen is reproduced in the IPAS.[67,68] On MRI, the lesion also closely follows the signal of the spleen on all acquisitions. This imaging feature although helpful is not definitive (**Fig. 15**).[69] There are several recent reports of associated epidermoid cysts within the IPAS, presenting an even more confusing picture.

Definitive diagnosis is made with scintigraphy using either technetium Tc 99m–labeled damaged red blood cell or technetium Tc 99m–sulfur colloid.[65,67,68] At present, many patients who are diagnosed with any type of pancreatic mass are referred for biopsy by EUS. Not surprisingly, the diagnosis of IPAS can only be suspected from the sonographic appearance alone. At biopsy, the cytopathologist should look for cytomorphologic features of splenic tissue, including endothelial cells and polymorphous lymphocytes admixed with neutrophils, eosinophils, plasma cells, histiocytes, and lymphoglandular bodies. Abundant large platelet aggregates are another distinguishing feature of splenic tissue.[70]

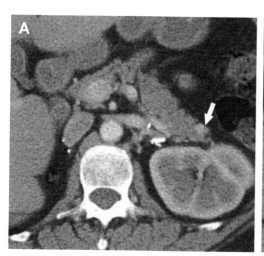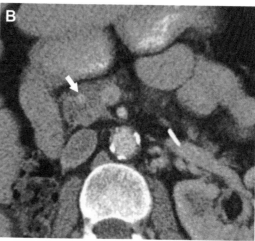

Fig. 14. (*A*) Metastatic RCC to the pancreas. Tiny hyperdense lesions appeared in the tail of the pancreas during surveillance follow-up for renal carcinoma (*arrow*). (*B*) Metastatic RCC to the pancreas, same patient as in (*A*). An additional hyperdense metastasis is seen in the pancreatic head (*arrow*).

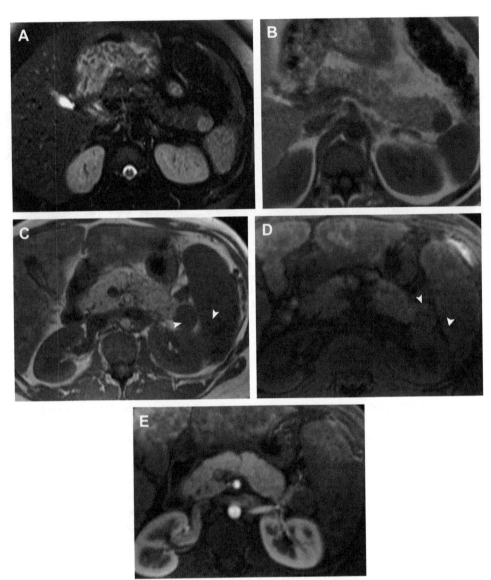

Fig. 15. IPAS. (*A*) T2-weighted magnetic resonance image reveals hyperintense lesion in the tail of pancreas. IPAS cannot be distinguished from PNET or even metastasis. (*B*) In-phase noncontrast T1-weighted image in the same patient as in (*A*) reveals on this and other sequences that the lesion has identical signal to spleen. (*C*) MRI appearance. The low signal lesion in the tail of the pancreas has identical signal compared with the spleen on the T1-weighted noncontrast image. (*D*) MRI appearance. On this fat-suppressed precontrast T1-weighted gradient-recall image, the similarity to splenic signal is again evident. The presence of Gamna-Gandy bodies in the spleen can be recognized in the IPAS (*arrowheads* in *C* and *D*). Note the cirrhotic changes in the liver. (*E*) MRI appearance. Following gadolinium, the signal remains the same as the spleen.

REFERENCES

1. Kloppel G, Solcia E, Longnecker DS, et al. Histologic typing of tumours of the exocrine pancreas. In: WHO, editor. International histological classification of tumours. 2nd edition. Berlin: Springer-Verlag; 1996.
2. Low G, Panu A, Millo N, et al. Multimodality imaging of neoplastic and nonneoplastic solid lesions of the pancreas. Radiographics 2011;31(4):993–1015.
3. Jensen RT, Norton JA. Endocrine tumors of the pancreas and gastrointestinal tract. In: Feldman M, Friedman LS, Brandt LJ, editors. Sleisenger and Fordtran's gastrointestinal and liver disease. 9th edition. Philadelphia: Saunders Elsevier; 2010. p. 491–522.
4. Capelli P, Zamboni G, Pesci A, et al. Pathology. In: Procacci C, Megibow AJ, editors. Imaging of the pancreas: cystic and rare tumors. Berlin; New York: Springer; 2003. p. 161–75.

5. Lewis RB, Lattin GE Jr, Paal E. Pancreatic endocrine tumors: radiologic-clinicopathologic correlation. Radiographics 2010;30(6):1445–64.

6. Metz DC, Jensen RT. Gastrointestinal neuroendocrine tumors: pancreatic endocrine tumors. Gastroenterology 2008;135(5):1469–92.

7. Solcia E, Capella C, Kloppel G, editors. Tumors of the pancreas. Washington, DC: Armed Forces Institute of Pathology; 1997.

8. Arva NC, Pappas JG, Bhatla T, et al. Well-differentiated pancreatic neuroendocrine carcinoma in tuberous sclerosis—case report and review of the literature. Am J Surg Pathol 2012;36(1):149–53.

9. Gusmini S, Nicoletti R, Martinenghi C, et al. Arterial vs pancreatic phase: which is the best choice in the evaluation of pancreatic endocrine tumours with multidetector computed tomography (MDCT)? Radiol Med 2007;112(7):999–1012.

10. Noone TC, Hosey J, Firat Z, et al. Imaging and localization of islet-cell tumours of the pancreas on CT and MRI. Best Pract Res Clin Endocrinol Metab 2005;19(2):195–211.

11. Hayashi D, Tkacz JN, Hammond S, et al. Gastroenteropancreatic neuroendocrine tumors: multimodality imaging features with pathological correlation. Jpn J Radiol 2011;29(2):85–91.

12. Powell AC, Hajdu CH, Megibow AJ, et al. Nonfunctioning pancreatic endocrine neoplasm presenting as asymptomatic, isolated pancreatic duct stricture: a case report and review of the literature. Am Surg 2008;74(2):168–71.

13. Kawamoto S, Shi C, Hruban RH, et al. Small serotonin-producing neuroendocrine tumor of the pancreas associated with pancreatic duct obstruction. AJR Am J Roentgenol 2011;197(3):W482–8.

14. Graziani R, Brandalise A, Bellotti M, et al. Imaging of neuroendocrine gastroenteropancreatic tumours. Radiol Med 2010;115(7):1047–64.

15. Buetow PC, Miller DL, Parrino TV, et al. Islet cell tumors of the pancreas: clinical, radiologic, and pathologic correlation in diagnosis and localization. Radiographics 1997;17(2):453–72.

16. Xue HD, Liu W, Xiao Y, et al. Pancreatic and peripancreatic lesions mimic pancreatic islet cell tumor in multidetector computed tomography. Chin Med J (Engl) 2011;124(11):1720–5.

17. Cirillo F, Falconi M, Bettini R. Clinical manifestations and therapeutic management of hyperfunctioning endocrine tumors. In: Procacci C, Megibow AJ, editors. Imaging the pancreas: cystic and rare tumors. Berlin; New York: Springer; 2003. p. 141–52.

18. Stabile BE, Morrow DJ, Passaro E Jr. The gastrinoma triangle: operative implications. Am J Surg 1984; 147(1):25–31.

19. Minter RM, Simeone DM. Contemporary management of nonfunctioning pancreatic neuroendocrine tumors. J Gastrointest Surg 2011;2011:19.

20. Khashab MA, Yong E, Lennon AM, et al. EUS is still superior to multidetector computerized tomography for detection of pancreatic neuroendocrine tumors. Gastrointest Endosc 2011;73(4):691–6.

21. Gouya H, Vignaux O, Augui J, et al. CT, endoscopic sonography, and a combined protocol for preoperative evaluation of pancreatic insulinomas. AJR Am J Roentgenol 2003;181(4):987–92.

22. Fidler JL, Fletcher JG, Reading CC, et al. Preoperative detection of pancreatic insulinomas on multiphasic helical CT. AJR Am J Roentgenol 2003; 181(3):775–80.

23. Fiebrich HB, van Asselt SJ, Brouwers AH, et al. Tailored imaging of islet cell tumors of the pancreas amidst increasing options. Crit Rev Oncol Hematol 2011;2011:24.

24. Thoeni RF, Mueller-Lisse UG, Chan R, et al. Detection of small, functional islet cell tumors in the pancreas: selection of MR imaging sequences for optimal sensitivity. Radiology 2000;214(2):483–90.

25. Carrasquillo JA, Chen CC. Molecular imaging of neuroendocrine tumors. Semin Oncol 2010;37(6): 662–79.

26. Oberg K, Castellano D. Current knowledge on diagnosis and staging of neuroendocrine tumors. Cancer Metastasis Rev 2011;30(Suppl 1):3–7.

27. Shi W, Johnston CF, Buchanan KD, et al. Localization of neuroendocrine tumours with [111In] DTPA-octreotide scintigraphy (Octreoscan): a comparative study with CT and MR imaging. QJM 1998;91(4): 295–301.

28. Krausz Y, Freedman N, Rubinstein R, et al. 68Ga-DOTA-NOC PET/CT imaging of neuroendocrine tumors: comparison with (1)(1)(1)In-DTPA-octreotide (OctreoScan(R)). Mol Imaging Biol 2011;13(3):583–93.

29. Lin XZ, Wu ZY, Tao R, et al. Dual energy spectral CT imaging of insulinoma—value in preoperative diagnosis compared with conventional multi-detector CT. Eur J Radiol 2011;2011:5.

30. Wang Y, Chen ZE, Yaghmai V, et al. Diffusion-weighted MR imaging in pancreatic endocrine tumors correlated with histopathologic characteristics. J Magn Reson Imaging 2011;33(5):1071–9.

31. Joseph S, Wang YZ, Boudreaux JP, et al. Neuroendocrine tumors: current recommendations for diagnosis and surgical management. Endocrinol Metab Clin North Am 2011;40(1):205–31.

32. Butte JM, Brennan MF, Gonen M, et al. Solid pseudopapillary tumors of the pancreas. Clinical features, surgical outcomes, and long-term survival in 45 consecutive patients from a single center. J Gastrointest Surg 2011;15(2):350–7.

33. Kloppel G, Solcia E, Longnecker DS, et al. World Health Organization International Classification of tumors. Histological classification of tumors of the exocrine pancreas. 2nd edition. Berlin: Springer-Verlag; 1996.

34. Buetow PC, Buck JL, Pantongrag-Brown L, et al. Solid and papillary epithelial neoplasm of the pancreas: imaging-pathologic correlation on 56 cases. Radiology 1996;199(3):707–11.

35. Martin RC, Klimstra DS, Brennan MF, et al. Solid-pseudopapillary tumor of the pancreas: a surgical enigma? Ann Surg Oncol 2002;9(1):35–40.

36. Lam KY, Lo CY, Fan ST. Pancreatic solid-cystic-papillary tumor: clinicopathologic features in eight patients from Hong Kong and review of the literature. World J Surg 1999;23(10):1045–50.

37. Yoon DY, Hines OJ, Bilchik AJ, et al. Solid and papillary epithelial neoplasms of the pancreas: aggressive resection for cure. Am Surg 2001;67(12):1195–9.

38. Yagi M, Shiraiwa K, Abiko M, et al. A solid and cystic tumor of the pancreas in a 10-year-old girl: report of a case and review of the literature. Surg Today 1994;24(9):826–8.

39. Horisawa M, Niinomi N, Sato T, et al. Frantz's tumor (solid and cystic tumor of the pancreas) with liver metastasis: successful treatment and long-term follow-up. J Pediatr Surg 1995;30(5):724–6.

40. Piatek S, Manger T, Rose I, et al. Solid pseudopapillary tumor of the pancreas. Int J Pancreatol 2000;27(1):77–81.

41. Matsunou H, Konishi F. Papillary-cystic neoplasm of the pancreas. A clinicopathologic study concerning the tumor aging and malignancy of nine cases. Cancer 1990;65(2):283–91.

42. Yao X, Ji Y, Zeng M, et al. Solid pseudopapillary tumor of the pancreas: cross-sectional imaging and pathologic correlation. Pancreas 2010;39(4):486–91.

43. Kim HH, Yun SK, Kim JC, et al. Clinical features and surgical outcome of solid pseudopapillary tumor of the pancreas: 30 consecutive clinical cases. Hepatogastroenterology 2011;58(107–108):1002–8.

44. Dong PR, Lu DS, Degregario F, et al. Solid and papillary neoplasm of the pancreas: radiological-pathological study of five cases and review of the literature. Clin Radiol 1996;51(10):702–5.

45. Choi BI, Kim KW, Han MC, et al. Solid and papillary epithelial neoplasms of the pancreas: CT findings. Radiology 1988;166(2):413–6.

46. Yu MH, Lee JY, Kim MA, et al. MR imaging features of small solid pseudopapillary tumors: retrospective differentiation from other small solid pancreatic tumors. AJR Am J Roentgenol 2010;195(6):1324–32.

47. Baek JH, Lee JM, Kim SH, et al. Small (<or=3 cm) solid pseudopapillary tumors of the pancreas at multiphasic multidetector CT. Radiology 2010;257(1):97–106.

48. Zinner MJ. Solid and papillary neoplasms of the pancreas. Surg Clin North Am 1995;75(5):1017–24.

49. Mao C, Guvendi M, Domenico DR, et al. Papillary cystic and solid tumors of the pancreas: a pancreatic embryonic tumor? Studies of three cases and cumulative review of the world's literature. Surgery 1995;118(5):821–8.

50. Willis R. The spread of tumors in the human body. 3rd edition. London: Butterworth; 1973. p. 216–7.

51. Cubilla A, Fitzgerald P. Surgical pathology of exocrine tumors of the pancreas. In: Moosa A, editor. Tumors of the pancreas. Baltimore: Williams and Wilkins; 1980. p. 159–93.

52. Muranaka T, Teshima K, Honda H, et al. Computed tomography and histologic appearance of pancreatic metastases from distant sources. Acta Radiol 1989;30(6):615–9.

53. Klein KA, Stephens DH, Welch TJ. CT characteristics of metastatic disease of the pancreas. Radiographics 1998;18(2):369–78.

54. Sohn TA, Yeo CJ, Cameron JL, et al. Renal cell carcinoma metastatic to the pancreas: results of surgical management. J Gastrointest Surg 2001;5(4):346–51.

55. Ferrozzi F, Bova D, Campodonico F, et al. Pancreatic metastases: CT assessment. Eur Radiol 1997;7(2):241–5.

56. Scatarige JC, Horton KM, Sheth S, et al. Pancreatic parenchymal metastases: observations on helical CT. AJR Am J Roentgenol 2001;176(3):695–9.

57. Merkle EM, Boaz T, Kolokythas O, et al. Metastases to the pancreas. Br J Radiol 1998;71(851):1208–14.

58. Palmowski M, Hacke N, Satzl S, et al. Metastasis to the pancreas: characterization by morphology and contrast enhancement features on CT and MRI. Pancreatology 2008;8(2):199–203.

59. Ballarin R, Spaggiari M, Cautero N, et al. Pancreatic metastases from renal cell carcinoma: the state of the art. World J Gastroenterol 2011;17(43):4747–56.

60. Alzahrani MA, Schmulewitz N, Grewal S, et al. Metastases to the pancreas: the experience of a high volume center and a review of the literature. J Surg Oncol 2011;2011(2):22009.

61. Ascenti G, Visalli C, Genitori A, et al. Multiple hypervascular pancreatic metastases from renal cell carcinoma: dynamic MR and spiral CT in three cases. Clin Imaging 2004;28(5):349–52.

62. Z'Graggen K, Fernandez-del Castillo C, Rattner DW, et al. Metastases to the pancreas and their surgical extirpation. Arch Surg 1998;133(4):413–7 [discussion: 8–9].

63. You DD, Choi DW, Choi SH, et al. Surgical resection of metastasis to the pancreas. J Korean Surg Soc 2011;80(4):278–82.

64. Goyal J, Lipson EJ, Rezaee N, et al. Surgical resection of malignant melanoma metastatic to the pancreas: case series and review of literature. J Gastrointest Cancer 2011;2011:13.

65. Guo W, Han W, Liu J, et al. Intrapancreatic accessory spleen: a case report and review of the literature. World J Gastroenterol 2009;15(9):1141–3.

66. Mortele KJ, Mortele B, Silverman SG. CT features of the accessory spleen. AJR Am J Roentgenol 2004; 183(6):1653–7.

67. Kawamoto S, Johnson PT, Hall H, et al. Intrapancreatic accessory spleen: CT appearance and differential diagnosis. Abdom Imaging 2011;2011:13.

68. Spencer LA, Spizarny DL, Williams TR. Imaging features of intrapancreatic accessory spleen. Br J Radiol 2010;83(992):668–73.

69. Hwang HS, Lee SS, Kim SC, et al. Intrapancreatic accessory spleen: clinicopathologic analysis of 12 cases. Pancreas 2011;40(6):956–65.

70. Conway AB, Cook SM, Samad A, et al. Large platelet aggregates in endoscopic ultrasound-guided fine-needle aspiration of the pancreas and peripancreatic region: a clue for the diagnosis of intrapancreatic or accessory spleen. Diagn Cytopathol 2011;2011(1):21832.

Imaging of Miscellaneous Pancreatic Pathology (Trauma, Transplant, Infections, and Deposition)

Nagaraj-Setty Holalkere, MD, DNB*, Jorge Soto, MD

KEYWORDS

- Pancreas • Trauma • Transplant • Tuberculosis
- Cystic fibrosis • Hemochromatosis • Fatty replacement
- Lymphoma

PANCREATIC TRAUMA

Although rare, with an incidence in blunt abdominal trauma ranging from 1% to 2%, pancreatic injuries are associated with significant morbidity and mortality.[1–3] Mortality rates in patients suffering pancreatic injuries from blunt trauma are reported to be as high as 30%, with the majority of deaths occurring within the first 48 hours of the inciting traumatic event.[4,5] When not recognized at admission, delayed complications (usually caused by unrecognized pancreatic ductal injuries) lead to further complications, such as the development of abscesses, fistulae, and pseudocysts as well as sepsis and multisystem organ failure.[5] Thus, a prompt diagnosis of pancreatic injury is critical in delivering appropriate and timely interventions and for minimizing the frequency and severity of delayed complications.

In blunt trauma to the anterior abdomen, the pancreas is vulnerable to crushing injuries from impact against the adjacent vertebral column. The majority (approximately two-thirds) of injuries to the pancreas after blunt trauma occur in the neck or body of the gland, whereas the remainder are equally distributed between the head and tail.[5] Significant forces are required to injure the pancreas; thus, isolated pancreatic trauma is rare. Concomitant injuries to other organs, especially the liver, spleen, stomach, and duodenum, occur in more than 90% of cases.[2] Common mechanisms of injury that can involve the pancreas include motor vehicle collisions and, in children, bicycle accidents and nonaccidental trauma.

Clinical symptoms and signs found in patients with pancreatic injuries are nonspecific and include fever, leukocytosis, and elevated serum amylase or lipase levels. The main cause of delayed complications from pancreatic trauma is disruption of the pancreatic duct. A disrupted pancreatic duct usually requires surgical or endoscopic interventions, whereas injuries that spare the duct are generally treated nonsurgically. The risks of abscess or fistula formation in patients with disruption of the pancreatic duct approach 25% and 50%, respectively.[3] Therefore, imaging studies specifically focus on assessing the integrity of the pancreatic duct.

CT is the imaging modality of choice in hemodynamically stable patients with blunt abdominal trauma.[6–8] On CT, direct signs of pancreatic injury include glandular contusion, laceration, and transection (if laceration involves the full thickness). Typically, contusions are ill-defined areas of low attenuation without discontinuity of the surface of the gland (Fig. 1). Lacerations are seen as low-attenuation linear defects in the parenchyma, typically oriented perpendicular to the axis of the gland (Fig. 2). Congenital clefts may be difficult

Department of Radiology, Boston Medical Center, 820 Harrison Avenue, FGH Building, 3rd Floor, Boston, MA 02118, USA
* Corresponding author.
E-mail address: Nagaraj.Holalkere@bmc.org

Radiol Clin N Am 50 (2012) 515–528
doi:10.1016/j.rcl.2012.03.011
0033-8389/12/$ – see front matter © 2012 Elsevier Inc. All rights reserved.

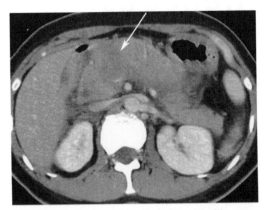

Fig. 1. Pancreatic contusion in a 36-year-old woman after a motor vehicle collision. Axial CT scan obtained with intravenous contrast material shows a large low-attenuation area in the head of the gland (*arrow*), representing a contusion/intraparenchymal hematoma.

to differentiate from a glandular laceration in the proper clinical setting.[9] Typical clefts are similar to lacerations in morphology and orientation but are usually better defined and contain fat (rather than fluid or blood, as is typical of lacerations). Fluid collections, such as hematomas, pseudocysts, and abscesses, are a common finding and may communicate with the pancreas at the site of transection or laceration. Focal enlargement of the pancreas and associated peripancreatic fluid are suggestive of pancreatic injury (contusion and intraparenchymal hematoma). Peripancreatic fat stranding, hemorrhage, and fluid located between the splenic vein and pancreas are useful secondary signs. Although CT may not always

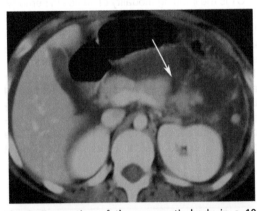

Fig. 2. Transection of the pancreatic body in a 10-year-old boy after a bicycle accident. Axial contrast-enhanced CT scan shows a complete fracture of the pancreatic body (*arrow*) with fluid and between the pancreatic fragments; the fluid also tracks into the lesser sac and peritoneal cavity.

directly demonstrate the pancreatic duct, injury to the duct can be predicted based on the degree of parenchymal injury. A CT grading scheme that classifies pancreatic injuries based on the depth of glandular involvement and likelihood of duct disruption has been devised, but it is only rarely used in clinical practice. In general, however, lacerations that involve 50% or more of the thickness of the gland have a high risk of involving the main duct.[10]

CT is less sensitive in identifying pancreatic injury than injury to all other solid abdominal organs. Pancreatic injuries tend to be subtle on CT, particularly within the first 12 hours after the traumatic event and, consequently, they can easily be overlooked.[2,6] Given the significance of pancreatic injuries, the best approach when faced with a questionable finding is to perform a repeat CT examination no later than 24 to 48 hours after admission. This should decrease the number of false-positive diagnoses. Magnetic resonance (MR) is an excellent alternative as a problem solver in cases of suspected pancreatic trauma. Historically, the sensitivity of CT (mostly performed with single-detector scanners) for the detection of pancreatic injuries has been reported to range from 60% to 70%.[2] With the continuously evolving multidetector CT technology and resulting improvements in image quality, it is expected that the sensitivity for detection of pancreatic injuries should improve. Published studies, however, have produced mixed results[6,11,12]; additional investigations are, therefore, warranted. The image quality afforded by multidetector CT may also permit an improved evaluation of the integrity of the main pancreatic duct.[13]

Evaluation of the pancreatic duct is essential following pancreatic injury since the main factor that determines the outcome is the integrity of the pancreatic duct. MR pancreatography has emerged as an attractive alternative to endoscopic retrograde cholangiopancreatography (ERCP) for direct imaging of the pancreatic duct.[13–15] MR pancreatography has the advantages of being noninvasive, faster, and more readily available than ERCP. The normal main pancreatic duct can be identified by MR pancreatography in the majority of patients. In addition, MR pancreatography may demonstrate abnormalities not visible at ERCP, such as fluid collections upstream of the site of duct transection, and is helpful in assessing parenchymal injury.[13–15] Recently, Gillams and colleagues[16] have shown that secretin MR cholangiopancreatography (MRCP) improves the detection of active leakage from the pancreatic duct disruption, which may further help in selection of interventional verus conservative treatment.

Finally, MR pancreatography can be helpful in directing ERCP-guided therapy. For assessing the glandular parenchyma, fat-suppressed T1-weighted (T1W) and T2-weighted (T2W) sequences are performed (**Fig. 3**). MR pancreatograms are acquired by using heavily T2W breath-hold or non–breath-hold sequences. Fast spin-echo (2-D or 3-D) and single-shot sequences performed in the oblique coronal and axial planes are usually sufficient.

ERCP remains important because of its potential to provide diagnostic images and to direct image-guided therapy. ERCP can direct appropriate surgical repair or be used for primary therapy by means of stent placement. Many studies have shown that mild pancreatic duct injuries, especially those shown at ERCP contained by the pancreatic parenchyma, may be treated with stent placement rather than surgical repair.[17]

PANCREATIC TRANSPLANTATION

Pancreas transplantation is a complex procedure that is increasingly performed for the management of advanced type 1 diabetes mellitus.[18–20] Pancreatic transplantation can be (1) pancreas transplant alone, performed in patients with diabetes and severe, frequent hypoglycemia but adequate kidney function; (2) simultaneous pancreas-kidney transplant, where pancreas and kidney are transplanted simultaneously from the same deceased donor; or (3) pancreas-after-kidney transplant, where a cadaveric or deceased donor pancreas transplant is performed after a previous and different living or deceased donor kidney

transplant. The majority (>80%) of pancreas transplantations are simultaneous pancreas-kidney transplantations.[20] The overall graft survival rates at 1 year in recent years is reported to be 86% for simultaneous pancreas-kidney transplant and 78% for pancreas-after-kidney transplant with a decrease in early technical graft loss rates to 8% to 9%, likely due to improvements in immunosuppressive therapy and surgical techniques.[19]

Typically, the pancreas transplantation is performed by harvesting the donor pancreas with a short segment of duodenum, containing the ampulla of Vater. Both the splenic artery and the proximal superior mesenteric artery (SMA) are preserved because the head is supplied by the inferior pancreaticoduodenal artery via the SMA, and the body and tail are supplied by the splenic artery. A Y-shaped graft from a segment of a donor's iliac artery bifurcation is connected to the superior mesenteric and splenic arteries to reconstruct a single common arterial conduit to be grafted to the recipient's artery. Venous drainage is provided by harvesting a segment of the portal vein, formed by the confluence of the splenic and superior mesenteric veins, with the pancreas allograft.[18,21] The donor pancreas is placed in the right pelvis laterally with the duodenal segment facing cephalad. The donor duodenum is anastomosed to the recipient's upper jejunum (rarely to the urinary bladder) and this allows drainage of the exocrine pancreatic secretions. The donor's arterial conduit is anastomosed to the recipient's right common iliac artery and the portal vein to the recipient's common iliac vein or IVC, rarely to superior mesenteric vein (**Fig. 4**).[22]

Various imaging modalities, such as sonography, CT, or MR imaging, can be used to image the pancreatic transplant and its potential complications. Ultrasound with Doppler is an easy bedside tool and has a high success rate in guiding biopsies of the pancreas allograft in cases of suspected rejection. Its utility, however, is limited in evaluation of the graft per se, due to technical challenges imposed by interposed bowel. In addition, the use of arterial resistive indices in pancreatic transplantation has not been helpful in the diagnosis of acute rejection.[23] In contrast, cross-sectional imaging with CT and MR imaging enables complete evaluation of the normal pancreatic graft, the vasculature, and the abdominal contents.[24–26] The main limitation with contrast-enhanced CT or MR imaging, however, is the concern for contrast-induced nephropathy or nephrogenic systemic fibrosis, especially in the cases of simultaneous pancreas-kidney transplants.

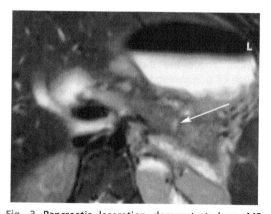

Fig. 3. Pancreatic laceration demonstrated on MR imaging in a 20-year-old man who was involved in a motor vehicle accident. Axial, fat-suppressed, T2W MR image shows a linear area of high signal intensity (*arrow*) in the tail of the pancreas.

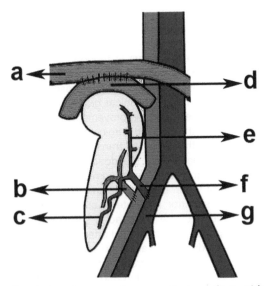

Fig. 4. Art diagram of pancreatic transplant with enteric drainage. The labeled letters corresponds to (a) recipient's jejunum, (b) donor portal vein, (c) donor splenic artery, (d) donor duodenum, (e) donor SMA, (f) Y-shaped graft, and (g) recipient's common iliac artery.

Imaging of Complications

Diagnostic imaging plays a crucial role in determining the appropriate treatment to maximize the chance of graft survival (Table 1). Clinical diagnosis of early graft failure remains difficult, because the signs and symptoms are nonspecific. The spectrum of clinical sequelae of graft failure includes pancreatic dysfunction, pancreatitis, infarction, and necrosis (Fig. 5).

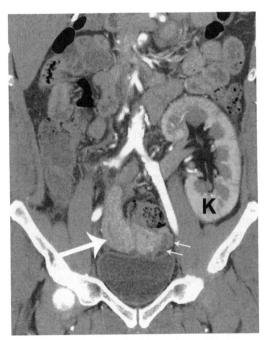

Fig. 5. A 40-year-old man with simultaneous pancreas (arrow) and kidney (K) transplant on postoperative day 5 developed clinical features of pancreatits. Coronal contrast-enhanced CT demonstrated minimal stranding around the pancreas with focal area of lack of enhancement (two small arrows), suggestive of mild necrotizing pancreatitis. Later, the pancreatitis resolved (not shown) with conservative management.

Acute immune-mediated allograft rejection and vascular thrombosis are the most common causes of early transplant failure. The incidence of acute rejection is decreasing with novel immunosuppression regimens.[27] The other complications are intrinsic pancreatic complications related to graft harvesting, post-transplantation lymphoproliferative disorder, and bowel-related complications from intra-abdominal surgery.

Vascular graft complications, both arterial and venous thromboses, occur in the postoperative period. These are the second most common cause of pancreatic transplant dysfunction after graft rejection, with a reported incidence of 2% to 19%.[28,29] Venous occlusion is more common than arterial occlusion, possibly secondary to slower flow on the venous side.[30] The compromised arterial or venous outflow may result in necrosis of the pancreatic graft, which often necessitates pancreatectomy. Imaging with contrast-enhanced CT and MR angiography helps to identify the thrombosis earlier. Graft salvage is dependent on prompt management with either anticoagulation or emergency surgical exploration. In addition, a confident diagnosis of vascular thrombosis can obviate an invasive

Table 1 Complication of pancreatic transplant	
Types of Complications	**Spectrum**
Vascular	Arterial/venous thrombosis, arterial dissection, stenosis at arterial anastomosis, arteriovenous fistula, pseudoaneurysm and Y-shaped graft kink
Enteric	Anastomotic leak, bowel obstruction, post-transplantation lymphoproliferative disorder
Graft	Pancreatitis, pseudocyst, acute rejection

percutaneous biopsy of the allograft to identify other causes of graft dysfunction, such as rejection, which requires an altogether different management strategy. Thrombus appears as an intraluminal filling defect in the allograft arteries or veins on contrast-enhanced CT and MR angiography.[31] Nonenhancement of some or all of the pancreatic graft can occur in the presence of complete donor arterial or venous occlusion. This suggests graft necrosis, which usually carries a poor prognosis for graft survival.[30] Less common vascular complications include arterial stenosis at the site of the anastomosis, pseudoaneurysm, arteriovenous fistulas, arterial dissection, and kinking of the arterial conduit Y-shaped graft (Fig. 6). These can be amenable to endovascular treatment with percutaneous transluminal angioplasty or stent placement.[31] Contrast-enhanced MR angiography and CT angiography are comparable in depicting the vascular complications. Nonenhanced MR angiography, however, using time-of-flight imaging help to identify the vascular complications in patients with renal dysfunction where both CT and MR imaging contrast are contraindicated. Alloimmune vasculitis, usually associated with acute graft rejection, can cause arterial small vessel occlusion progressing to proximal vessel occlusion. The imaging features are generally nonspecific and the vessels may appear normal or reduced in caliber. The pancreatic allograft can appear normal or edematous and demonstrate pancreatitis or decreased parenchymal enhancement (Fig. 7). The degree of parenchymal enhancement on dynamic contrast-enhanced MR imaging has been correlated with rejection and, although found highly sensitive, it remains nonspecific.[32] Chronic rejection results in an atrophic but normally enhancing graft with decreased parenchymal graft signal on T1W and T2W images. MR angiography helps distinguish the global effects of rejection from anastomotic strictures.

Pancreatic graft complications are a result of hypoxic injury inherent in cadaveric organ harvesting, a process that makes some degree of complication related to the pancreatic allograft itself almost expected. Such complications include pancreatitis, pseudocysts, and abscess formation. Pseudocysts form weeks after the onset of graft pancreatitis, often are large and complex, and often become infected (Fig. 8). Ultrasound or CT-guided percutaneous catheter drainage of pseudocysts are a treatment option. Enteric complications, such as mural thickening of bowel loops surrounding the graft, are common and resolve 3 to 4 weeks after transplantation.[33] Anastomotic leak at the duodenojejunostomy can result in peritonitis or localized abscess formation. Adhesions from intra-abdominal surgery are the most frequent cause of small bowel obstruction in pancreatic transplant patients. Internal hernia can occur secondary to the mesenteric defect created during surgery, which can allow internal herniation of jejunal loops posterior to the pancreas transplant. Other rare complications include post-transplantation lymphoproliferative disorder. Post-transplantation lymphoproliferative disorder should be suspected in patients with pancreatic allograft enlargement that does not respond to immunosuppression therapy and the presence of extraallograft masses or organomegaly.[34]

RARE PANCREATIC INFECTIONS
Tuberculosis

Pancreatic tuberculosis is caused by *Mycobacterium tuberculosis* and is exceedingly rare, due to

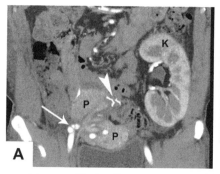
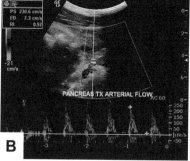

Fig. 6. A 32-year-old man with simultaneous pancreas (P) and kidney (K) transplant with recurrent episodes of abdominal pain underwent CT angiography (A) and Doppler ultrasonography (B). Coronal CT arteriography demonstrated kinking of the Y arterial graft at the site of iliac artery anastomosis (*arrow*). Radiodense suture lines are seen at the enteric anastomosis (*arrowhead*). On color and spectral Doppler ultrasound at the site of iliac artery and Y-shaped graft anastomosis, there is significant narrowing with high-velocity flow, suggestive of stenosis.

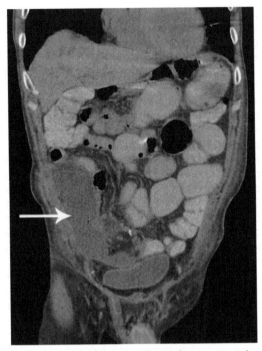

Fig. 7. A 48-year-old man at 2-month status post–isolated pancreatic transplant (*arrow*) developed acute graft rejection, which, on a nonenhanced coronal CT, was shown to be fluid density pancreas, suggestive of severe necrosis.

inherent antibacterial pancreatic factors. The most common sites of involvement in the abdomen include the mesentery, small bowel, peritoneum, liver, and spleen. Recently, there has been an increased incidence of tuberculosis in developed countries, likely due to both to the HIV pandemic

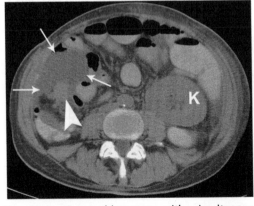

Fig. 8. A 43-year-old-woman with simultaneous pancreas and kidney (K) transplant on a nonenhanced axial CT showed a pseudocyst (*arrows*) around the transplant pancreas (*arrowhead*) after an episode of pancreatitis a week earlier (not shown).

that has produced a worldwide resurgence of *Mycobacterium tuberculosis* and to other immunocompromised conditions.[35] The clinical presentation of tuberculosis varies secondary to involvement of multiple systems. Patients may present with or without constitutional signs and symptoms related to tuberculosis or present with symptoms of tuberculosis elsewhere, such as in the lungs, brain, or bones. Typical symptoms and findings of pancreatic tuberculosis include intermittent or persistent vague upper abdominal pain, obstructive jaundice, portal vein obstruction, acute or chronic pancreatitis, gastrointestinal bleeding, ventral abdominal wall fistula with purulent discharge, and lymphadenopathy.[36]

Focal abscess, necrosis, or features of pancreatitis may be the initial manifestation pf pancreatic tuberculosis. The gland may be diffusely involved by the caseating granulomatous process or there may be a combination of granulomas and associated inflammation as the disease progress. The entire pancreas may have heterogeneous enhancement along with associated peripancreatic, mesenteric, and periportal lymphadenopathy. If untreated or drug resistant, TB can progress to involve bowel and may develop fistulas. Biliary obstruction is common either due to compression of the bile duct by lymphadenopathy or by direct involvement of the duct itself. The pancreatic parenchyma may atrophy; calcifications and pancreatic ductal stricture formation are common with treatment.[35–37]

Imaging plays an important role in establishment of early diagnosis and monitoring treatment response and complications. On noncontrast CT, the involved gland appears enlarged and hypodense. Focal areas of necrosis or abscess formation may result in a heterogeneous appearance. On contrast-enhanced CT, the lesion reveals peripheral enhancement with a nonenhancing central necrotic component.[38] Areas of central enhancement may result in a multiloculated appearance. Peripancreatic edema or collections may be seen. Peripancreatic, mesenteric, or periportal lymphadenopathy is more readily identified on CT. Lymphadenopathy may be homogeneous or may reveal necrotic foci.[38] Enterocutaneous or interloop fistulas can form, which are also better appreciated on CT when present. On MR imaging, the gland typically appears hypointense on T1W imaging and hyperintense or heterogeneous on T2W imaging. There may be heterogeneous enhancement or abscess-like enhancement, with a thick enhancing peripheral rim and central necrosis (**Fig. 9**). The abscess is best seen on postgadolinium MR imaging at portal venous or delayed phase of enhancement. The thick

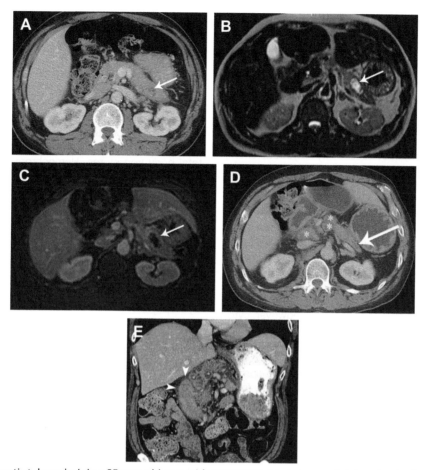

Fig. 9. Pancreatic tuberculosis in a 35-year-old man with recurrent pain abdomen. Axial contrast-enhanced CT (*A*) at the level of the pancreatic tail shows focal hypodensity (*arrow*) with peripancreatic stranding, suggestive of pancreatitis with small area of necrosis. Clinical symptoms were persistent after treatment for pancreatitis, however. Subsequently patient underwent abdominal MR imaging, which demonstrated a focal cystic area (*arrow*) on T2W axial image (*B*) with peripheral rind of enhancement (*arrow*) on postgadolinium T1W fat-saturated axial image (*C*). A diagnosis of possible pancreatic abscess or infected pseudocyst was made based on MR imaging findings. At this stage, patient was treated with broad-spectrum antibiotics because this small abscess was not amenable for drainage. Patient presented to the emergency department after 6 months with worsening pain and weight loss for which he underwent contrast-enhanced CT. Axial (*D*) and coronal (*E*) CT of the upper abdomen depicts atrophy of the tail of pancreas (*arrow*) with multiple enlarged lymph nodes with central low-density (*asterisks*) and periduodenal stranding (*arrowheads*). A diagnosis of pancreatic tuberculosis with associated duodenitis was made. The purified protein derivative (tuberculin) skin test and fine-needle aspiration of peripancreatic lymph node under endoscopic ultrasound guidance were positive for tuberculosis.

enhancing rim when present may be a useful imaging marker to identify an abscess and to differentiate it from a pseudocyst of typical pancreatitis. MRCP helps identify the site of biliary obstruction due to generalized pancreatic gland swelling. ERCP and endoscopic ultrasound–guided fine-needle aspiration are often required for establishment of diagnosis.[36] The disease can mimic acute or chronic pancreatitis and malignancy when there is diffusely altered anatomy.[35] Histologic diagnosis is required for appropriate medical therapy. Samples for cytology and culture

maybe obtained from either the pancreas or peripancreatic lymph nodes. CT-guided or ultrasound-guided percutaneous biopsy may not be feasible in all patients. Endoscopic ultrasound–guided fine-needle aspiration has shown promise as a minimally invasive technique for accurate diagnosis of pancreatic tuberculosis.[39] Rarely, surgical biopsy is required to make the diagnosis when image-guided biopsy results are negative in a setting of high clinical and radiologic suspicion. The samples are processed for acid-fast staining, culture, and polymerase chain reaction assay with acid-fast stating the least sensitive method and polymerase chain reaction the most sensitive method in diagnosis of tuberculosis.[35]

AIDS

AIDS patients can suffer opportunistic infections, drug-induced inflammation, or neoplasms of the pancreas in addition to the more typical pancreatic disorders seen in general population. Opportunistic infections may be caused by mycobacterium, Cryptococcus, Candida, Histoplasma, Aspergillus, Cryptosporidium, Cytomegalovirus, Herpesviruses, and others. Pancreatic involvement may present as signs and symptoms indistinguishable from other causes of pancreatitis. The clinical presentation ranges from asymptomatic pancreatitis to severe fulminant pancreatitis. The pancreas is often diffusely involved and imaging findings are indistinguishable from routine pancreatitis on ultrasound, CT, or MR imaging. If the pancreas is diffusely enlarged and boggy in appearance, however, cytomegalovirus infection should lead the differential. Likewise, hemorrhagic necrosis is often associated with herpes simplex infection (Fig. 10). Histologic evaluation may be necessary for organism-specific diagnosis. Special stains for mycobacteria, fungi, and viral inclusions after biopsy and serologic tests are required to establish a diagnosis.

DIFFUSE PANCREATIC DISEASES, INCLUDING DEPOSITION DISORDERS

Diffuse involvement of pancreas can occur with various inflammatory, infiltrative, or neoplastic disorders. The inflammatory deposition disorders, including autoimmune pancreatitis, are discussed in the article by Sahani and Perez-Johnston. In this section, other disorders of deposition and a few of the neoplastic processes that diffusely involve the pancreas are discussed. The deposition disorders include hemochromatosis, fatty replacement, and amyloidosis. The infiltrative disorders include cystic fibrosis, lymphoma, and metastatic deposition.

Hemochromatosis

Primary hemochromatosis is a disorder of abnormal iron deposition involving multiple organs and is characterized by a progressive increase in total body iron stores. Hemochromatosis affects men more often than women and is particularly common in whites of Western European descent. Patients usually present with abdominal pain, fatigue, joint pain, loss of body hair, weight loss, and loss of sexual desire.[40] Routinely, the diagnosis of hemochromatosis is established by buccal swab and genetic testing, biochemical analysis, and histologic examination of a liver biopsy. The assessment of the hepatic iron index by biopsy is considered the gold standard for diagnosis of hemochromatosis. Imaging is mainly used, however, for the diagnosis of iron deposition in various organs, to monitor the response to treatment noninvasively, and to diagnosis and manage complications, such as cirrhosis and hepatocellular cancer.

In primary hemochromatosis, iron is deposited in the parenchymal cells of the liver, pancreas, myocardium, and other organs. The spleen is not involved in primary hemochromatosis. Pancreatic involvement is uncommon in the absence of cirrhosis, and patients may develop type 1 diabetes mellitus. There is no correlation, however, between the amount of iron in the pancreas on imaging and pancreatic dysfunction or insufficiency. Alternatively, in hemosiderosis and secondary hemochromatosis, iron is deposited in the cells of the reticuloendothelial system (liver spleen lymph nodes and bone marrow) and

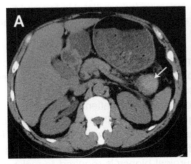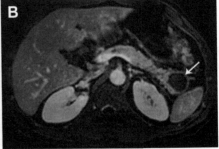

Fig. 10. A 28-year-old woman with AIDS and nontraumatic abdominal pain on nonenhanced axial CT (A) shows a focus of hemorrhage (arrow) in the tail of the pancreas without associated significant peripancreatic stranding. Same lesion on postgadolinium T1W image (B) shows lack of enhancement (arrow), suggestive of hemorrhagic necrosis. Although a definitive diagnosis was not established in his case, the findings resolved (not shown) with antiviral treatment and a presumptive diagnosis of herpes simplex hemorrhagic necrosis was made.

pancreatic parenchymal involvement occurs in later stages of the disease when the reticuloendothelial system is saturated with iron.[41,42] Contrast-enhanced CT is more useful for recognition of cirrhosis and hepatocellular cancer but limited for detection of iron deposition.[43] Increased pancreatic iron on nonenhanced CT demonstrates diffuse increased attenuation of the pancreas, usually greater than 75 Hounsfield units. CT is less sensitive and specific for detection of abnormal iron deposition compared with MR imaging. MR imaging measures tissue iron concentration indirectly via the detection of the paramagnetic influences of storage iron (ferritin and hemosiderin) on the proton resonance behavior of tissue water.[44] T2W and gradient-echo sequences are more sensitive for detection of iron compared with T1W and spin-echo sequences. Quantification of iron levels determined with MR imaging, especially from the liver, shows excellent correlation with that obtained from liver biopsy. MR imaging is emerging as an alternative to liver biopsy for quantification of liver iron load, mainly for follow-up after medical treatment.[45–47] The main advantage of MR imaging compared with biopsy is that MR imaging is a noninvasive technique and could be repeated to monitor the treatment response (**Fig. 11**).

Fatty Replacement of the Pancreas

Fat replacement, also termed lipomatosis, adipose atrophy, or fat infiltration of the exocrine pancreas, is commonly recognized on CT scans and often seen in obese and elderly patients. Most of the patients have no major clinical significance and findings on CT are considered a benign or normal finding.[48] Extreme degree of fat replacement of the pancreas is pathologic, however, and may be associated with significant depression of pancreatic function. Patients with cystic fibrosis, Cushing syndrome, adult-onset diabetes mellitus, chronic pancreatitis, hereditary pancreatitis, alcoholic hepatitis, malnutrition, Shwachman-Diamond syndrome, or long-term use of corticosteroids may have extreme lipomatosis.

On imaging, the fatty replacement may be of 3 types: (1) diffuse fatty replacement, which reveals separation of pancreatic parenchyma with prominence of lobulations; (2) asymmetric fatty replacement, where a part of pancreas, such as the head region is spared (often mistaken as tumor); and (3) fatty pseudohypertrophy, where the pancreas is massively enlarged due to fatty replacement.[49]

CT either with or without contrast is the best modality for identification of fatty replacement

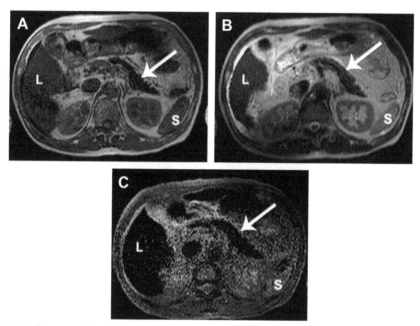

Fig. 11. A 55-year-old man with primary hemochromatosis on axial upper abdominal MR imaging using (*A*) T1 gradient-echo sequence (echo time [TE] = 4.6 ms, repetition time [TR] = 180 ms), (*B*) T2 spin-echo sequence (TE = 80 ms, TR = 270 ms), and (*C*) T2 gradient-echo sequence (TE = 14 ms, TR = 120 ms, flip angle 20) demonstrates iron deposition in cirrhotic liver (L) and pancreas (*arrow*) sparing the spleen (S). The decreased signal of pancreas and liver from iron deposition is more pronounced on T2 gradient-echo sequence (*C*) compared with T2 spin-echo sequence (*B*) and T1 gradient-echo sequence (*A*).

(Fig. 12). Although on ultrasound the fatty replaced pancreas may appear hyperecohic, the sensitivity is low due to overlying bowel gas and technical reasons. On T1W MR imaging, the pancreas appears homogenously hyperintense with loss of signal on fat-saturated T1W sequences. Both spared regions of fatty replacement and a small area of fatty infiltration may appear as tumor, also known as pseudotumor, on CT (Fig. 13). Chemical shift MR imaging is useful in these cases of patchy fatty infiltration because it has the advantage that the reduction in signal intensity of focal fatty replacement on opposed-phase images differentiates focal fatty replacement of the pancreas from true pancreatic tumors, which in general do not contain lipid.[50] The associated findings, if any, such as atrophy of the pancreas, ductal obstruction, or features of pancreatitis, can be seen on CT or MR imaging. Imaging can also be used in monitoring the response because fatty replacement is reversible in obese individuals after weight reduction, in patients treated for Cushing syndrome, or after discontinuation of corticosteroids.[48,51]

Cystic Fibrosis

Cystic fibrosis (CF) is the most common autosomal recessive disorder in humans. It mainly manifests as chronic obstructive lung disease and pancreatic disease. Pancreatic disease results in exocrine insufficiency, with clinically apparent dysfunction seen in 85% to 90% of patients.[52] Although endocrine pancreatic insufficiency is less common, nearly 1% to 2% of CF patients require insulin therapy.[53] The severity of manifestations increase with age. The main pathophysiology is due to a defective transmembrane ion transportation that leads to accumulation of thick, viscous pancreatic secretions in the pancreatic ducts, leading to ductal ectasia and acinar atrophy.[54] Inflammatory reaction, progressive fatty replacement, fibrosis, and sometimes calcification can occur.[54] Retention cysts may form in the pancreas from the inspissated secretions obstructing the small pancreatic ducts.[55]

On CT and MR imaging, the spectrum of pancreatic disease include (1) partial fibrofatty replacement, (2) complete fibrofatty replacement with enlargement of pancreas (lipomatous pseudohypertrophy), (3) pancreatic atrophy without evidence of fatty replacement, (4) diffuse pancreatic fibrosis, and (5) pancreatic cystosis.[51] Complete fatty replacement of pancreas is the most common imaging finding (see Fig. 12). MR imaging is most sensitive in detection of early fatty replacement in CF, with T1W MR imaging that shows high signal intensity. It has been demonstrated that the T1 signal intensity on MR imaging correlates well with the degree of clinical compromise due to exocrine insufficiency. The clinical utility of this observation is limited, however, because CF patients with a normal pancreas at MR imaging might also have clinically apparent exocrine insufficiency.[56–58]

Longstanding disease may produce atrophy, fibrosis, and calcifications. Pancreatic atrophy is the second most common finding reported and is seen in 27% to 35% of CF patients.[56,58] Atrophy can be seen on both CT and MR imaging. The findings of atrophy and fibrosis, however, overlap on CT and may be difficult to differentiate. Diffuse pancreatic fibrosis, although a rare finding, is reported to be seen on MR imaging where the pancreas is low in signal on all sequences.[57] Calcification is another finding that ranges from fine punctate concretions to granular or flecked areas of increased opacity; calcifications are generally found within dilated pancreatic ducts after ductal and ductular obstruction by calcium-rich inspissated material.[59] MR imaging is limited for evaluation of calcification. Pancreatic cysts are a common finding and probably occur secondary to duct obstruction by inspissated secretions. The cysts are typically small (1–3 mm) but can reach a diameter of several centimeters. Another rare manifestation is pancreatic cystosis where the entire pancreas is replaced by epithelium-lined cysts of varying size that may cause mass effect (Fig. 14).[60] Cyst formation and cystosis are seen on CT but better demonstrated on MR imaging. MRCP is helpful in evaluation of pancreatic duct. Typical abnormalities, such as narrowing, dilatation, stricture formation, and beading, are visualized better on ERCP (Fig. 15). These abnormalities are occasionally appreciated,

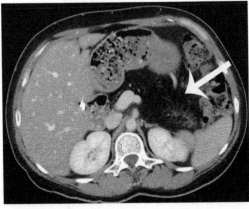

Fig. 12. A 22-year-old man with cystic fibrosis on axial contrast-enhanced CT of the abdomen shows diffuse replacement of the pancreas with fat (*arrow*).

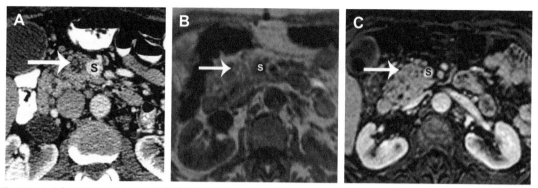

Fig. 13. Axial contrast-enhanced CT (*A*) in a 55-year-old-man for epigastric pain depicted a small hypodensity (*arrow*) in the head of the pancreas next to SMV (*S*). MR imaging was performed to rule out a neoplasm. On T1W in-phase axial image (*B*), the corresponding area (*arrow*) is hyperintense compared with the rest of the pancreas with no discrete mass on axial postgadolinium T1W image (*C*), suggestive of focal fatty infiltration.

however, on MRCP along with cysts related to the pancreatic duct.[53]

Diffuse Neoplastic Pancreatic Involvement

Diffuse involvement of the pancreas from malignancy can be seen with lymphoma, leukemia, and, rarely, carcinoma and metastases, with lymphoma the most common.

Pancreatic lymphoma
Pancreatic lymphoma is usually secondary to involvement of the pancreas by non-Hodgkin lymphoma. A rare type of primary pancreatic lymphoma (PPL) can also occur, however. Secondary involvement of pancreas innon-Hodgkin lymphoma is commonly associated with involvement of liver, spleen, bowel, and other retroperitoneal lymphadenopathy.[61,62] On CT, the pancreas is diffusely enlarged with low attenuation and mild enhancement (**Fig. 16**) and without any features of pancreatitis, such as peripancreatic stranding or fluid collections. Calcifications can occur after treatment. CT is helpful for assessment overall extent of disease. MR imaging is used as a problem-solving tool when a lesion is not completely characterized on CT. Typically on MR imaging, the pancreas is enlarged with low signal intensity on unenhanced T1W and T2W, with mild to moderate homogenous enhancement after gadolinium injection.[61]

PPL predominately presents with a pancreatic mass and involvement of only the peripancreatic lymph nodes, with no hepatic or splenic involvement, no other lymphadenopathy, and with a normal leukocyte count. Often the pancreas is focally involved with a bulky mass and without significant dilatation of the main pancreatic duct, which helps to differentiate PPL from adenocarcinoma. PPL on imaging, however, appears similar

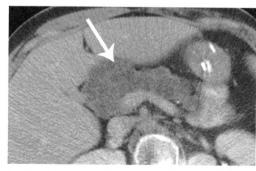

Fig. 14. Axial contrast-enhanced CT of the abdomen in a patient with cystic fibrosis demonstrates diffuse replacement of the pancreas with tiny cysts (*arrow*) consistent with pancreatic cystosis.

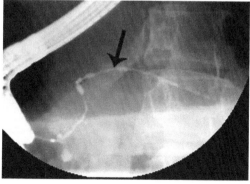

Fig. 15. ERCP in the same patient with cystic fibrosis as in Fig. 12 shows diffuse pancreatic ductal (*arrow*) narrowing with multiple beaded appearance and strictures.

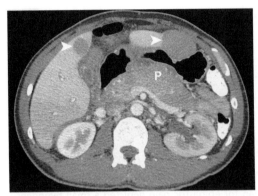

Fig. 16. Axial contrast-enhanced CT at pancreas in a patient with lymphoma demonstrates diffuse enlargement of the pancreas (P) with hypoenhancement, suggestive of pancreatic involvement. Focal hepatic masses of lymphoma (*arrowheads*) were also seen in this patient.

to adenocarcinoma and often the diagnosis is established by biopsy of the pancreatic mass.[62]

REFERENCES

1. Cirillo RL Jr, Koniaris LG. Detecting blunt pancreatic injuries. J Gastrointest Surg 2002;6(4):587–98.

2. Gupta A, Stuhlfaut JW, Fleming KW, et al. Blunt trauma of the pancreas and biliary tract: a multimodality imaging approach to diagnosis. Radiographics 2004;24(5):1381–95.

3. Akhrass R, Yaffe MB, Brandt CP, et al. Pancreatic trauma: a ten-year multi-institutional experience. Am Surg 1997;63(7):598–604.

4. Tyburski JG, Dente CJ, Wilson RF, et al. Infectious complications following duodenal and/or pancreatic trauma. Am Surg 2001;67(3):227–30 [discussion: 230–1].

5. Bradley EL 3rd, Young PR Jr, Chang MC, et al. Diagnosis and initial management of blunt pancreatic trauma: guidelines from a multiinstitutional review. Ann Surg 1998;227(6):861–9.

6. Teh SH, Sheppard BC, Mullins RJ, et al. Diagnosis and management of blunt pancreatic ductal injury in the era of high-resolution computed axial tomography. Am J Surg 2007;193(5):641–3 [discussion: 643].

7. Wong YC, Wang LJ, Fang JF, et al. Multidetector-row computed tomography (CT) of blunt pancreatic injuries: can contrast-enhanced multiphasic CT detect pancreatic duct injuries? J Trauma 2008; 64(3):666–72.

8. Venkatesh SK, Wan JM. CT of blunt pancreatic trauma: a pictorial essay. Eur J Radiol 2008;67(2): 311–20.

9. Brandon JC, Fields PA, Evankovich C, et al. Pancreatic clefts caused by penetrating vessels: a potential diagnostic pitfall for pancreatic fracture on CT. Emerg Radiol 2000;7(5):283–6.

10. Wong YC, Wang LJ, Lin BC, et al. CT grading of blunt pancreatic injuries: prediction of ductal disruption and surgical correlation. J Comput Assist Tomogr 1997;21(2):246–50.

11. Lee WJ, Foo NP, Lin HJ, et al. The efficacy of four-slice helical CT in evaluating pancreatic trauma: a single institution experience. J Trauma Manag Outcomes 2011;5(1):1.

12. Phelan HA, Velmahos GC, Jurkovich GJ, et al. An evaluation of multidetector computed tomography in detecting pancreatic injury: results of a multicenter AAST study. J Trauma 2009;66(3):641–6 [discussion: 646–7].

13. Linsenmaier U, Wirth S, Reiser M, et al. Diagnosis and classification of pancreatic and duodenal injuries in emergency radiology. Radiographics 2008;28(6):1591–602.

14. Soto JA, Alvarez O, Munera F, et al. Traumatic disruption of the pancreatic duct: diagnosis with MR pancreatography. AJR Am J Roentgenol 2001; 176(1):175–8.

15. Yang L, Zhang XM, Xu XX, et al. MR imaging for blunt pancreatic injury. Eur J Radiol 2010;75(2):e97–101.

16. Gillams AR, Kurzawinski T, Lees WR. Diagnosis of duct disruption and assessment of pancreatic leak with dynamic secretin-stimulated MR cholangiopancreatography. AJR Am J Roentgenol 2006;186(2): 499–506.

17. Kim HS, Lee DK, Kim IW, et al. The role of endoscopic retrograde pancreatography in the treatment of traumatic pancreatic duct injury. Gastrointest Endosc 2001;54(1):49–55.

18. Chandra J, Phillips RR, Boardman P, et al. Pancreas transplants. Clin Radiol 2009;64(7):714–23.

19. Gruessner AC. 2011 Update on pancreas transplantation: comprehensive trend analysis of 25,000 cases followed up over the course of twenty-four years at the International Pancreas Transplant Registry (IPTR). Rev Diabet Stud 2011;8(1):6–16.

20. Gruessner AC, Sutherland DE. Pancreas transplant outcomes for United States (US) and non-US cases as reported to the United Network for Organ Sharing (UNOS) and the International Pancreas Transplant Registry (IPTR) as of June 2004. Clin Transplant 2005;19(4):433–55.

21. Kelly WD, Lillehei RC, Merkel FK, et al. Allotransplantation of the pancreas and duodenum along with the kidney in diabetic nephropathy. Surgery 1967;61(6): 827–37.

22. Gruessner AC, Sutherland DE. Analyses of pancreas transplant outcomes for United States cases reported to the United Network for Organ Sharing (UNOS) and non-US cases reported to the International Pancreas Transplant Registry (IPTR). Clin Transplant 1999;51–69.

23. Nikolaidis P, Amin RS, Hwang CM, et al. Role of sonography in pancreatic transplantation. Radiographics 2003;23(4):939–49.

24. Freund MC, Steurer W, Gassner EM, et al. Spectrum of imaging findings after pancreas transplantation with enteric exocrine drainage: Part 2, posttransplantation complications. AJR Am J Roentgenol 2004;182(4):919–25.

25. Freund MC, Steurer W, Gassner EM, et al. Spectrum of imaging findings after pancreas transplantation with enteric exocrine drainage: Part 1, posttransplantation anatomy. AJR Am J Roentgenol 2004; 182(4):911–7.

26. Hagspiel KD, Nandalur K, Pruett TL, et al. Evaluation of vascular complications of pancreas transplantation with high-spatial-resolution contrast-enhanced MR angiography. Radiology 2007;242(2):590–9.

27. Gruessner AC, Sutherland DE. Pancreas transplant outcomes for United States (US) cases as reported to the United Network for Organ Sharing (UNOS) and the International Pancreas Transplant Registry (IPTR). Clin Transplant 2008;45–56.

28. Douzdjian V, Abecassis MM, Cooper JL, et al. Incidence, management and significance of surgical complications after pancreatic transplantation. Surg Gynecol Obstet 1993;177(5):451–6.

29. Sollinger HW, Knechtle SJ, Reed A, et al. Experience with 100 consecutive simultaneous kidney-pancreas transplants with bladder drainage. Ann Surg 1991; 214(6):703–11.

30. Eubank WB, Schmiedl UP, Levy AE, et al. Venous thrombosis and occlusion after pancreas transplantation: evaluation with breath-hold gadolinium-enhanced three-dimensional MR imaging. AJR Am J Roentgenol 2000;175(2):381–5.

31. Boeve WJ, Kok T, Tegzess AM, et al. Comparison of contrast enhanced MR-angiography-MRI and digital subtraction angiography in the evaluation of pancreas and/or kidney transplantation patients: initial experience. Magn Reson Imaging 2001;19(5): 595–607.

32. Krebs TL, Daly B, Wong-You-Cheong JJ, et al. Acute pancreatic transplant rejection: evaluation with dynamic contrast-enhanced MR imaging compared with histopathologic analysis. Radiology 1999;210(2):437–42.

33. Lall CG, Sandrasegaran K, Maglinte DT, et al. Bowel complications seen on CT after pancreas transplantation with enteric drainage. AJR Am J Roentgenol 2006;187(5):1288–95.

34. Meador TL, Krebs TL, Cheong JJ, et al. Imaging features of posttransplantation lymphoproliferative disorder in pancreas transplant recipients. AJR Am J Roentgenol 2000;174(1):121–4.

35. Woodfield JC, Windsor JA, Godfrey CC, et al. Diagnosis and management of isolated pancreatic tuberculosis: recent experience and literature review. ANZ J Surg 2004;74(5):368–71.

36. De Backer AI, Mortele KJ, Bomans P, et al. Tuberculosis of the pancreas: MRI features. AJR Am J Roentgenol 2005;184(1):50–4.

37. Pitchenik AE, Fertel D. Medical management of AIDS patients. Tuberculosis and nontuberculous mycobacterial disease. Med Clin North Am 1992; 76(1):121–71.

38. Schapiro RH, Maher MM, Misdraji J. Case records of the Massachusetts General Hospital. Case 3-2006. A 63-year-old woman with jaundice and a pancreatic mass. N Engl J Med 2006;354(4):398–406.

39. Itaba S, Yoshinaga S, Nakamura K, et al. Endoscopic ultrasound-guided fine-needle aspiration for the diagnosis of peripancreatic tuberculous lymphadenitis. J Gastroenterol 2007;42(1):83–6.

40. Dolbey CH. Hemochromatosis: a review. Clin J Oncol Nurs 2001;5(6):257–60.

41. Kawamoto S, Soyer PA, Fishman EK, et al. Nonneoplastic liver disease: evaluation with CT and MR imaging. Radiographics 1998;18(4):827–48.

42. Siegelman ES, Mitchell DG, Semelka RC. Abdominal iron deposition: metabolism, MR findings, and clinical importance. Radiology 1996;199(1):13–22.

43. Long JA Jr, Doppman JL, Nienhus AW, et al. Computed tomographic analysis of beta-thalassemic syndromes with hemochromatosis: pathologic findings with clinical and laboratory correlations. J Comput Assist Tomogr 1980;4(2):159–65.

44. Jensen PD. Evaluation of iron overload. Br J Haematol 2004;124(6):697–711.

45. Anderson LJ, Holden S, Davis B, et al. Cardiovascular T2-star (T2*) magnetic resonance for the early diagnosis of myocardial iron overload. Eur Heart J 2001;22(23):2171–9.

46. Ernst O, Sergent G, Bonvarlet P, et al. Hepatic iron overload: diagnosis and quantification with MR imaging. AJR Am J Roentgenol 1997;168(5):1205–8.

47. Gandon Y, Guyader D, Heautot JF, et al. Hemochromatosis: diagnosis and quantification of liver iron with gradient-echo MR imaging. Radiology 1994; 193(2):533–8.

48. Patel S, Bellon EM, Haaga J, et al. Fat replacement of the exocrine pancreas. AJR Am J Roentgenol 1980;135(4):843–5.

49. Matsumoto S, Mori H, Miyake H, et al. Uneven fatty replacement of the pancreas: evaluation with CT. Radiology 1995;194(2):453–8.

50. Kim HJ, Byun JH, Park SH, et al. Focal fatty replacement of the pancreas: usefulness of chemical shift MRI. AJR Am J Roentgenol 2007;188(2): 429–32.

51. Tham RT, Heyerman HG, Falke TH, et al. Cystic fibrosis: MR imaging of the pancreas. Radiology 1991;179(1):183–6.

52. Park RW, Grand RJ. Gastrointestinal manifestations of cystic fibrosis: a review. Gastroenterology 1981; 81(6):1143–61.

53. King LJ, Scurr ED, Murugan N, et al. Hepatobiliary and pancreatic manifestations of cystic fibrosis: MR imaging appearances. Radiographics 2000; 20(3):767–77.

54. Oppenheimer EH, Esterly JR. Pathology of cystic fibrosis review of the literature and comparison with 146 autopsied cases. Perspect Pediatr Pathol 1975;2:241–78.

55. Liu P, Daneman A, Stringer DA, et al. Pancreatic cysts and calcification in cystic fibrosis. Can Assoc Radiol J 1986;37(4):279–82.

56. Fiel SB, Friedman AC, Caroline DF, et al. Magnetic resonance imaging in young adults with cystic fibrosis. Chest 1987;91(2):181–4.

57. Murayama S, Robinson AE, Mulvihill DM, et al. MR imaging of pancreas in cystic fibrosis. Pediatr Radiol 1990;20(7):536–9.

58. Ferrozzi F, Bova D, Campodonico F, et al. Cystic fibrosis: MR assessment of pancreatic damage. Radiology 1996;198(3):875–9.

59. Iannaccone G, Antonelli M. Calcification of the pancreas in cystic fibrosis. Pediatr Radiol 1980; 9(2):85–9.

60. Berrocal T, Pajares MP, Zubillaga AF. Pancreatic cystosis in children and young adults with cystic fibrosis: sonographic, CT, and MRI findings. AJR Am J Roentgenol 2005;184(4):1305–9.

61. Merkle EM, Bender GN, Brambs HJ. Imaging findings in pancreatic lymphoma: differential aspects. AJR Am J Roentgenol 2000;174(3):671–5.

62. Grimison PS, Chin MT, Harrison ML, et al. Primary pancreatic lymphoma—pancreatic tumours that are potentially curable without resection, a retrospective review of four cases. BMC Cancer 2006;6:117.

Imaging After Pancreatic Surgery

Desiree E. Morgan, MD

KEYWORDS

- Pancreatic cancer • Pancreatic surgery • Pancreatitis
- Pancreatic imaging

Pancreatic surgery is performed for a number of clinical indications, and imaging serves both to aid in the planning of surgical therapy as well as to detect complications. Pancreatic resection provides the only treatment option that can lead to long-term survival in patients with pancreatic cancer or provides a potential for cure in various pancreatic neoplasms. Pancreatic resection also is used for the treatment of chronic pancreatitis, sometimes associated with islet cell transplantation. Pancreas transplantation has been successfully used to restore endocrine and exocrine function in diabetic patients. A variety of pancreatic drainage procedures, radiologic, endoscopic, and surgical, are available to aid in the treatment of patients with complications of acute and chronic pancreatitis. This article focuses on the common surgical procedures for treatment of pancreatic cancer and chronic pancreatitis.

Computed tomography (CT) is the imaging modality most often used to identify disease, plan surgical therapy, and evaluate for surgical complications.[1–6] After all types of pancreatic surgery, imaging for potential operative complications is typically indicated by the presence or development of persistent fever, elevated biliary enzymes or white blood cell count, elevated serum amylase, or significant abdominal distention and pain. In the longer term, assessment for local recurrence or distant metastatic disease in patients with resection for pancreatic neoplasms, or identification of complications, such as bilioenteric anastomotic stricture in patients following surgery for pancreatic inflammation or cancer, are well depicted by contrast-enhanced CT.[4–7] Suspected biliary complications also may be evaluated with magnetic resonance (MR) imaging using a hepatobiliary contrast agent.

In our practice, MR imaging is particularly useful if there is suspected obstruction of the pancreatic or bile ducts. Upper gastrointestinal (GI) series using water-soluble contrast media may be helpful in the assessment of leak of the gastrojejunal or duodenojejunal anastomoses, and has been used to evaluate gastric emptying.

CANCER OPERATIONS

Allen O. Whipple laid the foundation for modern pancreaticoduodenectomy. The Whipple procedure was first described in 1935,[8] and today is used for resection of pancreatic head tumors and periampullary lesions.[1,9,10] Although the first excisions of the pancreatic head region occurred in the late 1800s separately by both Codavilla and Halsted, and in the early 1900s by both Desjardens and Kausch, before Whipple's description in 1935 most surgeons did not conceive that the pancreas could be operated on without "disastrous results" for the patient.[11,12] Whipple's philosophy was to first relieve jaundice and improve nutritional intake, then address en bloc resection of the papillary region with permanent exclusion of the remaining pancreas. Initial mortality rates for the 2-stage operation reported by Whipple in 1940 approached 25%[13]; however, improved techniques and modification of the original Whipple procedure resulted in lower mortality rates after the 1970s, with high-volume centers now reporting perioperative mortality ranging from 1% to 3%.[10] The procedure (Fig. 1) consists of resection of the pancreatic head (divided at the neck), gastric antrum, duodenum, proximal 20 cm of jejunum, gallbladder, distal common bile duct, and lymph nodes. Three anastomoses are then created, and include Roux-en-Y

Department of Radiology, University of Alabama at Birmingham, 619 19th Street South, JT N452, Birmingham, AL 35249-6830, USA
E-mail address: dmorgan@uabmc.edu

Radiol Clin N Am 50 (2012) 529–545
doi:10.1016/j.rcl.2012.03.004
0033-8389/12/$ – see front matter © 2012 Elsevier Inc. All rights reserved.

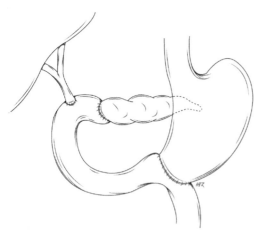

Fig. 1. Schematic of classic Whipple procedure.

pancreaticojejunostomy (Fig. 2), hepaticojejunostomy (Fig. 3), and gastrojejunostomy (Fig. 4).

The first pylorus-preserving pancreaticoduodenectomy was performed by Watson in 1944, then repopularized by Traverso and Longmire in 1978,[9,14] primarily for treatment of chronic pancreatitis. In this procedure (Fig. 5), the pylorus and first 2 cm of the duodenum are left intact, and a duodenojejunal Roux-en-Y anastomosis is performed (Fig. 6). This modification was devised to improve GI function and improve weight gain after surgery,[9] but in practice these outcomes have not been realized clinically.[1] In a prospective randomized multicenter comparison trial of 170 patients, the rate of pancreatic leakage/fistula, abscess, hemorrhage, and delayed gastric emptying was the same for classic Whipple and pylorus-preserving pancreaticoduodenectomy.[9]

With both the classic Whipple and pylorus-sparing modification, because the pancreatic neoplasms are located in the head, neck, or uncinate region, there may be involvement of the peripancreatic vessels. Involvement of the peripancreatic arteries typically renders a tumor nonresectable; however, when tumor invasion or encasement involves the portal or superior mesenteric veins, the lesions may be considered borderline resectable. Borderline resectable tumors can be

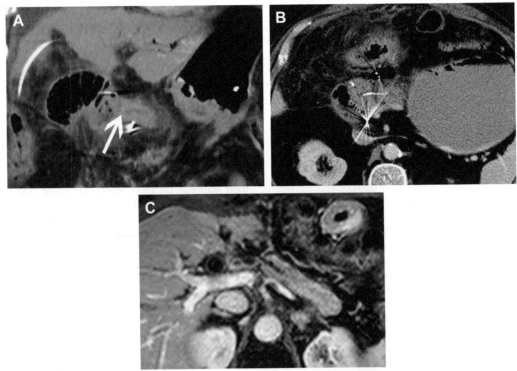

Fig. 2. Pancreaticojejunal anastomosis examples. (A) Axial contrast-enhanced CT image of a 68-year-old woman with history of classic Whipple procedure for ampullary adenocarcinoma demonstrates entrance of the remnant main pancreatic duct into the mucosal surface of the Roux jejunal limb (arrow). (B) Axial contrast-enhanced CT image of a 68-year-old man with pylorus-sparing pancreaticoduodenectomy for distal cholangiocarcinoma shows a temporary stent in the remnant pancreatic duct, which helps to identify the anastomosis with the jejunum. (C) Axial T1-weighted gadolinium-enhanced MR image of a 45-year-old man, who underwent pylorus-sparing pancreaticoduodenectomy for a T3 pancreatic adenocarcinoma, well depicts the entrance of the remnant pancreatic duct into the jejunum.

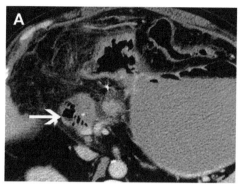
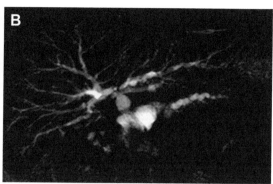

Fig. 3. Hepaticojejunal anastomosis examples. (A) Axial contrast-enhanced CT image of a 68-year-old woman status post classic Whipple (same patient as Fig. 2A) demonstrates the air-containing distal common bile duct (*arrow*) entering the jejunum. Note also the distended stomach in this patient who had delayed gastric emptying. (B) Pylorus-sparing pancreaticoduodenectomy of a 45-year-old man (same patient as Fig. 2C) for pancreatic adenocarcinoma. Magnetic resonance cholangiopancreatogram in oblique coronal projection demonstrates slightly dilated intrahepatic bile ducts and common hepatic duct entering the Roux jejunal limb.

successfully treated surgically if 2 conditions are met: the affected portion of the vein can be removed with the tumor, and the vein can be reconstructed. In general, when the affected portion of the vein involves a segment shorter than 2 cm in length, a primary end-to-end venous anastomosis can be achieved; if longer segments are involved or if tension is present on the venous anastomosis, a vein graft using the internal jugular vein or left renal vein[15,16] might be used. In the event that preoperative imaging fails to accurately depict vascular or hepatic involvement, despite state-of-the-art multiphasic multidetector CT or MR imaging, and a patient is found to be unresectable at surgery, a palliative gastrojejunostomy might be performed if gastrointestinal obstructive symptoms were present (Fig. 7) preoperatively. Palliative hepaticojejunostomies in the event of intraoperative discovery of unresectable disease are rarely performed at our institution in the era of metallic endoscopically placed biliary stents.

Occasionally, for pancreatic body/tail lesions that have undergone successful neoadjuvant treatment for peripancreatic vessel involvement by tumor, the Appleby procedure may be undertaken. With this procedure, en bloc celiac axis resection and accompanying distal pancreatectomy are performed.[17] Specifically, the celiac trunk, common hepatic artery, left gastric artery, and splenic artery are removed; the liver receives flow through retrograde perfusion of the gastroduodenal artery to the proper hepatic artery via the superior mesenteric artery. Care must be taken to not injure the gastroduodenal artery when the neck of pancreas is divided.

The central pancreatectomy, originally described in 1957 by Guillemin and Bessot,[18] is used to resect benign or low malignant-potential lesions in the neck

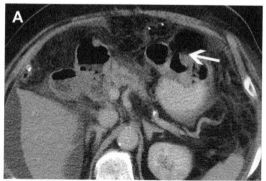
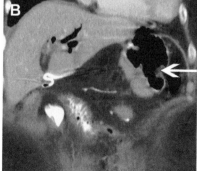

Fig. 4. Gastrojejunostomy examples. (A) Gastrojejunostomy of a 68-year-old woman who underwent Whipple procedure for ampullary adenoma (same patient as Fig. 2A). Axial contrast-enhanced CT image demonstrates the widely patent anastomosis anteriorly (*arrow*). (B) Gastrojejunostomy of a 75-year-old woman who underwent Whipple procedure to remove a 4.2-cm pancreatic adenocarcinoma. Coronal reformatted contrast-enhanced CT image reveals a predominantly gas-filled gastrojejunal anastomosis (*arrow*).

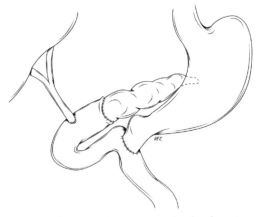

Fig. 5. Pylorus-sparing pancreaticoduodenectomy drawing.

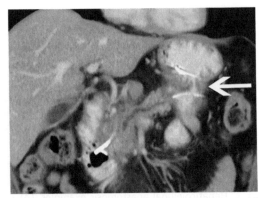

Fig. 7. Palliative gastrojejunostomy in unresectable pancreatic adenocarcinoma in 54-year-old man with gastrointestinal obstructive symptoms. Coronal reformatted contrast-enhanced CT image demonstrates the positive oral contrast-filled gastrojejunal anastomosis (arrow).

or body region of the pancreas. The operation was also originally performed for chronic pancreatitis. Operative candidates must have an adequate distal remnant to create a pancreaticoenteric anastomosis, and the lesion to be resected should be smaller than 5 cm.[19] The goal of central pancreatectomy is to preserve better postoperative endocrine and exocrine function by sparing the functional parenchyma upstream from the central lesion (that would otherwise be removed with a formal distal pancreatectomy), avoiding pancreatic enzyme supplementation and insulin administration.[1,19,20] In addition, preservation of the spleen is important to avoid risks associated with splenectomy sepsis or hematologic disorders.[20] With this procedure (Fig. 8), the distal pancreatic margin is anastomosed to a Roux-en-Y pancreaticojejunostomy, and the remnant of the head region is left in place but oversewn in a manner similar to a standard distal pancreatectomy (Fig. 9). Because there are 2 separate

suture lines oversewing the residual pancreatic tissue, there is a higher risk for fistula in these patients, and when the spleen is spared, care must be made to preserve the splenic artery and vein. With central pancreatectomy, if invasive ductal pathology is present on frozen section, larger resection is required to minimize rate of recurrence, sacrificing functionality of the pancreas preservation.[21]

Distal pancreatectomy is used to treat neoplastic lesions in the distal neck, body, or tail of the pancreas. With this procedure (Fig. 10), a varying amount of pancreas to the left of the portal confluence is resected along with en bloc removal of the spleen (Fig. 11). If the resectable lesion is thought to be of low malignant potential or if the distal pancreatectomy is performed for chronic pancreatitis with small duct disease, the spleen may be preserved.[22] Because adenocarcinomas in this

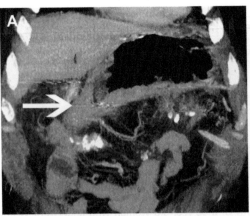
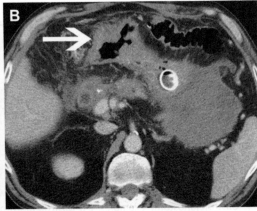

Fig. 6. Pylorus-sparing pancreaticoduodenectomy in 68-year-old man for distal cholangiocarcinoma (same patient as Fig. 2B). (A) Coronal and (B) axial contrast-enhanced CT images show the right-sided anastomosis. Note retrogastric hematoma (arrow) associated with placement of the percutaneous gastrostomy tube, which had been inserted to relieve delayed gastric-emptying symptoms.

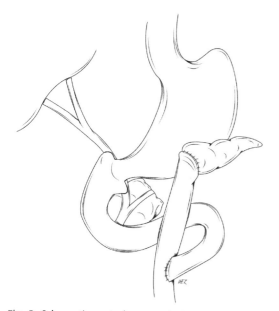

Fig. 8. Schematic central pancreatectomy.

region are often larger and are detected at a later stage than are lesions in the pancreatic head, approximately 20% of patients require multivisceral resections during a distal pancreatectomy[1] for that particular histology. In addition, lesions in the pancreatic body in proximity to the celiac axis and aorta may be found to be unresectable at surgery despite state-of-the-art preoperative imaging. Distal pancreatectomy may be performed with a laparoscopic approach. With this method, small lesions, such as functional pancreatic endocrine tumors, might have to be identified or have their locations confirmed with laparoscopic ultrasound, as tactile palpation of the mass is not possible. Specialized laparoscopic instruments are used to achieve resection, and the specimen is placed in a plastic bag before delivery through an enlarged port site.[1]

Total pancreatectomy was first performed by Billroth in 1884[23] and today is used to treat certain neoplastic conditions, such as multicentric or extensive endocrine tumors, nesidioblastosis, or multifocal intraductal papillary mucinous neoplasms. The procedure also is used for patients with familial

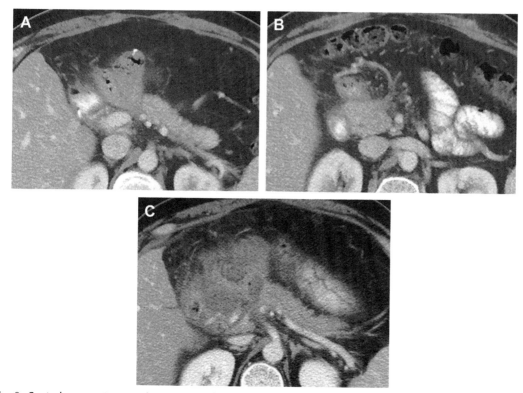

Fig. 9. Central pancreatectomy in a 47-year-old man who presented with symptomatic lymphoepithelial cyst at the pancreatic body/neck junction. (A) Axial contrast-enhanced CT image at the level of the resected central gland reveals filling of the defect by the Roux jejunal limb. (B) In the same examination more inferiorly, the normal pancreatic head is seen. (C) Perioperative period axial contrast-enhanced CT image of the same patient demonstrates inflammatory changes surrounding the Roux limb, owing to transient pancreatic fistula.

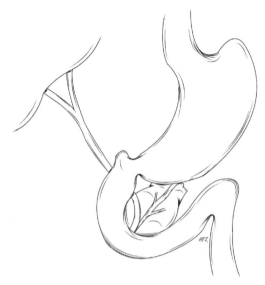

Fig. 10. Schematic distal pancreatectomy.

pancreatic cancer with premalignant lesions.[24] Total pancreatectomy (Fig. 12) involves removal of the entire pancreas, gastric antrum, duodenum, gallbladder, common bile duct, spleen, and lymph nodes. Anastomoses include Roux-en-Y gastrojejunostomy and end-to-side choledochojejunostomy (Fig. 13). When total pancreatectomy is performed for treatment of cancer, 5-year survival is approximately 9%.[25] Because morbidity and perioperative mortality are higher than for partial resections, this treatment option is not often used for sporadic pancreatic adenocarcinoma but is reserved for the familial type.

More commonly, patients undergo total pancreatectomy or completion total pancreatectomy for chronic pancreatitis, in which case the spleen and duodenum may be preserved.[26] When performed to treat chronic inflammation, islet cells from the resected pancreas are isolated and subsequently injected into the portal vein intraoperatively. Advances in autologous islet cell transplantation and insulin formation have improved blood glucose control in patients requiring total pancreatectomy. In the modern era, the University of Minnesota has the largest experience with total pancreatectomy with auto islet cell transplantation, reporting 70% of patients with significantly reduced pain and 72% of patients (without prior pancreatic resection) being insulin independent postoperatively.[27] For patients receiving allo islet cell transplantation, graft survival is reported at 77% at 3 years.

Enucleation is a surgical technique used for focal resection of low malignant-potential lesions or exophytic lesions,[5] and is typically used to resect insulinomas (Fig. 14). The lesion is dissected from the surrounding pancreatic parenchyma using a harmonic scalpel or electrocautery to seal small vessels and duct branches. During the procedure, if a significant ductal leak is seen following tumor removal, a formal pancreatectomy is often necessary to avoid complications of pancreatic fistula and abscess.

SURGERIES FOR CHRONIC PANCREATITIS

Longitudinal or lateral pancreaticojejunostomy (Puestow procedure) remains the preferred duct decompression procedure for patients with chronic pancreatitis where the main pancreatic duct is greater than or equal to 7 mm.[26,28] During this procedure (Fig. 15), the duct is incised longitudinally over the necessary length, stones are removed, and a side-to-side Roux-en-Y retrocolic pancreaticojejunostomy is created (Fig. 16). The surgery relieves pain in 65% to 93% of patients, and is associated with a 2% mortality and 20%

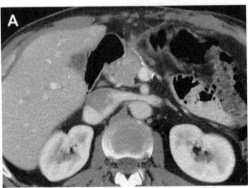
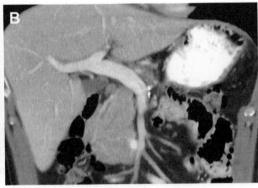

Fig. 11. Normal appearance of distal pancreatectomy in a 46-year-old woman who underwent resection of a unilocular serous cystadenoma. (A) Axial and (B) coronal contrast-enhanced CT images demonstrate the remnant gland in the pancreatic head with sharply marginated resection at midline.

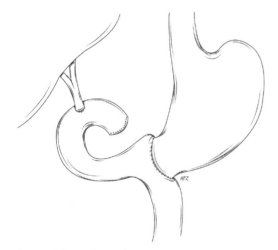

Fig. 12. Schematic total pancreatectomy.

perioperative morbidity. Up to 50% of patients will have recurrent symptoms.[26]

When chronic pancreatitis is head-dominant, pancreatic head resection is indicated because neural inflammation in the affected region likely contributes to pain.[29] Pancreatic resection leads to adequate pain control in most patients with chronic pancreatitis, with long-term outcome not dependent on the type of surgical procedure but more influenced by the severity of the disease preoperatively and by complications postoperatively.[30] In efforts to maintain GI function, preservation of the duodenum is important. The duodenum-preserving pancreatic head resection (Beger procedure) is indicated for the treatment of intractable pain in patients with chronic

pancreatitis who have head-dominant disease and small pancreatic ducts.[31] The procedure (Fig. 17) consists of ventral transection of the pancreatic neck along with Roux-en-Y pancreaticojejunostomies of both the remnant body/tail region and the rim of tissue along the inner surface of the C-loop of the duodenum. With this procedure, 91% of patients are reported pain-free at a median of 5 to 7 years with a hospital mortality of less than 1%.[31] The Frey procedure is used to treat intractable pain in patients with chronic pancreatitis with head-dominant disease and an enlarged pancreatic duct, and includes a subtotal duodenal-preserving pancreatic head resection combined with lateral pancreaticojejunostomy.[29] In this operation, the Roux-en-Y jejunal limb extends to the duodenum along the duct remnant, precluding the complicated portions of the Beger procedure and the creation of 2 separate pancreaticojejunal anastomoses. Pain relief was achieved in 75% of patients at 37 months, with perioperative morbidity of 22%.[29] Neither the Beger nor the Frey procedure should be undertaken if there is a high index of suspicion that pancreatic neoplasm is present in the pancreatic head[26]; rather, a standard pancreaticoduodenectomy or pylorus-preserving pancreaticoduodenectomy are indicated. Both of the duodenum-sparing procedures are more commonly used in Europe than in the United States.

Other surgical therapies for complications of chronic pancreatitis include resection of pseudocysts when septated or when associated with elevated carcinoembryonic antigen or cancer antigen (CA) 125 levels, cystogastrostomy when

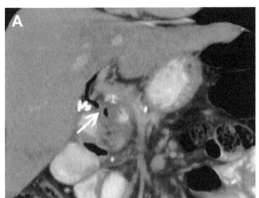
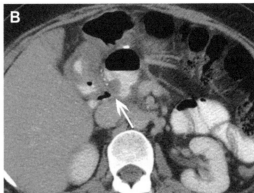

Fig. 13. Normal imaging appearance of total pancreatectomy in a 32-year-old woman who suffered multiple attacks of acute onset chronic pancreatitis and intractable pain. (A) Coronal reformatted contrast-enhanced CT image demonstrates absence of the pancreatic parenchyma. Note the pneumobilia, which well defines the location of the hepaticojejunal anastomosis (arrow). (B) Axial contrast-enhanced CT image of the same patient demonstrates absence of the pancreatic gland with contrast-filled duodenojejunal anastomosis (arrow). Note that there is a small amount of abnormal perioperative fluid adjacent to the vessels in this patient who underwent resection for inflammation. She also underwent concurrent autologous islet cell transplantation.

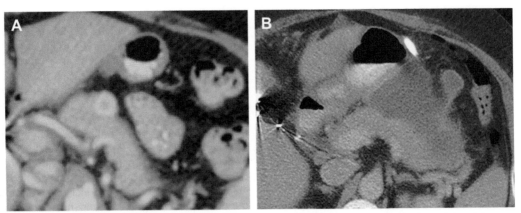

Fig. 14. Enucleation of small insulinoma in a 65-year-old woman with profound hypoglycemia. (*A*) Axial contrast-enhanced CT image through the pancreatic body before surgery reveals a 1.1-cm hyperenhancing mass in the anterior body. (*B*) Axial contrast-enhanced CT image at the same level postoperatively reveals focal parenchymal defect at the site as well as peripancreatic fluid accumulation owing to small-caliber pancreatic duct disruption not sealed over during enucleation.

the cyst is adherent to the posterior gastric wall, or Roux-en-Y cyst-jejunostomy if the cyst is not adherent to the stomach. Occasionally, if patients are symptomatic from left-sided portal hypertension attributed to chronic splenic vein thrombosis complicating chronic pancreatitis, splenectomy is indicated.

Similarly, surgical therapies for complications of acute pancreatitis have evolved over recent years, with modifications of formal necrosectomy, including minimally invasive transgastric or percutaneous retroperitoneal approaches, or standard cyst gastrostomy for mature collections.

NORMAL CT FINDINGS AFTER PANCREATIC SURGERY

After pancreaticoduodenectomy procedures, the pancreatic surgical bed is obscured by the presence of clips (**Fig. 18**) and beam-hardening artifact; this has been reported in up to 22% of patients[4,5] in the literature, but in our practice is seen in approximately 75% of patients. Another common postoperative finding is unopacified anastomotic bowel loops in the porta hepatis (69 of 82 scans),[5] described as a pseudomass[3] and varied in appearance depending on the degree of air within the Roux jejunal limb[12] (**Fig. 19**); administration of glucagon before CT can help fill the

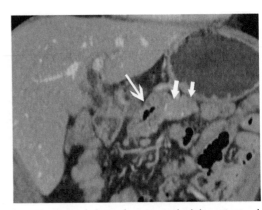

Fig. 16. Normal lateral pancreaticojejunostomy in a 46-year-old man with long-standing chronic pancreatitis and unrelenting pain. Coronal reformatted contrast-enhanced CT image demonstrates the Roux jejunal limb (*arrow*) adjacent to the body of the pancreas (*short arrows*). The main pancreatic duct is decompressed.

Fig. 15. Schematic lateral pancreaticojejunostomy.

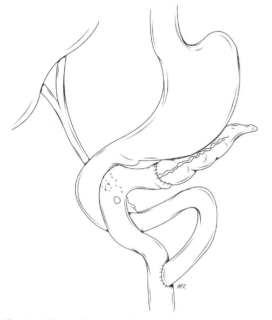

Fig. 17. Schematic of the Beger procedure.

Roux limb with oral contrast to better define the anatomy if needed.[32] A temporary stent may be placed across the pancreaticojejunal anastomosis during surgery, helping to identify the duct-to-mucosal communication with the pancreatic remnant on CT (Fig. 20). When a stent is not present, the pancreaticojejunal anastomosis can generally be localized anterior to the superior mesenteric artery at the level of the splenic vein.[2] Patency of the hepaticojejunostomy can be confirmed by the presence of biliary air (pneumobilia), another common postoperative finding seen in 67% to 80% of cases (see Fig. 4B; Fig. 13A; Fig. 19).[3,5–7] The duodenojejunal junction is located on the right side within the abdomen, usually inferior to the left hepatic lobe, whereas the gastrojejunal anastomosis in a classic Whipple is usually to the left of midline.[3] A small amount of surgical bed fluid is seen in 29% to 50% of patients[4–6] in the immediate perioperative period (Fig. 21), usually resolving spontaneously.[12] In addition, there may be soft tissue perivascular cuffing (see Figs. 4 and 13) that is not associated

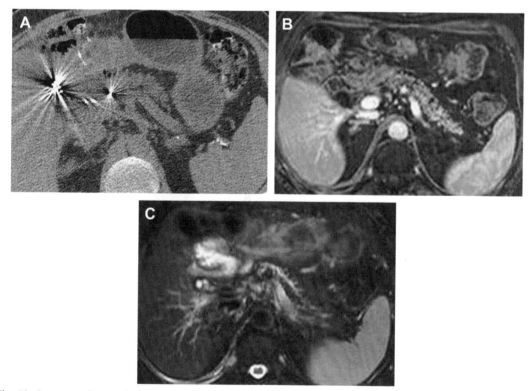

Fig. 18. Postoperative surgical clips in a 54-year-old man who underwent pylorus-sparing pancreaticoduodenectomy for a 2.0-cm moderately differentiated pancreatic adenocarcinoma. (A) Axial unenhanced CT image through the pancreatic bed reveals streak artifact from surgical clips obscuring detail. (B) Same patient, similar level as the CT scan, axial T1-weighted gadolinium-enhanced image better depicts the remnant pancreas and postsurgical anatomy. (C) Axial T2-weighted image, same level, of the same patient reveals the relationship of the remnant main pancreatic duct to the fluid-containing Roux jejunal limb. At 1.5 T, no significant clip-blooming artifact was noted in this patient.

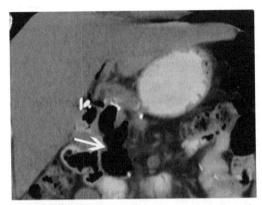

Fig. 19. Pneumobilia in a 32-year-old woman who underwent total pancreatectomy and auto islet cell transplantation (same patient as Fig. 13). Coronal re-formatted contrast-enhanced CT image well depicts the hepaticojejunal anastomosis without significant streak artifact from nearby clips. Note the gaseous distention of the gastrojejunal region (*arrow*), which also aids in identifying the postsurgical anatomy.

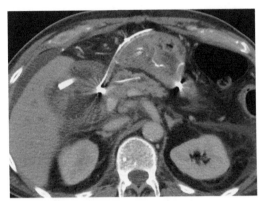

Fig. 21. Normal transient postoperative pancreatic bed fluid accumulation in a 65-year-old man who underwent classic Whipple after neoadjuvant chemo-radiation therapy for borderline pancreatic adenocarcinoma. Note the fluid in the portocaval space extending to the peripancreatic vessels, small amount of ascites, and fluid in the left anterior pararenal space.

with recurrent disease in 60% of patients, as well as reactive adenopathy in 32%.[2,6] These reactive lymph nodes regress rather than grow, helping to differentiate them from recurrence.[3] Likewise, the key to differentiating the perioperative perivascular soft tissue from recurrence is that it undergoes a gradual decrease, not increase, and was seen for a maximum duration of 13 months in one series.[3]

SURGICAL COMPLICATIONS

The morbidity of pancreaticoduodenectomy at high-volume centers is approximately 40%, and

mortality 2%.[31,33] In past years, the most common complication of pancreatic resection was the presence of early leakage from the pancreaticojejunal anastomosis, or fistula. The incidence of leak and fistula in more recent years is reported at 14% and 22%, respectively.[34] Leakage from the pancreaticoenteric anastomosis leads to breakdown

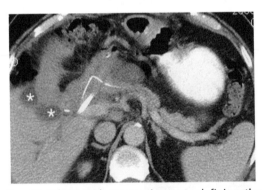

Fig. 20. Biliary and pancreatic stents defining the anastomotic region in a 74-year-old man who had a pylorus-sparing pancreaticoduodenectomy for distal common bile duct tubular adenoma. Note the smaller-caliber pancreatic stent denoting the pancreatic duct to mucosal anastomosis, and the larger-caliber biliary stent, in place to treat bilomas (*asterisks*).

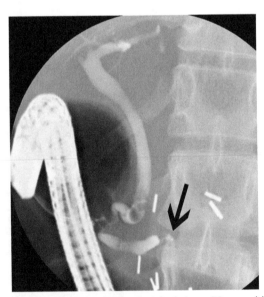

Fig. 22. Main pancreatic duct leak in a 36-year-old woman who underwent distal pancreatectomy to remove a 1.7-cm pancreatic endocrine tumor. Endoscopic retrograde cholangiopancreatography 2 weeks postoperative reveals filling of the bile and pancreatic duct to the resection margin, where a small leak (*black arrow*) was detected. A temporary pancreatic stent was inserted to resolve the leak.

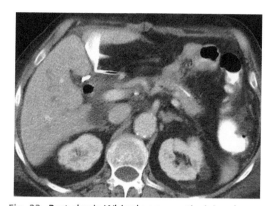

Fig. 23. Post classic Whipple pancreaticojejunal anastomotic leak in a 75-year-old woman who underwent resection for pancreatic adenocarcinoma. Axial contrast-enhanced CT image obtained 10 days after surgery reveals fluid surrounding the periportal region, extending back toward vessels. Note the presence of the right upper quadrant surgical drain through which amylase-rich secretions continued beyond postoperative day 10.

of the tissues at the anastomotic site and is related to the tissue characteristics of the remnant pancreas. For all pancreatic resections, when the parenchyma is soft, the anastomosis is harder to sew, and when there is a small duct, the anastomosis is more difficult to create; moreover, when there is a high degree of remnant function, there is more excretion and less healing. This is especially pertinent to distal pancreatectomies performed to resect neoplasms, where the remnant pancreatic tissue in the head is usually normal (Fig. 22). Various anastomotic surgical techniques have been used to reduce the incidence of pancreaticoenteric leaks over the years, including end-to-side, end invagination, and sealing the cut surface of the gland with glue. Clinically significant pancreaticoenteric leaks occur in from 0% to 13%[35] and require further therapy (Figs. 23 and 24). The use of octreotide to prevent fistulae in patients at high risk for leakage at the anastomosis is a point of discussion in much of the surgical

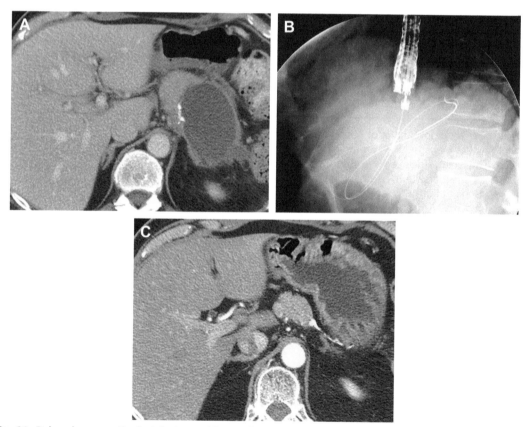

Fig. 24. Delayed pancreatic duct leak requiring endoscopic drainage in a 65-year-old man who underwent a hand-assisted distal pancreatectomy for cystic pancreatic endocrine tumor. (A) Axial contrast-enhanced CT image obtained 6 weeks postoperatively reveals a well-defined walled off fluid collection adjacent to the surgical material at the pancreatic resection margin. (B) Spot radiograph of the same patient during endoscopic transgastric drainage. Note the looped wire within the collection. (C) Same patient contrast-enhanced CT 6 months later demonstrates clean margin of retroperitoneal fat surrounding the suture material over the pancreatic stump.

literature. Typically, the fistula rate varies with the surgical indication. For patients having undergone resection for chronic pancreatitis, the fistula rate is 3% to 5%, for pancreatic adenocarcinoma is 12%, for periampullary lesions is 15%, and for distal bile duct carcinoma is 33%.[36]

Delayed gastric emptying (see **Fig. 2B**, **Fig. 6**), reported in 8% to 45% of patients,[35] is now the most common procedure-related morbidity because of the decline in incidence of leakage at the anastomosis over recent decades.[37,38] Perioperative hemorrhage is detected by the presence of high-density material in the surgical bed and is seen in 3% to 13% of resections (**Fig. 25**).[38–40] Hemorrhage is more common in duodenum-sparing procedures performed for chronic pancreatitis.[35] Another complication is acute pancreatitis of the remnant. The development of septic complications, especially intra-abdominal abscess, is seen in 1% to 12% of patients[35] and represents the most significant procedure-related morbidity of pancreatic resection (**Fig. 26**). The degree of destruction and inflammation in the retroperitoneum prognosticates patient outcome and determines the need for further operation.[35] Additional less common complications include pelvic abscess (because of the extensive intraperitoneal component of the surgery), hepatic infarct (**Fig. 27**) with or without abscess, bile duct injury and bile leak[12] (see **Fig. 20**), and anastomotic stricturing of the hepaticojejunal or pancreaticojejunal anastomoses.

Most clinical complications of pancreaticoduodenectomy are managed without radiologic intervention, including delayed gastric emptying (defined as the persistent need for nasogastric tube for longer than 10 days) seen in 11% to

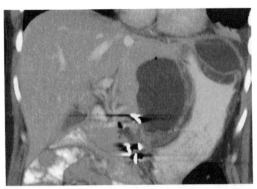

Fig. 26. Postoperative abscess in a 36-year-old woman (same patient as **Fig. 22**) who underwent distal pancreatectomy for pancreatic endocrine tumor. Coronal reformatted contrast-enhanced CT image reveals 2 uniformly homogeneous collections with well-defined walls. A single bubble of gas is seen within the larger collection. At endoscopic drainage, 300 mL of purulent material was removed.

29% of patients[37,41,42] (see **Fig. 2B**, **Fig. 6**); pancreatic fistula (defined as surgical drain output of amylase that exceeds greater than 50 mL per day at or beyond 7 to 10 days postoperative[37,43]) (see **Fig. 9C**); and wound infection (5% to 20%). The key to treatment of significant leaks is early detection with CT, and prompt external drainage.[12] The rates of postoperative collections requiring external drainage vary among institutions, but are generally less than 15%.[44,45] Zink and colleagues[46] reported a population of 373 patients with pancreaticoduodenectomy over 12 years (185 for pancreatic cancer). Eighty-three (22%) of 373 had image-guided drainage, and technical success was achieved in 98%, with

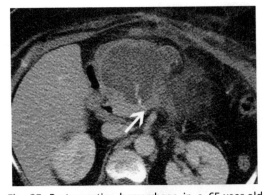

Fig. 25. Postoperative hemorrhage in a 65-year-old woman who underwent distal pancreatectomy to remove a 4.2-cm T2 pancreatic adenocarcinoma of the tail region. Axial contrast-enhanced CT scan 2 weeks after surgery reveals active extravasation (*arrow*) into the collection, which ultimately was drained surgically.

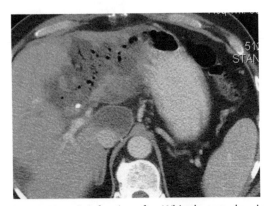

Fig. 27. Hepatic infarction after Whipple procedure in a 53-year-old man with pancreatic adenocarcinoma. Note the low-attenuation and scattered gas throughout the left lobe, with additional focal areas of diminished parenchymal attenuation in the caudate and right lobe periphery.

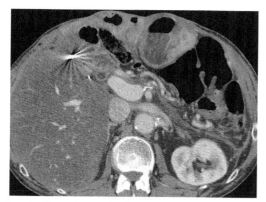

Fig. 28. Steatohepatitis after total pancreatectomy in a 48-year-old man with chronic pancreatitis. Note the absence of the anterior abdominal wall in this patient who developed postoperative abscesses and wound breakdown in the perioperative period.

overall drainage success of 80%. Forty-one percent of patients received a single drain, and 39 required multiple drains.

Most complications after total pancreatectomy and autologous islet cell transplantation are metabolic, and include development of steatohepatitis (Fig. 28), malabsorption, and marginal ulcers, owing to lack of bicarbonate excretion.[24] The latter can be overcome by the use of proton pump inhibitors. In an apancreatic state because of glycemic instability, patients often must eat 5000 calories per day.

Longer-term late postsurgical complications include chronic fistula and abscess, aneurysm or pseudoaneurysm formation, biliary anastomosis stenosis, perianastomotic ulceration, biloma, pseudocyst (Figs. 29 and 30), and tumor recurrence.

TUMOR SURVEILLANCE

When resections have been performed for cancer, because recurrent tumors grow rapidly, CT is usually performed at 3-month intervals. The accuracy of CT to detect recurrence after resection for pancreatic adenocarcinoma is 93.5%.[5] The most frequent sites of recurrence pancreatic cancer are the liver and pancreatic bed.[3,4,7] Hence, follow-up CT scans should be optimized to evaluation of the liver.[4] In 1 study, 4 of 19 patients had recurrent disease only in the liver, and an additional 4 had recurrence in the liver at the same time as local recurrence (Fig. 31).[3] In another study, there was no significant predilection for recurrence.[5] This phenomenon could in part be because of the difficulties involved in detecting subtle soft tissue recurrences in the pancreatic bed. Although collapsed Roux jejunal loops in the porta often obscure detection of local recurrence, an increase in the amount of soft tissue in the pancreatic bed or perivascular cuffing should raise suspicion for recurrence. The serum marker CA-19-9 might help differentiate postoperative increased attenuation from tumor recurrence. CA-19-9 is a tumor-associated antigen expressed

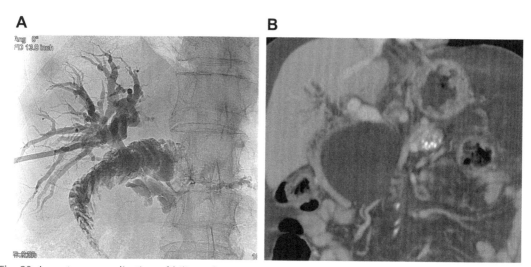

Fig. 29. Long-term complication of biliary obstruction caused by pseudocyst at the Roux limb in a 53-year-old woman who underwent pancreatic head resection for chronic pancreatitis. (A) Percutaneous transhepatic cholangiogram demonstrates moderate intrahepatic bile duct dilation, patent hepaticojejunostomy, and dilation of the Roux jejunal limb down to the point of narrowing several centimeters below the liver. (B) Coronal reformatted contrast-enhanced CT image of the same patient demonstrates the relationship of the large pseudocyst to the compressed Roux jejunal limb.

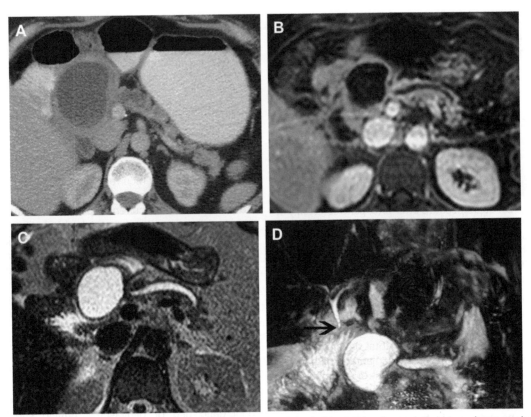

Fig. 30. Pseudocyst at pancreaticojejunal anastomosis in a 67-year-old woman who underwent a pylorus-sparing pancreaticoduodenectomy for pancreatic adenocarcinoma. (*A*) Axial contrast-enhanced CT image demonstrates the well-circumscribed pseudocyst adjacent to the dilated remnant main pancreatic duct. Note the importance of positive oral contrast administration to differentiate the pseudocyst from dilated Roux limb. (*B*) Axial T1-weighted gadolinium-enhanced MR image of the same patient demonstrates remnant pancreas with dilated main pancreatic duct leading toward the pseudocyst. No recurrent mass is noted. (*C*) Same-level single-shot fast spin-echo T2-weighted image and (*D*) coronal half-Fourier acquisition single-shot turbo spin-echo MR cholangiopancreatography image reveal the relationship of the pseudocyst to the dilated pancreatic remnant duct. Note the normal caliber of the bile duct emptying into the hepaticojejunal anastomosis (*arrow*).

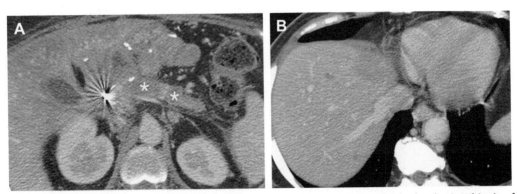

Fig. 31. Recurrence of the pancreatic resection margin in a 51-year-old woman who had a classic Whipple after neoadjuvant radiation and was receiving gemcitabine postoperatively. (*A*) Axial contrast-enhanced CT image superior to the pancreatic resection margin reveals recurrence in the pancreatic remnant (*asterisks*) and clip obscuring evaluation of the pancreatic relationship to the Roux jejunal limb. (*B*) The same examination more superiorly through the liver reveals 2 small hepatic metastases that developed 11 months after surgery.

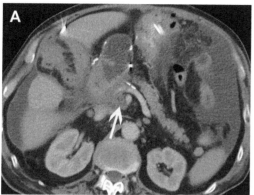 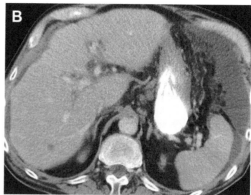

Fig. 32. Early recurrence in a 63-year-old man who underwent a pylorus-sparing pancreaticojejunostomy with R0 margins 4 months earlier. (*A*) Axial contrast-enhanced axial image through the surgical bed shows soft tissue attenuation surrounding the jejunal Roux limb and extending to the splenic vein, superior mesenteric vein, and superior mesenteric artery (*arrow*). Ascites is also a clue that recurrence has occurred. (*B*) The same examination more superiorly through the liver reveals a small hepatic metastasis, new gastrohepatic ligament adenopathy, and infiltration of the omentum in the left upper quadrant.

in 72% to 93% of malignant pancreatic tumors; however, it is also expressed in other GI tumors and is nonspecific. Recurrent tumor can obstruct the hepaticojejunal anastomosis and, therefore, the development of biliary dilation is an ominous sign. Detection of enlarging lymph nodes on serial examination may also indicate metastatic disease.

Liver metastases, lung metastases, and peritoneal carcinomatosis generally develop within a short interval after resection for pancreatic cancer, even when surgery is successful with an R0 margin, as median survival following resection ranges from 12 to 18 months.[47] Survival varies with resected tumor type, with one large observational study reporting 5-year actual survival rates

of 15% for pancreatic, 27% for distal bile duct, 39% for ampullary, and 59% for duodenal adenocarcinomas.[48] In a prospective, randomized, multicenter comparison trial of 170 patients, the rate of positivity of resection margins and positive lymph node rate was not different between classic Whipple and pylorus-preserving pancreaticoduodenectomy, and the median disease-free survival overall was similar as well.[9] Regarding timing of imaging-detected recurrence, one imaging-based review reported CT-detected recurrence in 15 (47%) of 32 patients after mean of 11 months (range 1 month to 3 years),[5] and another reported CT evidence of metastatic or recurrent disease in 5 (36%) of 14 patients after a mean of 11.8 months

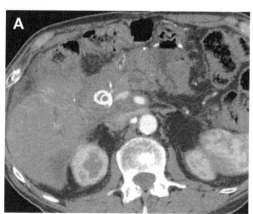 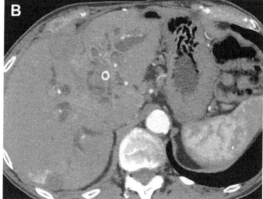

Fig. 33. Late recurrence in a 65-year-old man who underwent classic Whipple resection after successful downstaging with neoadjuvant chemoradiation for pancreatic adenocarcinoma 7 years earlier (same patient as Fig. 21). (*A*) Axial contrast-enhanced CT image through the same level as the perioperative fluid in Fig. 21 reveals replacement by soft tissue density, consistent with local recurrence in the surgical bed. (*B*) The same examination more superiorly demonstrates metastases in the porta surrounding metallic biliary stents, liver metastases, and ascites.

(range 5 to 32 months) following successful surgery.[7] Detection of generalized ascites more than 30 days after surgery was associated with tumor recurrence (**Fig. 32**), and is an ominous finding.[5] Patients with small tumors (smaller than 2 cm) limited to the pancreatic head region who undergo a Whipple have substantially improved survival, 30% at 5 years[49] (**Fig. 33**, same patient as **Fig. 21** 6 years earlier). Finally, patients often undergo surveillance CTs postoperatively at their local hospitals rather than tertiary care centers where most pancreaticoduodenectomies are performed; therefore, it is important for all radiologists to be aware of these patterns.

REFERENCES

1. Wolfgang CL, Corl F, Johnson PT, et al. Pancreatic surgery for the radiologist, 2011: an illustrated review of classic and newer surgical techniques for pancreatic tumor resection. AJR Am J Roentgenol 2011;197:1343–50.

2. Scialpi M, Scaglione M, Volterrani L. Imaging evaluation of post pancreatic surgery. Eur J Radiol 2005; 53(3):417–24.

3. Bluemke DA, Abrams RA, Yeo CJ, et al. Recurrent pancreatic adenocarcinoma: spiral CT evaluation following the Whipple procedure. Radiographics 1997;17:303–13.

4. Coombs RJ, Zeiss J, Howard JM, et al. CT of the abdomen after the Whipple procedure: value in depicting postoperative anatomy, surgical complications, and tumor recurrence. AJR Am J Roentgenol 1990;154:1011–4.

5. Mortele KJ, Lemmerling M, Hemptinne B, et al. Postoperative findings following the Whipple procedure: determination of prevalence and morphologic abdominal CT features. Eur Radiol 2000;10:123–8.

6. Lepanto L, Gianfelice D, Dery R, et al. Postoperative changes, complications, and recurrent disease after Whipple's operation: CT features. AJR Am J Roentgenol 1994;163:841–6.

7. Bluemke DA, Fishman EK, Kuhlman J. CT evaluation following Whipple procedure: potential pitfalls in interpretation. J Comput Assist Tomogr 1992;16:704–8.

8. Whipple AO, Parson N, Mullins C. Treatment of carcinoma of the ampulla of Vater. Ann Surg 1935; 102:763–79.

9. Tran KT, Smeenk HG, van Eijck CH, et al. Pylorus preserving pancreaticoduodenectomy versus standard Whipple procedure. A prospective, randomized, multicenter analysis of 170 patients with pancreatic and periampullary tumors. Ann Surg 2004;240(5):746–7.

10. Cameron JL. Long-term survival following pancreaticoduodenectomy for adenocarcinoma of the head of the pancreas. Surg Clin North Am 1995;75:939–51.

11. Shukla PJ, Barreto G, Shrikhande SV. The evolution of pancreatoduodenectomy. Hepatogastroenterology 2001;58:1409–12.

12. Gervais DA, Castillo CF, O'Neill MJ, et al. Complications after pancreatoduodenectomy: imaging and imaging-guided interventional procedures. Radiographics 2001;21:673–90.

13. Whipple AO. The rationale of radical surgery for cancer of the pancreas and ampullary region. Ann Surg 1941;114:612–5.

14. Traverso LW, Longmire WP. Preservation of the pylorus in pancreatoduodenectomy. Surg Gynecol Obstet 1978;146:959–64.

15. Smoot RL, Christein JD, Farnell MD. Durability of portal venous reconstruction following resection during pancreaticoduodenectomy. J Gastrointest Surg 2006;10(10):1371–5.

16. Smoot RL, Christein JD, Farnell MD. An innovative option for venous reconstruction after pancreaticoduodenectomy: the left renal vein. J Gastrointest Surg 2007;11:425–31.

17. Hirano S, Kondo S, Hara T, et al. Distal pancreatectomy with en bloc celiac axis resection for locally advanced pancreatic body cancer: long-term results. Ann Surg 2007;246:46–51.

18. Guillemin P, Bessot M. Pancreatite chronique calcifiante chez un tuberculeux rénal; pancreaticjejunostomie selon une technique originale. Mem Acad Chir 1957;83:869–71.

19. Christein JD, Kim AW, Golshan MA, et al. Central pancreatectomy for resection of benign or low malignant potential neoplasms. World J Surg 2003; 27:595–8.

20. Rotman N, Sastre B, Fagniez PL. Medial pancreatectomy for tumors of the neck of the pancreas. Surgery 1993;113:532–5.

21. Adham M, Giunippero A, Hervieu, et al. Central pancreatectomy: single-center experience of 50 cases. Arch Surg 2008;143(2):175–80.

22. Bruzoni M, Sasson AR. Open and laparoscopic spleen-preserving, splenic vessel-preserving distal pancreatectomy: indications and outcomes. J Gastrointest Surg 2008;12:1202–6.

23. Suave L. Des pancreatectemies et specialement de la pancreatectomie cephalique. Rev Chir 1908;37: 113–52.

24. Heidt DG, Burant C, Simeone DM. Total pancreatectomy: indications, operative technique, and postoperative sequelae. J Gastrointest Surg 2007;11:209–16.

25. Karpoff H, Klimstra DS, Brennan MF, et al. Results of total pancreatectomy for adenocarcinoma of the pancreas. Arch Surg 2001;136:44–7.

26. Gourgiotis S, Germanos S, Ridolfini MP. Surgical management of chronic pancreatitis. Hepatobiliary Pancreat Dis Int 2007;6(2):121–33.

27. Gruessner RW, Sutherland DE, Dunn DL, et al. Transplant options for patients undergoing total

pancreatectomy for chronic pancreatitis. J Am Coll Surg 2004;198:559–67.

28. Harrison JL, Prinz RA. The surgical management of chronic pancreatitis: pancreatic duct drainage. Adv Surg 1999;32:1–21.

29. Frey CF, Kathrin LM. Comparison of local resection of the head of the pancreas combined with longitudinal pancreaticojejunostomy (Frey procedure) and duodenum-preserving resection of the pancreatic head (Beger procedure). World J Surg 2003;27: 1217–30.

30. Riedeiger H, Adam U, Fischer E, et al. Long-term outcome after resection for chronic pancreatitis in 224 patients. J Gastrointest Surg 2007;11:949–60.

31. Beger HG, Scholosser W, Friess HM, et al. Duodenum-preserving head resection in chronic pancreatitis changes the natural course of the disease: a single-center 26-year experience. Ann Surg 1999;230:512–23.

32. Heiken JP, Balfe DM, Picus D, et al. Radical pancreatectomy: postoperative evaluation by CT. Radiology 1984;153:211–5.

33. Schafer M, Mullhaupt B, Clavian PA. Evidence-based pancreatic head resection for pancreatic cancer and chronic pancreatitis. Ann Surg 2002; 236:137–48.

34. Pessaux P, Tuech JJ, Arnaud JP. Prevention of pancreatic fistulas after surgical resection. A decade of clinical trials. Presse Med 2001;30(27): 1359–563.

35. Ho CK, Kleeff J, Friess H, et al. Complications of pancreatic surgery. Review article. HPB (Oxford) 2005;7:99–108.

36. Bartoli FG, Arnone GB, Ravera G, et al. Pancreatic fistula and relative mortality in malignant disease after pancreaticoduodenectomy. Review and statistical meta-analysis regarding 15 years of literature. Anticancer Res 1991;1:1831–48.

37. Yeo CJ, Cameron JL, Sohn TA, et al. Six hundred fifty consecutive pancreaticoduodenectomies in the 1990s: pathology, complications, and outcomes. Ann Surg 1997;226:248–57 [discussion: 257–60].

38. Büchler MW, Wagner M, Schmied BM, et al. Changes in mortality after pancreatic resection: towards the end of completion pancreatectomy. Arch Surg 2003;138:1310–4.

39. Suc B, Msika S, Piccinini M, et al. Octreotide in the prevention of intra-abdominal complications following elective pancreatic resection: a prospective, multicenter randomized controlled trial. Arch Surg 2004; 139:288–94.

40. Adam U, Makowiec F, Riediger H, et al. Risk factors for complications after pancreatic head resection. Am J Surg 2004;187:201–8.

41. Fernandez-del Castillo C, Rattner DW, Warshaw AL. Standards for pancreatic resection in the 1990's. Arch Surg 1995;130:295–300.

42. Barnes SA, Lillemoe KD, Kaufman HS, et al. Pancreaticoduodenectomy for benign disease. Am J Surg 1996;171:131–5.

43. Yeo CJ. Management of complications following pancreaticoduodenectomy. Surg Clin North Am 1995;75:913–24.

44. Suzuki Y, Fujino Y, Ajiki T, et al. No mortality among 100 consecutive pancreaticoduodenectomies in a middle-volume center. World J Surg 2005;29(11):1409–14.

45. Sohn TA, Yeo CJ, Camerson JL, et al. Pancreaticoduodenectomy: role of interventional radiologist in managing patients and complications. J Gastrointest Surg 2003; 7(2):209–19.

46. Zink SI, Soloff EV, White RR, et al. Pancreaticoduodenectomy: frequency and outcome of postoperative imaging-guided percutaneous drainage. Abdom Imaging 2009;34(6):767–71.

47. Glanemann M, Shi B, Liang F, et al. Surgical strategies for treatment of malignant pancreatic tumors: extended, standard or local surgery? World J Surg Oncol 2008;6:123.

48. Yeo CJ, Sohn TA, Cameron JL, et al. Periampullary adenocarcinoma: analysis of 5-year survivors. Ann Surg 1998;227:821–31.

49. Tsuchiya R, Noda T, Harada M, et al. Collective review of small carcinomas of the pancreas. Ann Surg 1986;203:77–81.

Update on Advanced Endoscopic Techniques for the Pancreas: Endoscopic Retrograde Cholangiopancreatography, Drainage and Biopsy, and Endoscopic Ultrasound

Linda S. Lee, MD*, Darwin L. Conwell, MD

KEYWORDS

- ERCP • EUS • Pancreas • Pancreas cyst • Pancreatitis
- Cystgastrostomy • Pancreatic disruption

Gastrointestinal endoscopy offers a comprehensive range of diagnostic and therapeutic options for a wide variety of pancreatic disorders from inflammatory conditions to cancer. Endoscopic retrograde cholangiopancreatography (ERCP) (Fig. 1) is a combined endoscopic and fluoroscopic procedure that was introduced in the early 1970s to allow access to the biliary and pancreatic ductal systems through their openings at the major or minor duodenal papillae. ERCP has evolved from a purely diagnostic technique performed by a few into a complex set of procedures integrating diagnosis and therapy for a wide variety of pancreatobiliary disorders offered in all major medical centers. Although it has become a highly successful therapeutic modality, ERCP also carries an overall morbidity of 7%, which includes acute pancreatitis (4%), hemorrhage (1%), cholangitis (1%), perforation (0.5%), and death (0.1%). With the advent of magnetic resonance cholangiopancreatography (MRCP) (Fig. 2), which safely and noninvasively images the pancreatic and biliary tracts, the need for purely diagnostic ERCP has diminished, whereas the demand for therapy has grown.[1]

Endoscopic ultrasound (EUS) has emerged as the premier tool for staging cancers and has revolutionized the role of gastrointestinal endoscopy in diagnostic imaging inside and outside the gastrointestinal tract. Similar to ERCP, EUS merges endoscopy, which is limited to visualizing the lumen of the gastrointestinal tract, with radiologic imaging and, specifically, ultrasonography, which allows imaging of the layers of the gastrointestinal wall and surrounding structures. Tissue diagnosis can be obtained with EUS-guided fine-needle aspiration (EUS-FNA), which uses a catheter with a retractable needle that can be advanced into visualized tissue. Exciting advances in the therapeutic application of EUS have begun with this technique, including the well-established endoscopic pseudocyst drainage and more recent endoscopic necrosectomy and rendezvous techniques with ERCP, as well as possibilities for EUS-guided fine-needle injection (EUS-FNI) therapy.

GALLSTONE PANCREATITIS

The goal of therapeutic ERCP in the setting of acute gallstone pancreatitis is to clear the bile duct of

Division of Gastroenterology, Hepatology, and Endoscopy, Brigham and Women's Hospital, Harvard Medical School, 75 Francis Street, Boston, MA 02115, USA
* Corresponding author.
E-mail address: lslee@partners.org

Radiol Clin N Am 50 (2012) 547–561
doi:10.1016/j.rcl.2012.03.002

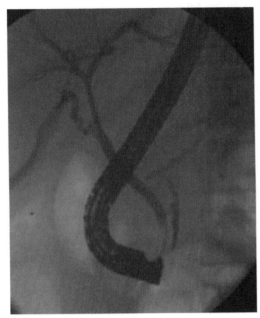

Fig. 1. ERCP radiograph showing standard endoscope position and normal biliary and pancreatic ductal systems.

stones that, if left in place, may worsen the severity of pancreatitis and increase the risk of further attacks. Urgent ERCP is indicated in patients with cholangitis and/or choledocholithiasis. Whether early ERCP benefits all other patients with acute gallstone pancreatitis has been investigated in multiple studies.[2–6] A recent meta-analysis of randomized controlled studies examining the role of urgent ERCP with biliary sphincterotomy (incision of the intraduodenal portion of the common bile duct sphincter muscle) compared with conservative management in acute gallstone pancreatitis

revealed no benefit in morbidity or mortality across all patients with early ERCP.[7] This study excluded a few trials that suggested urgent ERCP may improve morbidity in select patients with severe attacks but has little or no benefit in patients with mild pancreatitis because most of these patients pass the stones spontaneously and recover with supportive care. Cholecystectomy ideally should be planned for the same admission, if possible, but can be delayed following sphincterotomy because this confers a degree of protection from further pancreatitis and allows time for safe resolution of inflammation and fluid collections, making surgery less complicated.

Before ERCP is performed for select patients with gallstone pancreatitis, ascertaining the ongoing presence of choledocholithiasis is critical. For patients at low or high risk of choledocholithiasis, directly proceeding with conservative management or ERCP, respectively, is appropriate. However, intermediate-risk patients with mildly increased bilirubin, and/or alkaline phosphatase, and/or abnormal biliary system on radiology have about a 20% to 30% risk of choledocholithiasis. EUS has proved accurate and safe for detecting choledocholithiasis, and is the test of choice in these patients. A meta-analysis of randomized controlled blinded trials comparing EUS and MRCP with the gold standard of ERCP or intraoperative cholangiography in patients with suspected bile duct stones showed sensitivity for EUS and MRCP of 93% and 85%, with similar specificities of 96% and 93%, respectively.[8] A cost-analysis study indicated that initial EUS rather than MRCP had the greatest cost-utility by reducing unnecessary ERCP procedures.[9] EUS is also superior to MRCP for stones less than 4 mm and stones located near the ampulla.

IDIOPATHIC AND NONBILIARY ACUTE PANCREATITIS

EUS has proved helpful in cases of idiopathic acute pancreatitis with causes identified in 79% of these patients by EUS.[10] ERCP plays a role in delineating and treating those patients with pancreatic-type sphincter of Oddi dysfunction (SOD) presenting with unexplained pancreatitis and other rarer causes of pancreatitis, such as ampullary adenoma, pancreas divisum, autoimmune disease, rare tumors, and helminths if not detected by noninvasive imaging.

CHRONIC PANCREATITIS

Chronic pancreatitis is a progressive disease characterized by persistent inflammation, fibrosis,

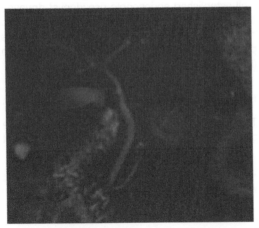

Fig. 2. MRCP image showing normal biliary and pancreatic ductal systems.

atrophy of the gland, and ductal abnormalities. Chronic pancreatitis causes significant morbidity related to chronic abdominal pain, loss of exocrine and endocrine function, and complications such as pancreatic stones, strictures, and fluid collections.

Pancreatic duct pressure may be increased secondary to strictures, stones, or outflow obstruction at the level of the major papilla. The goal of therapeutic ERCP is to decompress the pancreatic ductal system and relieve the obstruction with the hope of minimizing attacks of recurrent pancreatitis and alleviating chronic abdominal pain.

Benign strictures and stone disease of the main pancreatic duct (Figs. 3 and 4) can result in ductal hypertension, which may be the basis of relapsing pain and recurrent pancreatitis. Strictures are treated by balloon or catheter dilation and insertion of 1 or more plastic stents that are exchanged every 2 to 4 months for up to 1 year. Stone extraction is technically feasible if the stones are small, few in number, located in the head of the pancreas, and not impacted. A pancreatic sphincterotomy is usually required, and the stones are removed with a basket or balloon similar to bile duct stones. Stones located in the upstream duct proximal to a stricture require stricture dilation before extraction. Direct pancreatoscopy and electrohydraulic lithotripsy of pancreatic duct stones offers an additional option, although extracorporeal shock wave lithotripsy alone seems as effective as combined therapy with ERCP for pancreatic duct stones.[11] Although most studies have shown overall long-term pain relief in about 67% of patients who undergo endoscopic therapy, surgery seems to offer more durable pain relief with fewer procedures.[12–14]

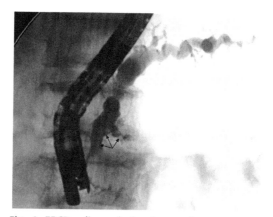

Fig. 4. ERCP radiograph showing small stones in main pancreatic duct of head and side branch with diffusely dilated main pancreatic duct and clubbed side branches. Arrows point to stones.

Although severe cases of chronic pancreatitis offer a therapeutic but not necessarily a diagnostic challenge, diagnosing milder forms of chronic pancreatitis remains difficult, especially because there is no defined gold standard. Histology may be considered the true gold standard; however, it is available in a minority of patients, sampling error may occur if only a core biopsy specimen is obtained, and there is no consensus on a histologic grading scale for severity of chronic pancreatitis. ERCP is less attractive as a diagnostic modality because of its potential complications and decreased sensitivity for early-stage chronic pancreatitis. In addition, the Cambridge classification for endoscopic retrograde pancreatography (ERP) changes in chronic pancreatitis was based on expert consensus and has not been validated. A few older studies compared pancreatic functional studies with histology, and found accuracy of the functional test to be approximately 81%.[15,16]

EUS is an attractive alternative diagnostic possibility because of its low morbidity and ability to assess both parenchymal and ductal features. EUS criteria for chronic pancreatitis include the following parenchymal and ductal changes: hyperechoic foci, hyperechoic strands, lobulation, cysts, calcifications, main-duct dilatation, main-duct irregularity, hyperechoic walls of the main duct, and visible side branches (Fig. 5). A retrospective study noted that the presence of 4 or more EUS criteria had 91% sensitivity and 86% specificity for diagnosing chronic pancreatitis using histology as the gold standard.[17] The threshold for diagnosing chronic pancreatitis can be varied depending on whether the intention is to establish or exclude the diagnosis. Certain features including calcification and lobulation more strongly indicate

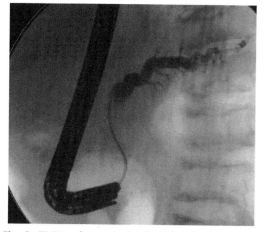

Fig. 3. ERCP radiograph showing chronic pancreatitis with dilated main pancreatic duct, ectatic side branches, and stones in pancreatic head.

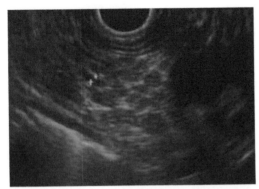

Fig. 5. EUS image of chronic pancreatitis showing lobularity and hyperechoic pancreatic duct walls.

chronic pancreatitis, and recently a weighted scoring system termed the Rosemont classification accounting for these factors has been proposed.[18] Addition of FNA does not seem to increase diagnostic yield for chronic pancreatitis.

A study comparing EUS and MRCP using the gold standards of ERP, histology, or long-term clinical follow-up of a median of 15 months showed higher sensitivity, of 93%, for EUS compared with 65% sensitivity for MRCP, and similar specificity of 90% to 93%. The combination of both studies yielded higher sensitivity and specificity of 98% and 83%.[19] Therefore, the less invasive modalities of EUS and MRCP have largely supplanted ERCP in the diagnosis of chronic pancreatitis. More recent studies suggest that the addition of endoscopic pancreatic function testing, which can be performed during routine endoscopy or EUS, may enable earlier diagnosis of chronic pancreatitis.[20,21]

PANCREATIC DUCTAL DISRUPTION AND FLUID COLLECTIONS

Pancreatic duct disruption and fluid collections may result from acute or chronic pancreatitis. Ongoing pancreatic duct disruption can be healed

in 78% to 92% of cases with stent placement across the disruption (Fig. 6); success rates plummet to 23% to 44% with transpapillary stents that do not bridge the leak.[22,23] A pseudocyst is a collection of amylase-rich pancreatic juice enclosed by a wall of nonepithelialized, fibrous, or granulation tissue. Pancreatic pseudocysts are the most common type of nonneoplastic pancreatic cysts, and studies suggest that even large pseudocysts greater than 6 cm can be followed conservatively until symptoms develop or the cyst further increases in size. Surgical drainage had been the standard of care but carries a 10% morbidity rate and a 1% mortality; therefore, radiologic and endoscopic drainage have replaced surgical drainage as initial treatment options.

Endoscopic drainage of pancreatic pseudocysts can be performed by using transpapillary or transmural (transgastric, transduodenal) placement of endoprostheses. The transpapillary approach is used for pseudocysts communicating with the main pancreatic duct, with the tip of the stent positioned in the cyst cavity after a pancreatic sphincterotomy. Fluid collections not clearly communicating with the pancreatic duct are drained using the transmural approach. The goal is to establish a communication between the cyst cavity and gastric or duodenal lumen for continuous drainage of pancreatic juice. Traditionally, endoscopic cystgastrostomy was performed by piercing the endoscopically visible bulge. Access to the pseudocyst can be achieved by using a needle knife with electrocautery or the Seldinger technique, which advances a guidewire through a 19-gauge needle. Retrospective studies suggest that the rate of bleeding is reduced to 4.6% using the Seldinger technique compared with 15.7% using the needle knife. After establishing access to the cavity, the opening is dilated with a balloon followed by placement of several pigtail stents.

Major prerequisites for such a procedure are an interval of at least 4 to 6 weeks from onset of acute

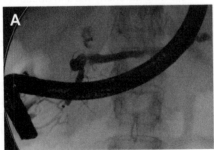
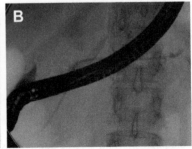

Fig. 6. (A) ERCP image showing pancreatic duct leak from neck region. (B) ERCP image with stent bridging across pancreatic duct disruption.

pancreatitis to allow development of a mature pseudocyst wall, a distance between the cyst and gastrointestinal tract of 10 mm or less, and lack of intervening blood vessels, with the second and third findings best determined during EUS. EUS also allows drainage of pseudocysts that do not create a visible bulge and has changed the management of about 25% of patients undergoing endoscopic pseudocyst drainage. Recent randomized studies suggest that technical success and, potentially, morbidity are improved with EUS-guided drainage compared with the non–EUS-guided approach.[24,25] Complications of endoscopic pseudocyst drainage include early bleeding, perforation of adjacent structures, and infection.

EUS also allows characterization of pancreatic and peripancreatic fluid collections. The presence of necrotic debris within a (peri)pancreatic collection necessitates either surgical debridement and/or aggressive percutaneous or endoscopic drainage techniques, termed endoscopic necrosectomy, which involve entering the cavity with the endoscope and removing necrotic debris with a variety of accessories. A retrospective study suggested that, for patients with walled-off pancreatic necrosis, endoscopic necrosectomy led to superior rates of resolution of necrosis with decreased need for adjunctive surgical or percutaneous drainage and recurrence compared with simple endoscopic cystgastrostomy.[26] The technique of endoscopic necrosectomy is still evolving (**Fig. 7**A–E), is available in only select major academic centers, and needs to be compared with surgical management.

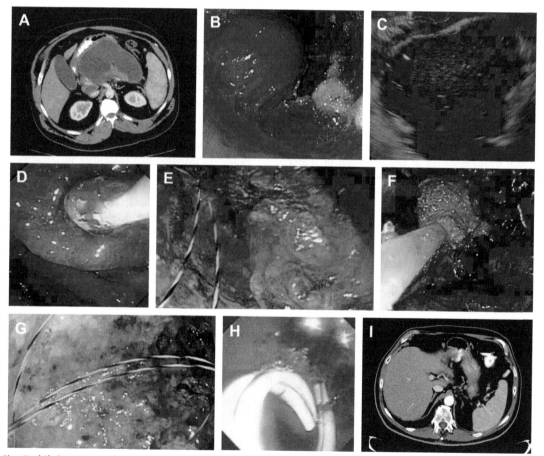

Fig. 7. (*A*) Sequence of endoscopic necrosectomy with computed tomography (CT) scan showing retrogastric walled-off pancreatic necrosis. (*B*) Endoscopic image of extrinsic compression in stomach by walled-off pancreatic necrosis. (*C*) EUS image of walled-off pancreatic necrosis. (*D*) Balloon dilation of cystgastrostomy track. (*E*) Endoscopic appearance of walled-off pancreatic necrosis cavity that has been entered by the endoscope and contains Jagwire and necrotic tissue. (*F*) Endoscopic removal of necrotic tissue that is deposited in the stomach lumen before more debris is removed from the cavity. (*G*) Endoscopic appearance of cavity after debridement. (*H*) Double pigtail stents across cystgastrostomy stoma. (*I*) Follow-up CT scan showing resolution. (*Courtesy of* Dr Christopher C. Thompson.)

PANCREAS DIVISUM

Pancreas divisum, the failure of fusion of dorsal and ventral pancreatic ductal systems during embryogenesis, is the most common variant of pancreatic ductal anatomy and occurs in about 10% of individuals (**Fig. 8**). The relationship between pancreas divisum and pancreatitis remains controversial, but endoscopic therapy in patients with acute recurrent pancreatitis and a normal dorsal duct is intended to decompress the dorsal pancreatic duct by minor papillotomy and temporary stent insertion for a few weeks (**Fig. 9**), with greater than 80% long-term success.[27] These patients were the first group shown to develop ductal changes resulting from stent therapy, and care must be taken to avoid this complication by not leaving stents in place for longer than necessary.

PANCREATIC CYSTS

Pancreatic cysts are discovered more often since abdominal imaging studies have improved in quality and have become more frequently used. These lesions are often of unclear clinical significance and pose a diagnostic dilemma. An increasing number of pancreatic cysts are pancreatic cystic neoplasms, which may be benign serous cystadenomas or premalignant or malignant mucinous lesions that include mucinous cystic neoplasms or intrapapillary mucinous neoplasm (IPMN). Therefore, it is important to differentiate these different cysts.

Serous cystadenomas occur anywhere throughout the pancreas, typically in women more than 60 years of age. On radiology or EUS imaging, they usually appear microcystic and, less commonly, macrocystic or even solid because of the presence of numerous microcysts that give the appearance of a homogeneous hypoechoic mass. A central calcification is pathognomonic but is only seen in about 10% of serous cystadenomas. Malignant transformation is exceedingly rare, and these cysts can typically be followed.

Mucinous cystic neoplasms are premalignant lesions that generally occur in women between 40 and 50 years old. They typically appear macrocystic in the body and tail of the pancreas with rare peripheral eccentric calcification. IPMN is also a mucinous cyst that involves the main pancreatic duct, side branches, or both (**Fig. 10**A, B). It is characterized by intraductal growth of mucin-producing epithelium, segmental or diffuse ductal dilatation, and, when the tumor is in the head of the pancreas, a gaping or fish-mouth papilla from which large amounts of mucus flow (**Fig. 11**). IPMN occurs more commonly in elderly men who may present with recurrent pancreatitis and/or diabetes. Jaundice and weight loss can be the presenting symptoms in cases with malignant transformation. About 40% of main-duct IPMNs contain malignancy at the time of diagnosis. Features that suggest malignancy in branch duct IPMNs include presence of a mass, mural nodules, dilated main pancreatic duct, and cyst size greater than 3 cm, although a recent study showed the rare presence of malignancy in smaller cysts.[28]

Accurate preoperative diagnosis of pancreatic cystic neoplasms is difficult. Imaging alone, including EUS, is often not sufficient to diagnose pancreatic cystic lesions; accurate diagnosis is possible in only about 40% to 60% of cystic lesions. EUS-FNA probably improves diagnostic yield for pancreatic cystic lesions; however, the optimal cyst fluid markers remain unknown. Current evidence suggests that carcinoembryonic antigen (CEA) may be most useful, whereas

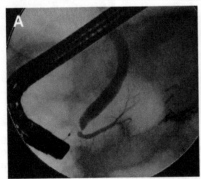 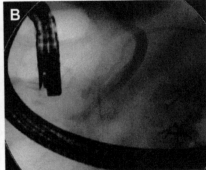

Fig. 8. (*A*) ERCP image of complete pancreas divisum with ventral pancreatic duct injection. (*B*) ERCP image showing injection into dorsal pancreatic duct of complete pancreas divisum. Note the long duodenoscope position required to gain access into the minor papilla located more proximal to the major papilla along the medial wall of the descending duodenum.

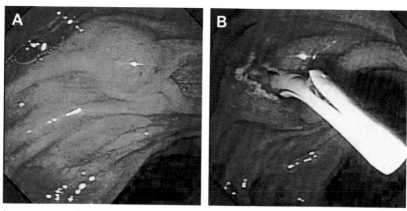

Fig. 9. (A) Endoscopic view of native minor papilla in pancreas divisum. (B) Minor papilla sphincterotomy with temporary stent placement.

cytology has poor sensitivity and accuracy in differentiating mucinous from nonmucinous lesions as well as benign from malignant or premalignant lesions (Table 1).[29,30] Molecular analysis of pancreatic cyst DNA for mutations, including early k-ras mutation followed by allelic loss, has been similarly disappointing in differentiating mucinous from nonmucinous cystic lesions. It is highly specific for differentiating malignant from nonmalignant cysts.[31] Further work is necessary to discover new and more accurate markers of malignancy and mucinous cystic lesions, because pancreatic cystic lesions are increasingly uncovered incidentally on imaging studies.

Although ERCP is not useful in the diagnosis of most pancreatic cystic lesions, it can provide valuable information in IPMNs. A pancreatogram is usually remarkable for dilated pancreatic ducts, intraluminal filling defects, and mural nodules. During ERCP, pancreatic juice can be aspirated for cytology, and transpapillary brushings and biopsies can be obtained from suspicious lesions seen on pancreatography. Direct pancreatoscopy involves the use of an ultrathin endoscope of

10-French diameter or less introduced through the working channel of a duodenoscope and advanced into the pancreatic duct through the major papilla. The ductal epithelium can be examined, and directed biopsies of suspicious mural nodules or masses can be performed. Pancreatoscopy has been increasingly used as an adjunct to other imaging modalities for diagnosing and determining the extent of IPMN, because the tumor is easily seen as a cluster-of-eggs appearance when it affects the main duct (Fig. 12), and surgical resection is currently designed to be as conservative as possible.[32] A recent study suggests that intraductal ultrasound during ERCP may also prove useful at defining the extent of IPMN before surgery.[33]

PANCREATIC CANCER

The role of EUS in pancreatic cancer includes diagnosis (Fig. 13) and staging. Tissue diagnosis is important to confirm malignancy and rule out metastatic lesions to the pancreas, which comprised 11% of masses referred for EUS-FNA in

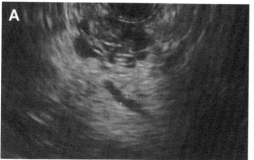
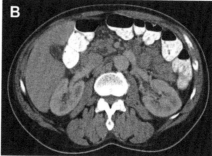

Fig. 10. (A) EUS image of intraductal papillary mucinous neoplasm with multiple thin septations and irregular border. (B) CT image of the intraductal papillary mucinous neoplasm seen in (A).

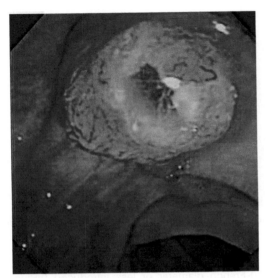

Fig. 11. Fish-mouth papilla showing mucus emerging from major papilla. (*Courtesy of* Dr Christopher C. Thompson.)

one study. EUS-FNA is the most accurate diagnostic modality, with 80% to 95% sensitivity and near 100% specificity compared with computed tomography (CT)–guided or ultrasound-guided FNA, which have sensitivity ranging from 62% to 81%.[34] Other studies suggest that EUS-FNA and CT-guided FNA have comparable diagnostic accuracy regardless of mass size.[35] Diagnostic sensitivity diminishes to 73% in the setting of chronic pancreatitis.[36] Presence of an onsite cytopathologist increases diagnostic accuracy and reduces procedure time, number of needles

used, and overall procedure cost. EUS-FNA is favored because of its accurate detection of small lesions less than 1.5 cm, and because the needle tract along which seeding can theoretically occur is resected for lesions in the pancreatic head. Tumor spread along the needle tract was suspected in one case report of a patient who developed recurrent cancer within the gastric wall 3 years after complete resection of a T2N0M0 pancreatic tumor located in the pancreatic body.[37] Therefore, for potentially resectable tumors located in the pancreatic body or tail, the options of proceeding directly to surgery without a tissue diagnosis versus EUS-FNA should be carefully considered.

The best outcome in pancreatic cancer occurs in patients without nodal, vascular, or systemic metastases (5-year survival up to 25%). More accurate patient selection could reduce unnecessary surgeries in patients with unresectable tumors. A recent review of studies comparing EUS and CT for preoperative staging of pancreatic cancer concluded that it is unclear which modality is superior for both tumor and nodal staging.[38] EUS criteria for vascular invasion include abnormal vessel contour, loss of hyperechoic interface between the tumor and blood vessel, tumor in the vessel lumen, and presence of collateral vessels in the absence of a main vascular structure. Presence of any of these criteria indicates vascular invasion. A recent meta-analysis examining the accuracy of these EUS criteria for assessing vascular invasion showed 73% sensitivity and 90% specificity.[39] EUS is more reliable for evaluating invasion into the portal vein and splenic confluence than the superior mesenteric artery or vein. With recent advances in multidetector-row CT and magnetic resonance imaging, these modalities will most likely surpass EUS for vascular staging.

Pancreatic endocrine tumors (PETs) are notoriously difficult to diagnose, and EUS is particularly helpful in evaluating these tumors (**Fig. 14**).[40] In an older series of 82 patients with suspected pancreatic endocrine tumor based on clinical, biochemical, or radiologic evidence, the sensitivity, specificity, and accuracy of EUS imaging for localizing PET were 93%, 95%, and 93%, respectively.[41] Other studies have reported sensitivity of EUS for detecting these lesions ranging from 83% to 94%.[42,43] When a lesion is not visualized on CT scan in patients with PET, sensitivity of EUS-FNA for diagnosing a PET is 70%.[44]

Despite EUS and improved radiologic imaging, small PETs may be difficult to localize in the operating room. Intraoperative palpation combined with intraoperative ultrasound is more than 95%

| Table 1 |
| Diagnostic markers for pancreatic cysts |

Marker	Sensitivity (%)	Specificity (%)
Cytology	27	100
CEA <5 ng/mL (serous vs other lesions)	100	86–93
CEA >192 ng/mL (mucinous vs other lesions)	73	84
Amylase >5000 units/mL (pseudocyst vs other lesions)	61–94	58–74
k-ras mutation + allelic loss (malignant vs nonmalignant)	37	93

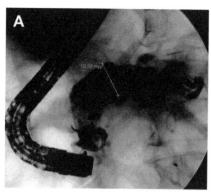 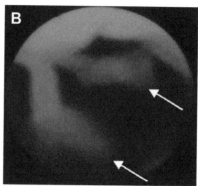

Fig. 12. (*A*) ERCP in a patient with main-duct IPMN with massively dilated main pancreatic duct and mucus filling defect. (*B*) Direct pancreatoscopy showing the ductal tumor, which appears as villous projections indicated by the 2 arrows.

sensitive; however, it prolongs operative time, rarely has been associated with splenic vessel rupture from manipulation of the pancreas, and is not practical with laparoscopic resections.[45] Tattooing the lesion during EUS seems feasible and safe in small case series. The agents injected into the pancreas have included presterilized, diluted, and filtered India ink, indocyanine green, methylene blue, and sterile purified carbon particles.[46,47] EUS-fine-needle injection with sterile purified carbon particles lasted up to 69 days after injection and operative time was significantly reduced in tattooed patients.[40]

EUS has revolutionized staging of many cancers including pancreatic cancer, and it may allow more directed, and potentially more efficacious, anticancer treatments. Case series have shown the feasibility and safety of EUS-guided placement of inactive radiographic markers, termed fiducials, which serve as targets for image-guided radiation therapy (IGRT).[48] Fiducials have traditionally been placed surgically or percutaneously. IGRT delivers high doses of precisely targeted, small beams of radiation using real-time image guidance. This technique reduces radiation exposure of surrounding organs, the total time of radiation treatment, and side effects compared with conventional radiotherapy.

SOD

The sphincter of Oddi is a complex muscular structure that surrounds the distal pancreatic duct, bile duct, and ampulla of Vater. This sphincter mechanism lies mostly within the duodenal wall and measures 6 to 10 mm in length. The sphincter of Oddi is functionally independent from the duodenal smooth muscle system. It serves to prevent reflux of duodenal contents into the ductal system and controls the flow of bile and pancreatic juice into the duodenum.

SOD describes an abnormality within the sphincter, either motility related (dyskinesia or

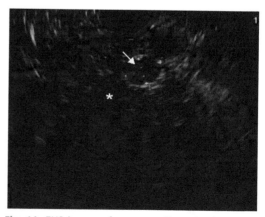

Fig. 13. EUS image of a pancreatic mass that appears homogeneous, hypoechoic, with irregular border and a small amount of normal pancreatic parenchyma surrounding the mass.

Fig. 14. EUS image of a pancreatic endocrine tumor that appears homogenous, hypoechoic, round, and well defined. Arrow points to the tumor and asterisk indicates area of normal pancreatic parenchyma.

spasm) or structural (stenosis), and can involve the biliary sphincter, the pancreatic sphincter, or both. In pancreatic-type SOD, patients typically present with episodic pancreatic-type epigastric pain radiating to the back and associated with pancreatic enzyme abnormalities or frank acute pancreatitis. Pancreatic SOD has 3 subtypes:

- Pancreatic type I SOD: patients have typical pancreatic pain, increased pancreatic enzymes 1.5 to 2 times the upper limit, and dilated pancreatic duct greater than 5 mm
- Pancreatic type II SOD: patients have pancreatic pain and 1 or 2 of the criteria listed earlier
- Pancreatic type III SOD: patients have only pancreatic-type pain

Sphincter function can be evaluated by noninvasive methods that include hepatobiliary scintigraphy, ultrasound assessment of pancreatic duct after secretin or cholecystokinin stimulation, and secretin-stimulated MRCP. However, the gold standard diagnostic test for SOD is manometric assessment of basal sphincter pressure during ERCP by sphincter of Oddi manometry (SOM). This test involves the use of solid-state or perfusion low-compliance catheters that can measure the biliary and pancreatic sphincter pressures through ports located at the distal end (**Fig. 15**). Multiple station pull-throughs are performed and graphic recording of the pressures are displayed on a dedicated workstation. The patient must be sedated for the procedure but narcotics and smooth muscle relaxants are usually avoided because they may interfere with the recordings. A basal sphincter pressure more than 40 mm Hg greater than duodenal pressure is considered abnormal, and sphincterotomy is the current standard treatment of choice for SOD in the appropriate clinical setting. Limited data suggest that the overall sustained response rate is approximately 69% in patients with abnormal pancreatic SOM.[49] The rate of complications is high in patients with suspected SOD undergoing ERCP, with pancreatitis being most common and occurring in up to 20% to 40%. The risk of pancreatitis is reduced by temporary stenting of the pancreatic duct.

AUTOIMMUNE PANCREATITIS

The first case of chronic inflammatory sclerosis of the pancreas with possible underlying autoimmune mechanism was reported in 1961, but the term autoimmune pancreatitis (AIP) was not proposed until 1995. The epidemiology of AIP is not well known but a prevalence of 5% has been reported among patients with chronic pancreatitis. The name of the HISORT diagnostic criteria is an acronym for (1) histopathologic examination of the pancreas showing fibrotic changes with lymphocyte and plasma cell infiltration, (2) pancreatic imaging studies showing diffuse narrowing of the main pancreatic duct with irregular walls and diffuse enlargement of the pancreas (**Fig. 16**), (3) laboratory serology data showing abnormally increased levels of serum γ-globulin, or immunoglobulin G fraction 4 (IgG4; increased to >2 times the upper limit of normal), or the presence of autoantibodies, (4) other organ involvement, and (5) response to steroid therapy in select patients. For diagnosis of AIP, various combinations of these criteria are used in the Mayo Clinic, Japan Pancreas Society, and Korean criteria. ERCP is used in non-Western countries for diagnosis of

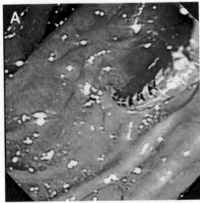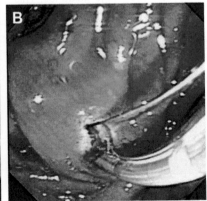

Fig. 15. (*A*) SOM with endoscopic view of perfusion catheter in pancreatic duct. (*B*) Pancreatic sphincterotomy in a patient who had increased pancreatic sphincter pressure on SOM.

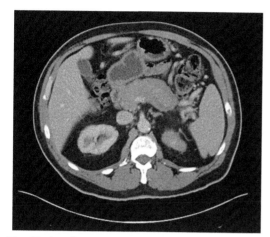

Fig. 16. Autoimmune pancreatitis manifesting as diffusely swollen pancreas on abdominal CT imaging.

AIP with findings including diffuse irregular narrowing of the main pancreatic duct and segmental narrowing with only mild upstream dilatation of the main pancreatic duct.[50]

AIP can be difficult to diagnose and often mimics pancreatic cancer in presentation with a pancreatic mass (Fig. 17). Findings of hyperechoic foci within a hypoechoic mass and the duct-penetrating sign on EUS suggest AIP rather than pancreatic cancer. Histology, and not cytology, is a diagnostic criterion for AIP, and use of a 19-gauge Trucut needle has been reported in small case series to yield histologic diagnosis of AIP.[51] Ampullary biopsy for IgG4 staining may also aid in diagnosis (Fig. 18). Although EUS and EUS-FNA currently have a limited role in diagnosing AIP, appreciation of a diffusely hypoechoic, enlarged pancreas with chronic inflammatory cells on cytology should raise the concern for AIP. A 2-week trial of steroids followed by reimaging is an alternative method for distinguishing AIP from pancreatic cancer. The lesion should diminish in size in AIP, but persists in pancreatic cancer.

EUS-GUIDED CELIAC PLEXUS NEUROLYSIS AND BLOCK

Celiac plexus neurolysis (CPN) refers to the permanent destruction of the celiac plexus using absolute ethanol. Temporary block of the plexus with corticosteroid injection is termed celiac plexus block (CPB). The celiac plexus predominantly controls pancreatic pain. CPN using surgical and transcutaneous approaches has been used for many years; however, major complications including paralysis can occur in about 1% of cases, which makes the endoscopic approach a potentially more attractive option.

The EUS technique involves first flushing a 22-gauge needle with normal saline to clear the needle of air, followed by insertion of the needle 1 cm cranial and anterior to the take-off of the celiac artery and aspiration to ensure that no blood returns. There has been recent interest in injecting the celiac ganglia visible during EUS; however, further research is necessary to validate this approach. For CPN, 10 mL of 0.25% bupivacaine is injected, followed by 20 mL of 98% absolute ethanol. For CPB, 20 mL of 0.25% bupivacaine is injected followed by 80 mg of triamcinolone, although a recent randomized study suggests that the addition of triamcinolone does not increase efficacy in chronic pancreatitis.[52] This technique is safe, without reported incidences of paralysis. Minor complications include transient diarrhea in 4% to 15% of patients, transient increase in pain in 9%, and transient orthostasis in 1%. Normal saline is administered during the procedure, and patients should be monitored for orthostasis for 2 hours after the procedure. Major complications include retroperitoneal bleed and peripancreatic abscess.

A recent meta-analysis suggests that EUS-CPN offers safe and effective pain relief for patients with pancreatic cancer and chronic pancreatitis.[53] Nearly 80% of patients with pancreatic cancer experience pain relief, whereas the response rate and durability are lower in chronic pancreatitis, with an initial 55% response rate that decreases to 10% at 24 weeks. Pain reduction lasts about 20 weeks following EUS-CPN in pancreatic cancer, compared with 2 weeks for chronic pancreatitis with EUS-CPB.

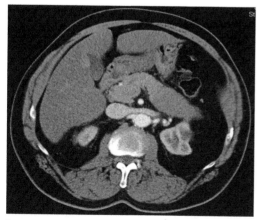

Fig. 17. Autoimmune pancreatitis appearing as a homogeneously hypodense mass in tail of pancreas.

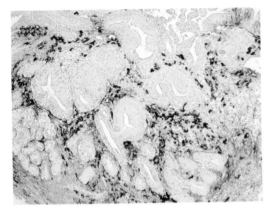

Fig. 18. Ampullary biopsy in a patient with autoimmune pancreatitis showing IgG4 staining shown by brown pigmentation.

EUS-GUIDED ANTEGRADE CHOLANGIOPANCREATOGRAPHY

Endoscopic decompression of biliary and pancreatic obstruction has traditionally been performed via ERCP, with greater than 90% success in biliary drainage and lower success rates for pancreatic procedures by skilled endoscopists. Unsuccessful endoscopic drainage results from surgically altered anatomy, tumor invasion, periampullary diverticulum, endoscopist inexperience, or other causes.

EUS-guided antegrade cholangiopancreatography (EACP) refers to 2 different approaches to pancreatic drainage: EUS-rendezvous ERCP or direct EUS-intervention with the creation of an EUS-guided enterobiliary or enteropancreatic fistula (Fig. 19). During a rendezvous procedure, a 19-gauge or 22-gauge needle is used to access the pancreatic duct transgastrically under EUS guidance. A guidewire is then advanced into the duodenum, followed by exchange of the echoendoscope for a duodenoscope to complete the ERCP procedure. Successful pancreatic drainage occurred in 56% of these patients in a recent study.[54]

Another EUS-guided technique involves creating an enterobiliary or enteropancreatic fistula. The pancreatic duct is punctured with a 19-gauge needle followed by guidewire placement, dilation of the puncture tract to 4 to 6 mm, and placement of plastic stents. This approach had a 71% success rate. Complications occurred in 16% of patients, and included self-limited pneumoperitoneum, mild

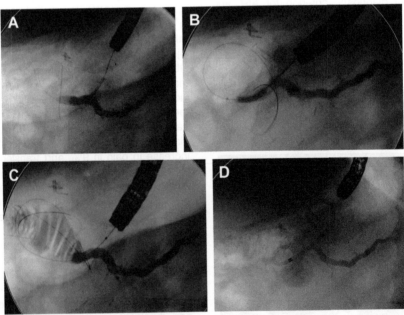

Fig. 19. (A) EUS-guided antegrade pancreatography of a patient who underwent a Whipple operation for chronic pancreatitis and developed an anastomotic stricture at the pancreaticojejunostomy. Transgastric access of the pancreatic duct was achieved with a wire advanced antegrade into the jejunum. (B) Balloon dilation of anastomotic stricture. (C) Contrast-filling jejunum following balloon dilation. (D) Placement of pigtail stent spanning pancreaticojejunostomy and enteropancreatic fistula that was created to enable transgastric access to the pancreatic duct. (Courtesy of Dr Christopher C. Thompson.)

pancreatitis, and severe pancreatitis requiring surgical management.

SUMMARY

ERCP and EUS provide a wide array of diagnostic and therapeutic opportunities in managing the spectrum of pancreatic disorders from pancreatitis to pancreatic cancer. ERCP and EUS often offer complementary approaches to patients with pancreatic disorders.

REFERENCES

1. Baron T, Kozarek RA, Carr-Locke DL. ERCP. Elsevier, Philadelphia: Saunders; 2007.
2. Oria A, Cimmino D, Ocampo C, et al. Management in patients with acute gallstone pancreatitis and biliopancreatic obstruction: a randomized clinical trial. Ann Surg 2007;245:10–7.
3. Neoptolemos JP, Carr-Locke DL, London NJ, et al. Controlled trial of urgent endoscopic retrograde cholangiopancreatography and endoscopic sphincterotomy versus conservative treatment for acute pancreatitis due to gallstones. Lancet 1988;2:979–83.
4. Fan ST, Lai EC, Mok FP, et al. Early treatment of acute biliary pancreatitis by endoscopic papillotomy. N Engl J Med 1993;328:228–32.
5. Nowak A, Marek TA, Nowakowska-Dulawa E, et al. Biliary pancreatitis needs endoscopic retrograde cholangiopancreatography with endoscopic sphincterotomy for cure. Endoscopy 1998;30:A256–9.
6. Folsch UR, Nitsche R, Ludtke R, et al. Early ERCP and papillotomy compared with conservative treatment for acute biliary pancreatitis. The German Study Group on Acute Biliary Pancreatitis. N Engl J Med 1997;336:237–42.
7. Petrov MS, van Santvoort HC, Besselink MG, et al. Early endoscopic retrograde cholangiopancreatography versus conservative management in acute biliary pancreatitis without cholangitis: a meta-analysis of randomized trials. Ann Surg 2008;247:250–7.
8. Verma D, Kapadia A, Eisen G, et al. EUS vs. MRCP for detection of choledocholithiasis. Gastrointest Endosc 2006;64:248–54.
9. Arguedas MR, Dupont AW, Wilcox CM. Where do ERCP, endoscopic ultrasound, magnetic resonance cholangiopancreatography, and intraoperative cholangiography fit in the management of acute biliary pancreatitis? A decision analysis model. Am J Gastroenterol 2001;96:2892–9.
10. Vila JJ, Vicuna M, Irisarri R, et al. Diagnostic yield and reliability of endoscopic ultrasonography in patients with idiopathic acute pancreatitis. Scand J Gastroenterol 2010;45:375–81.
11. Dumonceau JM, Costamagna G, Tringali A, et al. Treatment for painful calcified chronic pancreatitis extracorporeal shock wave lithotripsy versus endoscopic treatment: a randomized controlled trial. Gut 2007;56:545–52.
12. Rosch T, Daniel S, Scholz M, et al. Endoscopic treatment of chronic pancreatitis: a multicenter study of 1000 patients with long-term follow-up. Endoscopy 2002;34:765–71.
13. Cahen DL, Gouma DJ, Nio Y, et al. Endoscopic versus surgical drainage of the pancreatic duct in chronic pancreatitis. N Engl J Med 2007;356:676–84.
14. Dite P, Ruzicka M, Zboril V, et al. A prospective, randomized trial comparing endoscopic and surgical therapy for chronic pancreatitis. Endoscopy 2003;35:553–8.
15. Hayakawa T, Kondo T, Shibata T, et al. Relationship between pancreatic exocrine function and histological changes in chronic pancreatitis. Am J Gastroenterol 1992;87:1170–4.
16. Heij HA, Obertop H, van Blankenstein M, et al. Relationship between functional and histological changes in chronic pancreatitis. Dig Dis Sci 1986;31:1009–13.
17. Varadarajulu S, Eltoum I, Tamhane A, et al. Histopathologic correlates of noncalcific chronic pancreatitis by EUS: a prospective tissue characterization study. Gastrointest Endosc 2007;66:501–9.
18. Catalano MF, Sahai A, Levy M, et al. EUS-based criteria for the diagnosis of chronic pancreatitis: the Rosemont classification. Gastrointest Endosc 2009;69:1251–61.
19. Pungapong S, Wallace M, Woodward T, et al. Accuracy of endoscopic ultrasonography and magnetic resonance cholangiopancreatography for the diagnosis of chronic pancreatitis: a prospective comparison study. J Clin Gastroenterol 2007;41:88–93.
20. Stevens T, Conwell DL, Zuccaro G, et al. A prospective crossover study comparing secretin-stimulated endoscopic and Dreiling tube pancreatic function testing in patients evaluated for chronic pancreatitis. Gastrointest Endosc 2008;67:458–66.
21. Albashir S, Bronner MP, Parsi MA, et al. Endoscopic ultrasound, secretin endoscopic pancreatic function test, and histology: correlation in chronic pancreatitis. Am J Gastroenterol 2010;105:2498–503.
22. Telford JJ, Farrell JJ, Saltzman JR, et al. Pancreatic stent placement for duct disruption. Gastrointest Endosc 2002;56:18–24.
23. Varadarajulu S, Noone TC, Tutuian R, et al. Predictors of outcome in pancreatic duct disruption managed by endoscopic transpapillary stent placement. Gastrointest Endosc 2005;61:568–75.
24. Park DH, Lee SS, Moon SH, et al. Endoscopic ultrasound-guided versus conventional transmural drainage for pancreatic pseudocysts: a prospective randomized trial. Endoscopy 2009;41:842–8.

25. Varadarajulu S, Christein JD, Tamhane A, et al. Prospective randomized trial comparing EUS and EGD for transmural drainage of pancreatic pseudocysts. Gastrointest Endosc 2008;68:1102–11.

26. Gardner TB, Chahal P, Papachristou GI, et al. A comparison of direct endoscopic necrosectomy with transmural endoscopic drainage for the treatment of walled-off pancreatic necrosis. Gastrointest Endosc 2009;69:1085–94.

27. Gerke H, Byrne MF, Stiffler HL, et al. Outcome of endoscopic minor papillotomy in patients with symptomatic pancreas divisum. JOP 2004;5:122–31.

28. Tanaka M, Chari S, Adsay V, et al. International consensus guidelines for management of intraductal papillary mucinous neoplasms and mucinous cystic neoplasms of the pancreas. Pancreatology 2006;6: 17–32.

29. Brugge WR, Lewandrowski K, Lee-Lewandrowski E, et al. Diagnosis of pancreatic cystic neoplasms: a report of the cooperative pancreatic cyst study. Gastroenterology 2004;126:1330–6.

30. Van der Waaij LA, van Dullemen HM, Porte RJ. Cyst fluid analysis in the differential diagnosis of pancreatic cystic lesions: a pooled analysis. Gastrointest Endosc 2005;62:383–9.

31. Khalid A, Zahid M, Finkelstein SD, et al. Pancreatic cyst fluid DNA analysis in evaluating pancreatic cysts: a report of the PANDA study. Gastrointest Endosc 2009;69:1095–102.

32. Yasuda K, Sakata M, Ueda M, et al. The use of pancreatoscopy in the diagnosis of intraductal papillary mucinous tumor lesions of the pancreas. Clin Gastroenterol Hepatol 2005;3:S53–7.

33. Cheon YK, Cho YD, Jeon SR, et al. Pancreatic resection guided by preoperative intraductal ultrasonography for intraductal papillary mucinous neoplasm. Am J Gastroenterol 2010;105:1963–9.

34. Turner BG, Cizginer S, Agarwal D, et al. Diagnosis of pancreatic neoplasia with EUS and FNA: a report of accuracy. Gastrointest Endosc 2010;71:91–8.

35. Erturk SM, Mortelé KJ, Tuncali K, et al. Fine-needle aspiration biopsy of solid pancreatic masses: comparison of CT and endoscopic sonography guidance. Am J Roentgenol 2006;187:1531–5.

36. Krishna NB, Mehra M, Reddy AV, et al. EUS/EUS-FNA for suspected pancreatic cancer: influence of chronic pancreatitis and clinical presentation with or without obstructive jaundice on performance characteristics. Gastrointest Endosc 2009; 70:70–9.

37. Ahmed K, Sussman JJ, Wang J, et al. A case of EUS-guided FNA-related pancreatic cancer metastasis to the stomach. Gastrointest Endosc 2011;74: 231–2.

38. Dewitt J, Devereaux BM, Lehman GA, et al. Comparison of endoscopic ultrasound and computed tomography for the preoperative evaluation of pancreatic cancer: a systematic review. Clin Gastroenterol Hepatol 2006;6:717–25.

39. Puli SR, Singh S, Hagedorn CH, et al. Diagnostic accuracy of EUS for vascular invasion in pancreatic and periampullary cancers: a meta-analysis and systematic review. Gastrointest Endosc 2007;65: 788–97.

40. Lee LS. Diagnosis of pancreatic neuroendocrine tumors and role of endoscopic ultrasound. Gastroenterol Hepatol 2010;6:520–2.

41. Anderson MA, Carpenter S, Thompson NW, et al. Endoscopic ultrasound is highly accurate and directs management in patients with neuroendocrine tumors of the pancreas. Am J Gastroenterol 2000;95:2271–7.

42. Gouya H, Vignaux O, Augui J, et al. CT, endoscopic sonography and a combined protocol for preoperative evaluation of pancreatic insulinomas. AJR Am J Roentgenol 2003;181:987–92.

43. Ardengh JC, Rosenbaum P, Ganc AJ, et al. Role of EUS in the preoperative localization of insulinomas compared with spiral CT. Gastrointest Endosc 2000;51:552–5.

44. Pais SA, Al-Haddad M, Mohamadnejad M, et al. EUS for pancreatic neuroendocrine tumors: a single-center, 11-year experience. Gastrointest Endosc 2010;71:1185–93.

45. Wong M, Isa SH, Zahiah M, et al. Intraoperative ultrasound with palpation is still superior to intra-arterial calcium stimulation test in localizing insulinoma. World J Surg 2007;31:586–92.

46. Gress FG, Barawi M, Kim D, et al. Preoperative localization of a neuroendocrine tumor of the pancreas with EUS-guided fine needle tattooing. Gastrointest Endosc 2002;55:594–7.

47. Lennon AM, Newman N, Makary MA, et al. EUS-guided tattooing before laparoscopic distal pancreatic resection. Gastrointest Endosc 2010;72: 1089–94.

48. Sanders MK, Moser AJ, Khalid A, et al. EUS-guided fiducial placement for stereotactic body radiotherapy in locally advanced and recurrent pancreatic cancer. Gastrointest Endosc 2010;71:1204–10.

49. Sgouros SN, Pereira SP. Systematic review: sphincter of Oddi dysfunction - non-invasive diagnostic methods and long-term outcome after endoscopic sphincterotomy. Aliment Pharmacol Ther 2006;24:237–46.

50. Kamisawa T, Anjiki H, Takuma K, et al. Endoscopic approach for diagnosing autoimmune pancreatitis. World J Gastrointest Endosc 2010;16(2):20–4.

51. Mizuno N, Bhatia V, Hosoda W, et al. Histological diagnosis of autoimmune pancreatitis using EUS-guided Trucut biopsy: a comparison study with EUS-FNA. J Gastroenterol 2009;44:742–50.

52. Stevens T, Costanzo A, Lopez R, et al. Adding triamcinolone to endoscopic ultrasound-guided celiac

plexus blockade does not reduce pain in patients with chronic pancreatitis. Clin Gastroenterol Hepatol 2012;10(2):186–91, 191.e1.

53. Puli SR, Reddy JB, Bechtold ML, et al. EUS-guided celiac plexus neurolysis for pain due to chronic pancreatitis or pancreatic cancer pain: a meta-analysis and systematic review. Dig Dis Sci 2009; 54:2330–7.

54. Shah JN, Marson F, Weilert F, et al. Single-operator, single-session EUS-guided antegrade cholangio-pancreatography in failed ERCP or inaccessible papilla. Gastrointest Endosc 2012;75:56–64.

Index

Printed and bound by CPI Group (UK) Ltd, Croydon, CR0 4YY

03/10/2024

01040359-0020